Combined Survey Sampling Inference

Weighing Basu's Elephants

Ken Brewer
Australian National University

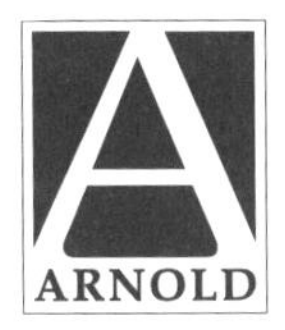

A member of the Hodder Headline Group
LONDON
Distributed in the United States of America by
Oxford University Press Inc., New York

First published in Great Britain in 2002 by
Arnold, a member of the Hodder Headline Group,
338 Euston Road, London NW1 3BH

http://www.arnoldpublishers.com

Distributed in the United States of America by
Oxford University Press Inc.,
198 Madison Avenue, New York, NY10016

British Library Cataloguing in Publication Data
A catalogue record for this book is available from the British Library

Library of Congress Cataloging-in-Publication Data
A catalog record for this book is available from the Library of Congress

ISBN 0 340 692294 (pb)

1 2 3 4 5 6 7 8 9 10

Production Editor: James Rabson
Production Controller: Iain McWilliams
Cover Design: Terry Griffiths

Typeset in 10.5/12 pt Times New Roman by Charon Tec Pvt. Ltd, Chennai, India
Printed and bound in Malta by Gutenberg Press Ltd

What do you think about this book? Or any other Arnold title?
Please send your comments to feedback.arnold@hodder.co.uk

Dedication

To Maggie

Contents

	Acknowledgements	**xi**
	Prologue: Hints on How to Read this Book	**1**
1	**Simple Random Sampling with Equal Weights**	**4**
	Narrator's Introduction	4
	Simple Random Sampling without Replacement	8
	Simple Random Sampling with Replacement	14
	Simple Random Sampling: the Prediction-Based Theory	18
	An Excursus on Independence, Exchangeability and Non-informative Sampling	22
	Prediction-Based Theory (Continued)	23
	Summary	26
	Exercises	27
2	**Stratification and Poststratification**	**29**
	Stratifying the Population	29
	Poststratified Estimation	29
	Designing a Stratified Sample	34
	Summary	37
	Exercises	38
3	**Ratio Estimation (Design-Based)**	**40**
	Finding a Supplementary Variable	40
	The Classical Ratio Estimator under Design-Based Inference	41
	Exact Bias of Ratio Estimator	43
	Asymptotic Approximations to the Relative Design Bias and Relative Design Variance of the Ratio Estimator	44
	Asymptotic Approximations to the Actual Design Bias and Actual Design Variance of the Ratio Estimator	46
	Numerical Results	48
	Across-Stratum (or Combined) Ratio Estimation	52
	Exercises	57

4 Ratio Estimators for Unequal Probability Samples 60
Facing the Dilemma 60
The Lahiri–Midzuno Unbiased Ratio Estimator 60
The Horvitz–Thompson and Hansen–Hurwitz Estimators of Total 63
Poisson Sampling 74
Exercises 79

5 Ratio Estimation (Prediction-Based) 80
Understanding the Difference 80
The Ratio Prediction Model 83
Exercises 93

6 The Reporting 95
Report to Supervisor 95
Draft of a Report for the Circus Owner 98
Comments from Supervisor 98
Action Consequential on Supervisor's Comments 99
Randomization-Based and Prediction-Based Sampling Inferences are Complementary 101
More about the Background to Our Assignment 104

7 The Simple Regression Estimator and Synthetic Estimation 107
Report for Supervisor: Introduction 107
Circumstances Favourable for Simple Regression Estimation 108
Questionable Reasons for Using Simple Regression Estimation 109
Properties of the Simple Regression Estimator 112
Some Empirical Evidence 119
Summary 121
Conclusions 121
Response from Supervisor 121
Exercises 121

8 Regression Estimation with More Than One Supplementary Variable 123
Report for Supervisor: Introduction 123
Combining the Inferences When Using Simple Random Sampling without Replacement 123
Combining the Inferences When Sampling with Unequal Probabilities 127
Generalization to *p* Regressor Variables 128
The Problem of Unacceptably Small Case Weights 133
Design Variance and Anticipated Variance of any Generalized Regression Estimator 135

Prediction Variance of any Prediction-Unbiased Linear Estimator Based on a Probability Sample 138
Estimation of the Prediction Variances of Individual Sample Units 139
Response from Supervisor 143
Exercises 143

9 Short-Cut Variance Estimation for the Horvitz–Thompson and Generalized Regression Estimators 146
Report for Supervisor: Introduction 146
Some Approximate Formulae for the Design Variance of the Horvitz–Thompson Estimator 148
A Model-Assisted Check on the Usefulness of the Approximate Horvitz–Thompson Estimator's Design Variance Formulae 154
Sample Estimators of the High-Entropy Anticipated Variance of the Horvitz–Thompson Estimator 156
Sample Estimators of the Design Variance of the Horvitz–Thompson Estimator Suitable for Use with Ordered Systematic Sampling 159
Adaptation to Estimating the Design Variance of a Generalized Regression Estimator 161
Some Empirical Results 163
Response from Supervisor 167
Postscripts 167
Exercises 172

10 Multistage Area Sampling for Household Surveys: Sampling with Replacement 174
Report for Supervisor: Introduction 174
How a Multistage Equal Probability Sample Can Be Selected 177
Selecting Persons Associated with Dwellings: Eligibility and Coverage 183
Survey Coverage and Survey Scope 185
The Self-Weighting Nature of an Equal Probability Multistage Sample 186
Estimation Formulae for Multistage Samples 188
Variance Estimation Formulae for Multistage Samples 191
Estimating the Total Variance 196
Estimating the Individual Stages of Variance 197
Optimal Levels of Clustering 199
The Variance Components Reconsidered 199
The Cost Parameters 203
Equations for Optimum Clustering 204
A Quick Fix 205
Acknowledgement from Supervisor 208
Exercises 208

11 Multistage Area Sampling for Household Surveys: Sampling without Replacement **209**
Report for Supervisor: Introduction 209
Selecting a Multistage Equal Probability Sample of Dwellings without Replacement 209
Estimation Formulae for Multistage Samples Selected without Replacement 212
Variance Estimation Formulae for Multistage Samples Selected without Replacement 214
Estimating $Y^*_{\bullet\bullet}$ Using Combined Design-Based and Prediction-Based Inference 219
Estimating the Prediction-Based, Design-Based and Anticipated Variances of $\hat{Y}^*_{\bullet\bullet}$ (Totals and Components) 223
Estimation of Variance Using Jackknife, Bootstrap and Other Resampling Methods 228
Response from Supervisor 229
Exercises 229

12 Multiphase Sampling, Repeated Sampling and Non-response **231**
Introduction 231
Report on Non-response and Related Topics 231
Response from Supervisor 244
Exercises 244

13 Tracking and Rotating Samples **246**
Introduction 246
Permanent Random Number Sampling 247
Bernoulli Sampling 247
Poisson Sampling 248
Rotation and Control of a Poisson Sample 248
The Problem with Having a Random Sample Size 251
Estimation and Variance Estimation for a Poisson Sample 252
Two Ways of Viewing the Horvitz–Thompson Ratio Estimator 254
Alternatives to Poisson Sampling 256
Response from Supervisor 266
Exercises 266

14 Coping with Extreme Values and Other Unusual Features **268**
Report for Supervisor: Introduction 268
Relevant and Recognizable Subsets 268
Stratification and Selection of Atypical Units 270
Spurious Extreme Values 271
Genuine Extreme Values 272

Winsorization 274
Spreading the Estimated Bias Back 278
Summary and Concluding Remarks 280
Response from Supervisor 281
Exercises 282

15 Resampling Methods of Variance Estimation: the Jackknife and the Bootstrap 283
Report to Supervisor: Introduction 283
Jackknifing the Variance 284
Bootstrapping the Variance 285
Some Semi-empirical and Empirical Findings 286
Response from Supervisor 287
Exercise 287

Epilogue: The Most Important Topic Left Out 288
The Other Statistical Inference Controversy 288
Statistical Inference under Tractable Distributions 288
The Inference Problem When the Distributions are Intractable 291

Postscript: Bayesian Methods for Estimation 293

Appendices
A Basu's Original Elephant Fable 297
B The Circus's 50 Indian Elephants 298
C Details of Calculations in the Postscript 299

References 303

Index 310

Acknowledgements

I am deeply indebted to all the following, many of whom, alas, will not have lived to be able to read this tribute:

Miss Leonard, who taught mathematics so expertly at the combined Coopers-Coborn School in Bow, 1943–45; E.G. Bowley, her successor at Coopers and a nephew of the pioneer sampling statistician A.L. Bowley, who gave me my first taste of statistics; G.A. Barnard whose lectures led me to realise that I had some aptitude for the subject; Miss Lorna Colwell, who at a low ebb in my life found me a job at the Australian Bureau of Statistics (ABS); E.K. (Ken) Foreman A.M., to whom I pay a fuller tribute in the Prologue; Betty Hanslow (neé Walls), Digby Pridmore, John Carroll A.M. and all the other fine people who subsequently worked with and for Ken in the Sampling and Methodology areas of the ABS during 1954–74; E.J. (Ted) Hannan, Ray Byron, Sleeba John, C.E.V. Leser and others who belatedly filled some of the gaps in my formal statistical education; J.N.K. Rao, who was the first person outside my immediate circle to recognise that I might have something substantial to contribute to survey sampling methodology, and who raised my profile accordingly; R.L. (Ray) Chambers, who took the risk of bringing me back into statistics at another difficult stage in my career; J. Neyman, M.H. Hansen and W.N. Hurwitz on the one hand, and R.M. Royall on the other, who demonstrated so cogently the need to use randomization based and prediction based inference respectively; C.-E. (Carl) Särndal, whose innovative ideas, more than anyone else's, have so often inspired me to exploit them; V.P. Godambe, who seminally suggested at I.S.I., New Delhi 1977, that what we really needed were estimators that made sense in both approaches; Ray Chambers (again) for being such an invaluable PhD supervisor and sparring partner, and Alan Welsh for competently taking over those roles when Ray left for fresher pastures.

The following have been more directly involved in the preparation of this book:

Maggie, my wife, without whose urging and constant encouragement it would never have been written, started, or even thought of; Terry O'Neill, Michael Martin, Steve Stern and their colleagues at the Australian National University for providing an ideal milieu for writing it, and doing all sorts of clever things with their computers for me; the students in my 2001–02 classes who kindly put up with the many imperfections in the then current drafts of the book, and equally kindly pointed many of them out; Bill Gross, Matthew Cronin and those other staff at the ABS who generously provided information on its operations (and who cannot be held responsible if I have misrepresented them); Phil Kott, Tim

Gregoire and Martin Donadio, who made substantial contributions to Chapters 8 and 9; Stephen Horn and Phil Kokic who gave helpful comments on Chapters 12 and 14 respectively; Borek Puza who wrote the Bayesian Postscript; and not least my publishers, who put up so graciously with my many requests for extensions of time and changes to already composite material.

My apologies also to the many others who have substantially influenced my thinking for good over the course of a long career. Their absence from the above lists is more likely to be attributable to a failing memory than anything else.

Ken Brewer
School of Finance and Applied Statistics
Australian National University, Canberra
June 2002

Prologue

Hints on How to Read this Book

> The circus owner is planning to ship his 50 adult elephants and so he needs a rough estimate of the total weight of the elephants. As weighing an elephant is a cumbersome process, the owner wants to estimate the total weight by weighing just one elephant. Which elephant should he weigh?

With these words, Basu (1971) introduced his famous elephant fable. If this book is indeed your own personal introduction to survey sampling, it is sadly too soon to expose you to the rest of it. Suffice to say that in 1971 it called into question the entire basis of sampling inference as then understood. But because it is such a good story and carries such a profound moral, it also provides us with a convenient context within which to explore the fundamentals of survey sampling. In it, Basu's circus statistician stuck too closely to the then current textbook theory of survey sampling, and paid the price by losing his job. In this book you are invited to follow the adventures of two relatively inexperienced survey statisticians from an outside agency who have been assigned the same task: to find a rough estimate of the total weight of the elephants.

I realized when the book was nearly complete that one of these novices (the narrator) was a personification of the logical side of my own character, and that his female Australian colleague was a personification of its intuitive side. So in the early chapters I am pretty much reporting the debate that was going on inside my own head in the 1960s and 1970s. Their supervisor, not surprisingly, is an alter ego of my own supervisor at the time, Ken Foreman. Ken had two great virtues. He knew far more about the practicalities of sampling than I did, and he knew how to bring out the best in his subordinates, including myself. He allowed me, from time to time, to sit back and think about what we were doing and why, whether it was necessary, how to do it better and (in due course) what allowed us to make any inferences at all from the sample to the population, and how different possible answers to that question were affecting the ways we made those inferences. Eventually that led to my advocating an inferential system that drew on randomization and prediction at the same time.

The reader should be cautioned that there is no consistent chronology built into the early chapters, or indeed the entire book. Ideally it would have to take place at a time before the weighing of elephants had ceased to be cumbersome and after the introduction of certain quite subtle techniques in the field of survey sampling. No real time interval corresponds to the intersection of these two requirements. On the one hand, it has long been possible to weigh an elephant by weighing an empty van on a weighbridge, coaxing the elephant into it, and weighing it again. On the other hand, some of the sampling techniques in this book were devised in the course of its writing. The reader must construct an imaginary time – or, better still, a complex time containing a real and an imaginary component. For those who have enjoyed stories in which human beings coexist with dinosaurs, as they do in the *Flintstones*, this should provide no serious problem.

Another and perhaps a more serious problem arises where considerations of convenience require the narrator in the latter part of this book to refer to results and equations from earlier chapters that in his life story would not actually have been written down. It seems inescapable that, with this style of writing, not only time becomes fuzzy but the whole environment in which the characters operate has to have its own peculiar dream logic, as does *South Park*, where Kenny has almost always been killed by the end of each episode, but is still able to reappear none the worse for wear in each succeeding one. The dream logic of this book is therefore one that allows the narrator to refer to earlier chapters wherever it suits the reader's convenience for him to do so, and even to refer to the present author's other writings as though he were a character in his own book.

The subject matter of the surveys in this book also goes through a rather abrupt transition after the end of Chapter 6, the elephants yielding centre stage to more mundane populations such as businesses, trees and households. The elephants are there, of course, to sugar-coat the pill in the initial chapters, but they also serve a practical purpose in illustrating the problems that occur when dealing with very small samples. The sample surveys of businesses, trees and the like are not only more realistic; the samples drawn for them are typically much larger, and present problems entirely different from and more realistic than those faced by the narrator and his colleague in the elephant circus.

Finally, two liberties have been taken with Basu's original fable. According to that source, the circus owner 'discovers a list of the elephants' weights taken 3 years ago [and] finds that Sambo, the middle sized elephant, was the average (in weight) elephant in the herd. He checks with the elephant trainer who reassures him (the owner) that Sambo may still be considered to be the average elephant in the herd.' As you can guess, the owner wants to weigh Sambo, but events move swiftly and the circus statistician is sacked before Sambo (or any other elephant) is weighed. That list of the elephants' weights taken 3 years ago would have made our heroes' task too easy. They are not provided with any such list and have to find a suitable substitute.

The other liberty is the division of the herd into a bulls' stratum and a cows' stratum. There had to be a reason for using stratified sampling, and this was the obvious way to provide one. But then there could not be a single 'average elephant in the herd'. Sambo retains his place as the average bull, but there is now also an average cow, and her name is Kara.

This second liberty was rather more difficult to accommodate to Basu's account of events. There were basically two possibilities. Either Sambo had to be the average *bull*, or else he would have to be treated *mistakenly* as the average elephant. Following the first of these options, two elephants would need to have been weighed, creating an awkward duplication, and substantial changes to the second half of Basu's text would have been needed.

The second option allowed the original text to be followed more closely, but required a plausible explanation of how the mistake could have been made. Any such explanation had inevitably to rely on some human frailty, and this had to be built either into the circus owner, or else into the elephant trainer, or possibly into both. With some reluctance, the second of these three options has been adopted. I have no reason to believe that circus folk are particularly prone to these particular frailties; they just happen to be the statisticians' clients in this story, and the mistakes they make are of the same kind as all human beings are prone to make when dealing with such subtle semantic concepts as 'average'.

Apart from the liberties taken with the list and the division between bulls and cows, the events recorded in Basu's fable provide the immediate past history in the context of which our narrator and his colleague are called upon to do their work. If you are really desperate to read the rest of Basu's fable, you will find it in Appendix A; otherwise, from now on, the story is in the hands of the narrator.

1

Simple Random Sampling with Equal Weights

Narrator's Introduction 4
Simple Random Sampling without Replacement 8
Simple Random Sampling with Replacement 14
Simple Random Sampling: the Prediction-Based Theory 18
An Excursus on Independence, Exchangeability and Non-informative Sampling 22
Prediction-Based Theory (Continued) 23
Summary 26
Exercises 27

Narrator's Introduction

1.1 According to what we have been told, the circus owner originally wanted to weigh only one elephant. This is too restrictive a condition for our purposes, but it reminds us that sampling is all about using resources efficiently. We must work out how to estimate the total weight for him as economically as possible, achieving the best balance between accuracy and cost. We will start by considering the most basic sampling strategy of all, simple random sampling with equal weights.

First, however, we must know what we are sampling from. We start by compiling a list of the 50 (Indian) elephants. Basu's elephants had names like Sambo and Jumbo, which are very convenient identifiers, so we list these names in some convenient order. Here we will use alphabetical order: 1. Amanda, 2. Anembo, 3. Bembo, 4. Brenda, etc. (see Appendix B).

Secondly, we have to decide on a sample size. More will be said about this later, but since a sample of one would allow us no basis for estimating the accuracy of our estimate, we already know that two is the absolute minimum. A *sample fraction* of 0.1 (one elephant in ten) will give us a sample of five. This will probably still be too small, but it is generally a good idea to select a small 'pilot' sample first to get a feel for the problem.

Thirdly, we need a random selection procedure. Most personal computers can be used to produce pseudo-random numbers that repeat the same pattern only after an extremely long sequence. Alternatively, we could use a book like the Rand Corporation's *Million Random Digits* (Rand Corporation, 1955), the entries in which were carefully screened to ensure that they were random for all practical purposes. The last few digits of the listed numbers in a large alphabetically listed telephone directory could also be used, but only with caution. There are certain discernibly non-random patterns that can be detected there. Switchboards are the most obvious example, but others can be found, with persistence.

Suppose, then, that we decide to use published tables of random numbers. It is common practice to choose the starting point by some chance or quasi-chance process to begin with, in order to avoid using the same random numbers over and over again. For instance, the date and time of day can be used to determine which page, which column and how far down the column we begin to read. As an additional precaution, those that we use on each occasion can be marked off, to ensure that they are not used in future.

Since there are fifty elephants, we need to consider digits in pairs. Suppose that the first five pairs we find are 31, 24, 36, 61 and 74. The first three selections are straightforward. We are selecting the 31st elephant at the first draw, the 24th at the second draw and the 36th at the third draw. When we come to the entry 61, we might decide to skip, because there are only 50 names on the list, but it is a more economical use of the directory to interpret the numbers from 51 to 99 as referring to the 1st to 49th elephants, respectively, by 'casting out' the unwanted 50. (An entry of 00 would, of course, refer to the 50th elephant.) So we in fact take the fourth entry, 61, to mean that the 11th elephant is to be selected at the fourth draw.

Applying the same procedure to the fifth entry, 74, we interpret this as referring to the 24th elephant. Now, however, we have to make another decision. The 24th elephant was already selected as a result of the second entry. Do we include it twice, or do we skip and go on until we get a fifth distinct sample elephant?

Actually, both procedures are permissible. Including the 24th elephant twice (at the second and fifth draws) would imply that we had opted for *simple random sampling with replacement*, often abbreviated to *srswr*. Passing it over until we find a fifth distinct sample elephant is the correct procedure for *simple random sampling without replacement*, or *srswor*. Using traditional methods of sampling analysis, *srswr* is slightly simpler to handle, but *srswor* provides estimators with lower mean squared errors, and is generally considered preferable. In this case, we decide to use *srswor*, so we skip the fifth entry and take the sixth, which is 55, to mean that the 5th elephant on the list is also the fifth and last to be included in the sample.

1.2 Our sample therefore consists of elephant numbers 5, 11, 24, 31, and 36: Combo, Flimbo, Linda, Pamela and Sara. The next task is to weigh them. This presents an immediate practical problem. The circus owner, you will remember, had wanted to weigh only one elephant. He is naturally taken aback when we inform him that we now want to weigh five, and that they will only be a pilot sample! He needs to be convinced that this is really necessary. We ask him how accurately he wants to know their combined weight. He says he would be satisfied if he knew it within 10% either way. We explain that it would be impossible to be certain of being within 10% of the true value and ask how confident he needs to be that the estimate we give him lies within 10% of the true value. (This is not a book about statistical inference in general, but there is a short note about confidence intervals and Bayesian credibility intervals in the Epilogue.) If he wants to be absolutely certain we will have to weigh perhaps not all, but certainly most of the elephants, a fact which helps him appreciate the need not to demand too much certainty. He is prepared to settle for 99% confidence.

In order to find the estimated variance corresponding to a two-sided 99% confidence interval, we make the assumption that the weights of our elephants are normally distributed. This would be a totally unrealistic and catastrophically unwise assumption to make if we were dealing with any kind of economic population (which is why most sampling statisticians, when they deal with confidence intervals at all, limit themselves to statements about estimates based on very large samples, where the central limit theorem ensures that these estimates will have distributions that are nearly normal). Elephants, however, are not economic but biological entities, and the normal distribution (or something very like it) is what we would expect to find for their weights.

We cannot, however, assume from this that the sampling distribution of our estimate of the total weight of the herd will be normally distributed. We have at present only five elephants in our sample, and we don't want to weigh any more if we can avoid it. So even given the assumption that our elephant weights are normally distributed, our estimate of the average weight of the elephants (and therefore also our estimate of the total weight of the herd) will follow not a normal but a t distribution with $5 - 1 = 4$ degrees of freedom.

For four degrees of freedom, both the classical two-sided 99% confidence interval and the corresponding 99% Bayesian credibility interval (based on a uniform prior) extend to 4.60 standard deviations either side of the best point estimate. (The comparable figure for the normal distribution is 2.58 standard deviations.) So if we aim for the standard error to be $10\% \div 4.60$ or a little more than 2% of the sample estimate of total, we should be just about right. When we explain to the circus owner what this means, he is ready to accept that we clearly need a sample substantially larger than a single elephant, but he practically begs us to do our best with just the original five in sample, and if at all possible avoid the need for weighing any more.

1.3 So the five elephants we selected are now being weighed. My colleague and I are both present and have been co-opted into the weighing. Basu had not exaggerated when he described it as a cumbersome business. Perhaps it would be easier if the elephant trainer were here, but his last-minute stand-in (who, like ourselves, is on contract) seems to know what he is about and tells us it is always like this. It is not so much that the elephants are actively uncooperative as that they have no idea in this context what co-operation would involve. We just have to wait for a moment when the one we are currently working on is still and in the right position, then make the most of it: act very quickly, record his or her weight, and bring on the next one. Although we take it in turns to keep vigil, by the end of the day we are all thoroughly exhausted. No wonder the circus owner was so keen to weigh just a single elephant and no wonder he is so reluctant for us to weigh any more after these five. We would be just as reluctant ourselves!

To add to our misery, we lost the use of our laptop while I was seeing to the fourth of the five weighings. The opportunity arrived to weigh Pamela, and immediately I started to do so, injudiciously leaving our computer on the floor while I did. But Combo, the only elephant still unattended on, thereupon decided that this weighing business was worth inspecting at close quarters; so he just ambled across and planted his great hind foot on it. I know what this will mean. Until I can afford to pay for the repairs, all our calculations will have to be done with a hand-held calculator, and there will be rounding errors all over the place.

Actually, this will not be without its compensations. My colleague will now be checking my arithmetic at every turn, and it will do her good to 'get her hands dirty with a few X_{ij}s', as Ken Foreman used to put it. (To be fair, though, I suppose I shall be checking hers too, and that will be equally good for me.)

Incidentally, when the elephant trainer rang in sick this morning he seemed a little cagey as to what was wrong with him. He simply said he was 'indisposed'. We wonder now whether he was simply indisposed to be present. If only we had known, we might have been 'indisposed' ourselves. But that is just one of those things about being a statistician, and perhaps particularly a survey statistician. One never knows what one might be called upon to do next.

1.4 Well, at least the elephants are now weighed. Their weights in kilograms are as follows: Combo 4675, Flimbo 3032, Linda 3328, Pamela 3427 and Sara 2910. The sum of these numbers (the *sample total* or *sample take*) is 17 372, and the *sample mean* is 3474.4. Since there are 50 elephants in total, the assumption that the *population mean* is equal to the sample mean yields an estimate of their total weight that is $50 \times 3474.4 = 173\,720$ kg.

So far so good, but how accurate is that estimate? One way to look at that question is to say that we can make five estimates of total, each based on a sample of one elephant. The estimate based on Combo's weight alone is $50 \times 4675 = 233\,750$ kg, and the others are 151 600, 166 400, 171 350 and 145 500 kg. Our population could provide at the most 50 distinct single-elephant estimates, but it will be simpler for the moment if we can imagine that our five are taken from a hypothetical infinite population. To estimate its *population variance* we divide the mean-corrected sum of squares by $(5 - 1) = 4$, the 1 being subtracted to allow for the degree of freedom taken up by the mean.

Deliberately using a slightly roundabout way of calculating the mean-corrected sum of squares (in order to highlight the different sizes of contributions from the individual elephants), we find it to be

$$
\begin{aligned}
&(233\,750 - 173\,720)^2 + (151\,600 - 173\,720)^2 + (166\,400 - 173\,720)^2 \\
&\quad + (171\,350 - 173\,720)^2 + (145\,500 - 173\,720)^2 \\
&\quad = 60\,030^2 + (-22\,120)^2 + (-7320)^2 + (-2370)^2 + (-28\,220)^2 \\
&\quad = 4\,948\,463\,000\ \text{kg}^2,
\end{aligned}
$$

and the resulting estimate of the population variance is therefore $4\,948\,463\,000 \div 4 = 1\,237\,115\,750\ \text{kg}^2$. The square root of this quantity, 35 173 kg to the nearest whole kilogram, therefore estimates the *population standard deviation* of the hypothetically infinite number of single-elephant estimates. (It is also, of course,

50 times the estimated population standard deviation of the theoretically infinite herd of the elephants themselves.) On the assumption that our five single-elephant estimates are independent of each other, the estimated variance of our estimate of total herd weight is therefore 1 237 115 750 $\div$ 5 or 247 423 150 kg^2, and a rounded estimate of its standard error is 15 730 kg.

1.5 This answer is not the best that can be obtained, because it ignores the additional accuracy that we have actually achieved by sampling without replacement from a finite population of 50 elephants. It is not immediately obvious that the appropriate adjustment to our estimated variance is to reduce it by the factor 'one minus the sample fraction', in our case $1 - 0.1 = 0.9$, but this rule will be derived in the next section. Applying it now, we find that the appropriate sample estimate of the variance (of our sample estimate of the total weight of the 50 elephants, 173 720 kg) is 247 423 150 $\times$ 0.9 = 222 680 835 kg^2. The rounded estimate of its standard deviation is thus 14 922 kg, or 8.6% of the estimate.

For convenience, we will round still further and describe our estimate of total herd weight as 174 ± 15 tonnes. What does this tell us about the adequacy of the sample size? If the elephants' weights are normally distributed (a strong assumption for elephants and an even stronger one for most economic variables) our estimator of standard error will be distributed as t with four degrees of freedom. The top end of its two-sided 99% confidence interval is therefore $174 + 4.60 \times 15$ or 243 tonnes, corresponding to an average weight of 4860 kg per elephant. Since this is not far off the average weight of a full-grown Indian bull, and since there are fairly obviously quite a few cows in the herd, for which the average weight is appreciably lower, we are not yet telling the circus owner anything of value that he did not know before. We must improve on this estimate, either by increasing the sample size or by using a better sampling methodology, if we want him to hire us again! Some of these better methodologies will be found in succeeding chapters, but in the meantime it will be useful to formalize our knowledge about what we have done already.

Simple Random Sampling without Replacement

1.6 In the previous section, the individual population values were the weights of elephants. Now we will denote them by the symbols Y_i, $i = 1, 2, \ldots, N$, where N is the number of units in the population (elephants in the herd). So Amanda's weight will be symbolized by Y_1, Flimbo's weight by Y_{11} and so on. The *indicator variate* (or indicator random variable) δ_i will take the value 1 if the ith population unit is in sample and 0 if it is not. Amanda is not in sample, so in our case the realized value of δ_1 is 0; but Flimbo is in sample, so the realized value of δ_{11} is 1. The Y_i are not themselves variates but fixed values. Their population total will be denoted by $Y_{\bullet}$ and their population mean by $\bar{Y} = N^{-1} Y_{\bullet}$.

We will be assuming throughout that the weighing process is accurate and that no mistakes are made. It would have been somewhat safer had we chosen to write, 'the value that would have been obtained if the entire population had been in sample', rather than 'the population total' or 'its true value', but that would not have made for easy reading. We will therefore also assume that the reader is capable of making this qualification without constantly needing to be reminded of it.

The operators E(·), V(·) and C(·, ·) will denote *design expectation*, *design variance* and *design covariance*, respectively. By design expectation (or design variance or covariance), we will mean the expectation (or variance or covariance) over all possible samples defined by a given sample design; for instance, over all samples of a given number of units selected using *srswor*. The operator $\sum_{i=1}^{N}$, or more briefly $\sum_i$, will denote summation over all N population units. Thus the population total is $Y_{\bullet} = \sum_{i=1}^{N} Y_i = \sum_i Y_i$.

The sample size, or number of units included in sample, will be denoted by $n = \sum_i \delta_i$. The operator $\sum_{i \in s}$, or simply $\sum_s$, will denote summation over all the units included in sample. Here $s = \{s_1, \ldots, s_n\}$ denotes the set of subscripts identifying the n sample units in population order. For instance, our recently drawn sample of elephants is $s = \{5, 11, 24, 31, 36\}$ and the corresponding set of y-values is $\{Y_5, Y_{11}, Y_{24}, Y_{31}, Y_{36}\}$.

The sample mean will sometimes be denoted by $\bar{Y}_s$ but, when it is being used as an estimator of the population mean, $\bar{Y}$, it will usually be written $\hat{\bar{Y}}$. Thus $\hat{\bar{Y}} = \bar{Y}_s = n^{-1} \sum_i \delta_i Y_i = n^{-1} \sum_s Y_i$. In our example, since $\delta_i = 1$ for the five elephants in sample and $\delta_i = 0$ for the remaining 45 elephants,

$$\begin{aligned} \bar{Y}_s &= 5^{-1}(Y_5 + Y_{11} + Y_{24} + Y_{31} + Y_{36}) \\ &= 5^{-1}(4675 + 3032 + 3328 + 3427 + 2910) \\ &= 3474.4. \end{aligned}$$

Another way we will sometimes write the sample mean is $\bar{y} = n^{-1} \sum_{i=1}^{n} y_i$ where y_i is the value for the ith sample unit in population order, which can also be written Y_{s_i}. In our example, for instance, $y_1 = Y_{s_1} = Y_5 = 4675, y_2 = Y_{s_2} = Y_{11} = 3032$, etc.

We define the *expansion estimator* of $Y_{\bullet}$ as N times the sample mean and denote this estimator by $\hat{Y}_{\bullet}$. Thus $\hat{Y}_{\bullet} = N\hat{\bar{Y}} = Nn^{-1} \sum \delta_i Y_i = Nn^{-1} \sum_s Y_i = Nn^{-1} \sum_{i=1}^{n} y_i$.

Note that since $\bar{Y}_s$ and $\hat{Y}_{\bullet}$ are functions of the δ_i, they are *random variables* rather than fixed numbers.

The operator $\sum_{i(\neq j)=1}^{N}$ will denote summation over all the N population units other than the jth, and $\sum_{i(\neq j)=1}^{n}$ will denote summation over all n sample units other than the jth. Thus in our example, $\sum_{i(\neq 3)=1}^{N} Y_i = Y_{\bullet} - Y_3$ and $\sum_{i(\neq 3)=1}^{n} = y_1 + y_2 + y_4 + y_5$.

1.7 The standard *paradigm*, or procedure under which design-based inference usually operates, requires us first to find estimators of the population mean and total that are design-unbiased, that is, estimators for which the design expectations are equal to the population values. Next, expressions have to be found for the design variances of those estimators. Finally, estimators must be constructed for the design variances themselves, and those estimators will also ideally be design-unbiased.

To prove that $\hat{\bar{Y}}$ and $\hat{Y}_\bullet$ are design-unbiased estimators of $\bar{Y}$ and $Y_\bullet$, respectively, we first need to prove:

Lemma 1.7.1 Under *srswor*, $\mathrm{E}\delta_i = N^{-1}n$ for all $i = 1, 2, \ldots, N$.

Proof. Since sampling is without replacement, $\mathrm{E}\delta_i$ is the sum of the probabilities of selection of the ith population unit over all n sample draws. Its probability of selection at the first draw is N^{-1}. At the second draw, its probability of selection is the product of its probability of non-selection at the first draw, $1 - N^{-1}$, and its probability of selection at the second draw conditional on its non-selection at the first, $(N - 1)^{-1}$. That product is also N^{-1}. By a straightforward extension of the same kind of reasoning, the ith population unit's probability of selection can be shown to be N^{-1} at each of the n draws. The sum of its selection probabilities at these n draws is therefore $N^{-1}n$. Hence $\mathrm{E}\delta_i = N^{-1}n$ for all $i = 1, 2, \ldots, N$. ◇

Theorem 1.7.1 Under *srswor*, $\hat{\bar{Y}}$ and $\hat{Y}_\bullet$ are design-unbiased estimators of $\bar{Y} = N^{-1}\sum_i Y_i$ and $Y_\bullet = \sum_i Y_i$, respectively; that is, $\mathrm{E}\hat{\bar{Y}} = \bar{Y}$ and $\mathrm{E}\hat{Y}_\bullet = Y_\bullet$.

Proof. $\mathrm{E}\hat{\bar{Y}} = \mathrm{E}(n^{-1}\sum_i \delta_i Y_i) = n^{-1}\sum_i \mathrm{E}\delta_i Y_i$. But by Lemma 1.7.1, $\mathrm{E}\delta_i = N^{-1}n$ for all $i = 1, 2, \ldots, N$. Hence $\mathrm{E}\hat{\bar{Y}} = N^{-1}\sum_i Y_i = \bar{Y}$. Multiplying through by N, $\mathrm{E}\hat{Y}_\bullet = \sum_i Y_i = Y_\bullet$. ◇

It follows from Theorem 1.7.1 that $\hat{Y}_\bullet$ (the expansion estimator) was not merely the obvious one to use, but one that would have tended to average out to the true value had the processes of selecting five units by *srswor* and taking 50 times the sample mean been repeated a large number of times. It would also have averaged out to the true value exactly if we had painstakingly selected every possible distinct sample of five out of the 50 elephants and averaged out the 2 118 760 estimates. (The same result could of course have been obtained less laboriously by taking any ten mutually exclusive samples of five, or equivalently, a single 'sample' of 50 units selected by *srswor*, but neither of these last two results is directly related to the design-unbiasedness of $\hat{Y}_\bullet$.)

To find expressions for the variances of $\hat{\bar{Y}}$ and $\hat{Y}_\bullet$, we require two further lemmas.

Lemma 1.7.2 Under *srswor*, $\mathrm{E}\delta_i^2 = N^{-1}n$ for all $i = 1, 2, \ldots, N$.

Proof. Under *srswor*, δ_i can take only one of two values, 0 or 1. But $0^2 = 0$ and $1^2 = 1$; hence $\delta_i^2 = \delta_i$ for all $i = 1, 2, \ldots, N$. Finally, by Lemma 1.7.1, $\mathrm{E}\delta_i = N^{-1}n$ for all $i = 1, 2, \ldots, N$. Hence $\mathrm{E}\delta_i^2 = \mathrm{E}\delta_i = N^{-1}n$ for all $i = 1, 2, \ldots, N$. ◇

To prove the next lemma, which derives a corresponding expression for $\mathrm{E}(\delta_i\delta_j)$, we shall appeal to a particular form of symmetry known as *exchangeability*. In **1.6** we wrote the set of the n sample units in population order as $s = \{s_1, \ldots, s_n\}$ and therefore (implicitly) the vector of the corresponding y-values as $(Y_{s_1}, \ldots, Y_{s_n})$. We will now write the set that defines the same n sample units, but this time in the order of their selection, as $s' = \{s'_1, \ldots, s'_n\}$ and the vector of the corresponding y-values therefore as $(y_{s'_1}, \ldots, y_{s'_n})$. Each of the $y_{s'_i}$, $i = 1, 2, \ldots, n$, is then a random variable and has its own sampling distribution, as does the vector $(y_{s'_1}, \ldots, y_{s'_n})$ itself.

Now the sampling distributions of the $y_{s'_i}$ are not independent, because if a particular unit is selected at the ith draw, it cannot be selected at any subsequent draw. It is nevertheless possible to show that their distributions are exchangeable, where *exchangeability* is defined as the property of variables $U_{s'_1}, \ldots, U_{s'_n}$ for which the joint distribution of the vector $(U_{s'_1}, \ldots, U_{s'_n})$ remains unchanged under any permutation of the subscripts $s'_1, \ldots, s'_n$.

In order to prove the exchangeability of the variables $y_{s'_1}, \ldots, y_{s'_n}$ in our particular case, we need to show that the probability of obtaining our sample, $s = (5, 11, 24, 31, 36)$, in *any* particular permutation order, was the same as the probability of obtaining it in our actual order, which was 31, 24, 36, 11, 5. This is easy, as the probability of selecting the same five sample units in any given order, such as $Y_{24}, Y_{11}, Y_{36}, Y_5, Y_{31}$, is clearly $50^{-1} \times 49^{-1} \times 48^{-1} \times 47^{-1} \times 46^{-1}$. In the general case, that probability is the reciprocal of the number of different orders (or *permutations*) in which n units selected out of N using *srswor* can be listed. This probability may be written $(N!)^{-1}(N - n)!$, where for instance $N!$ (pronounced 'N factorial') denotes the product $N \times (N - 1) \times \cdots \times 3 \times 2 \times 1$.

Lemma 1.7.3 Under *srswor*,

$$E(\delta_i\delta_j) = N^{-1}(N - 1)^{-1}n(n - 1) \text{ for all } i, j = 1, 2, \ldots, N \text{ such that } j \neq i.$$

Proof. Under *srswor*, $E(\delta_i\delta_j) = \Pr(\delta_i = 1, \delta_j = 1)$ is the joint inclusion probability, or joint probability of inclusion in sample, for the ith and jth population units. (The ith unit may be selected at any draw and the jth unit at any other draw.)

The joint probability of selecting the ith population unit at the first draw and the jth at the second draw is $N^{-1}(N - 1)^{-1}$.

By exchangeability, it is also $N^{-1}(N - 1)^{-1}$ for each of the other $n(n - 1) - 1$ possible ordered pairs of draws.

Since selection is *srswor*, neither the ith nor the jth population unit can be selected more than once, so their joint selection probabilities at the $n(n - 1)$ possible ordered pairs of draws are additive, and the total of these is their joint inclusion probability.

Hence the joint probability of selecting the ith population unit at any draw and the jth at any other draw is

$$\begin{aligned} E(\delta_i\delta_j) &= \Pr(\delta_i = 1)\Pr(\delta_j = 1 | \delta_i = 1) \\ &= N^{-1}(N - 1)^{-1}n(n - 1) \quad \text{for all } i, j = 1, 2, \ldots, N \text{ such that } j \neq i. \quad \diamond \end{aligned}$$

In the next theorem we shall show that the expression for the variance of the estimated sample mean, $\hat{\bar{Y}}$, is $V\hat{\bar{Y}} = N^{-1}(N - n)n^{-1}S^2$ and that the corresponding expression for the variance of the estimated sample total, $\hat{Y}_{\bullet}$, is $V\hat{Y}_{\bullet} = N(N - n)n^{-1}S^2$, where $S^2 = (N-1)^{-1}NS^2_{\infty}$ and $S^2_{\infty} = N^{-1}\sum_i (Y_i - \bar{Y})^2$ is the *population variance*.

The interrelationship between these expressions may be understood as follows. The true population variance of a population of size N is, by definition, $S^2_{\infty} = N^{-1}\sum_i (Y_i - \bar{Y})^2$. Thus if a sample of a single unit is selected from a population of size N, and its y-value is treated as an estimator of the population mean, $\bar{Y}$, the variance of that estimator is S^2_{∞}.

Next, if a sample of n units is selected from the same population using *srswr*, the variance of the sample mean, $\hat{\bar{Y}}$, again regarded as an estimator of the population mean, $\bar{Y}$, is $n^{-1}S^2_{\infty}$. If, however, that sample is selected using *srswor*, the sample mean is somewhat more accurate as an estimator of $\bar{Y}$, and its variance is in fact $\{(N - n)/(N - 1)\}n^{-1}S^2_{\infty}$.

However, since in practice sampling is almost always without replacement, it is convenient to write $\{(N-n)/(N-1)\}n^{-1}S^2_{\infty}$ more compactly as $N^{-1}(N-n)n^{-1}S^2$, where $S^2 = (N-1)^{-1}NS^2_{\infty}$ may be referred to as the *adjusted population variance*. And, finally, since $\hat{Y}_{\bullet}$ is simply $N\hat{\bar{Y}}$ and N is a fixed number, the variance of $\hat{Y}_{\bullet}$ is N^2 times that of $\hat{\bar{Y}}$, i.e. $V\hat{Y}_{\bullet} = N(N - n)n^{-1}S^2$.

Theorem 1.7.2 Under *srswor*, the design variances of $\hat{\bar{Y}}$ and $\hat{Y}_{\bullet}$ are $V\hat{\bar{Y}} = N^{-1}(N - n)n^{-1}S^2$ and $V\hat{Y}_{\bullet} = N(N - n)n^{-1}S^2$, respectively.

Proof. Under *srswor*, $\hat{\bar{Y}}$ is a design-unbiased estimator of $\bar{Y}$ and its variance may therefore be written as

$$V\hat{\bar{Y}} = E(\hat{\bar{Y}} - \bar{Y})^2 = E\hat{\bar{Y}}^2 - 2\bar{Y}E\hat{\bar{Y}} + \bar{Y}^2 = E\hat{\bar{Y}}^2 - \bar{Y}^2$$

$$= n^{-2}E\left(\sum_i \delta_i^2 Y_i^2 + \sum_i \sum_{j \neq i} \delta_i \delta_j Y_i Y_j\right) - \bar{Y}^2.$$

Applying Lemmas 1.7.2 and 1.7.3, we obtain

$$V\hat{\bar{Y}} = N^{-1}n^{-1}\sum_i Y_i^2 + N^{-1}(N - 1)^{-1}n^{-1}(n - 1)\sum_i \sum_{j \neq i} Y_i Y_j - \bar{Y}^2.$$

But $\sum_i \sum_{j \neq i} Y_i Y_j = -\sum_i Y_i^2 + N^2\bar{Y}^2$, so that

$$V\hat{\bar{Y}} = \left\{N^{-1}n^{-1} - N^{-1}(N - 1)^{-1}n^{-1}(n - 1)\right\}\sum_i Y_i^2$$

$$+ \left\{N^{-1}(N - 1)^{-1}n^{-1}(n - 1)N^2 - 1\right\}\bar{Y}^2$$

$$= (N - n)n^{-1}(N - 1)^{-1}\left(N^{-1}\sum_i Y_i^2 - \bar{Y}^2\right).$$

Also $N^{-1}\sum_i Y_i^2 - \bar{Y}^2 = N^{-1}(N-1)S^2$, so

$$\mathrm{V}\hat{\bar{Y}} = (N-n)n^{-1}(N-1)^{-1}N^{-1}(N-1)S^2 = N^{-1}(N-n)n^{-1}S^2.$$

Finally, multiplying through by N^2,

$$\mathrm{V}\hat{Y}_{\bullet} = N(N-n)n^{-1}S^2. \qquad \diamond$$

Corollary 1.7.1 When $n=1$, $\mathrm{V}\hat{\bar{Y}} = N^{-1}(N-1)S^2 = N^{-1}\sum_i Y_i^2 - \bar{Y}^2$ and

$$\mathrm{V}\hat{Y}_{\bullet} = N(N-1)S^2 = N\sum_i Y_i^2 - Y_{\bullet}^2.$$

This corollary will be useful when we start to consider the theory of *srswr*. (When $n=1$, there is no difference between sampling with and without replacement.)

The last part of the paradigm for *srswor* is the construction of design-unbiased estimators for $\mathrm{V}\hat{\bar{Y}}$ and $\mathrm{V}\hat{Y}_{\bullet}$. Since N and n are known, the only quantity requiring estimation is the adjusted population variance, $S^2 = (N-1)^{-1} \times \sum_i (Y_i - \bar{Y})^2$. An obviously promising estimator of S^2 is the *sample variance*, $\hat{S}^2 = (n-1)^{-1}\sum_i \delta_i(Y_i - \hat{\bar{Y}})^2$, and the following lemma shows that it is in fact design-unbiased.

Lemma 1.7.4 Under *srswor*, $\mathrm{E}\hat{S}^2 = S^2$.

Proof.

$$\begin{aligned}
E\hat{S}^2 &= (n-1)^{-1}\mathrm{E}\left\{\sum_i \delta_i(Y_i - \hat{\bar{Y}})^2\right\}\\
&= (n-1)^{-1}\mathrm{E}\left\{\sum_i \delta_i[(Y_i - \bar{Y}) - (\hat{\bar{Y}} - \bar{Y})]^2\right\}\\
&= (n-1)^{-1}\mathrm{E}\left\{\sum_i \delta_i(Y_i - \bar{Y})^2 - 2(\hat{\bar{Y}} - \bar{Y})\sum_i \delta_i(Y_i - \bar{Y})\right.\\
&\qquad\left. + (\hat{\bar{Y}} - \bar{Y})^2\sum_i \delta_i\right\}\\
&= (n-1)^{-1}\mathrm{E}\left\{\sum_i \delta_i(Y_i - \bar{Y})^2 - n(\hat{\bar{Y}} - \bar{Y})^2\right\}\\
&= (n-1)^{-1}\left\{N^{-1}n\sum_i (Y_i - \bar{Y})^2 - n\mathrm{V}(\hat{\bar{Y}})\right\}\\
&= (n-1)^{-1}\left\{N^{-1}n(N-1)S^2 - nN^{-1}(N-n)n^{-1}S^2\right\}\\
&= S^2.
\end{aligned} \qquad \diamond$$

Theorem 1.7.3 Under *srswor*, design-unbiased estimators of $\mathrm{V}\hat{\bar{Y}}$ and $\mathrm{V}\hat{Y}_\bullet$ are $\hat{\mathrm{V}}\hat{\bar{Y}} = N^{-1}(N-n)n^{-1}\hat{S}^2$ and $\hat{\mathrm{V}}\hat{Y}_\bullet = N(N-n)n^{-1}\hat{S}^2$, respectively.

Proof. This follows immediately from Theorem 1.7.2 and Lemma 1.7.4.

Given our five observations of elephant weights in kilograms, which were 4675, 3032, 3328, 3427 and 2910, with mean 3474.4, our value of $\hat{S}^2$ is 494 846.8, the value of $N(N-n)n^{-1}$ is 450 and $\mathrm{V}\hat{Y}_\bullet = N(N-n)n^{-1}\hat{S}^2 = 222\,681\,038$. The estimated standard deviation of $\hat{Y}_\bullet$ is therefore 14 922 kg, confirming the earlier calculations that were carried out in a different but equivalent fashion.

1.8 In summary, the three important results for *srswor* are as follows:

Result 1.8.1 If our estimators of the population mean, $\bar{Y} = N^{-1}\sum_i Y_i$, and the population total, $Y_\bullet = \sum_i Y_i$, are $\hat{\bar{Y}} = n^{-1}\sum_i \delta_i Y_i$ and $\hat{Y}_\bullet = N\hat{\bar{Y}} = Nn^{-1}\sum_i \delta_i Y_i$, respectively, then $\mathrm{E}\hat{\bar{Y}} = \bar{Y}$ and $\mathrm{E}\hat{Y}_\bullet = Y_\bullet$; thus $\hat{\bar{Y}}$ and $\hat{Y}_\bullet$ are design-unbiased.

Result 1.8.2 The design variances of $\hat{\bar{Y}}$ and $\hat{Y}_\bullet$ are $\mathrm{V}\hat{\bar{Y}} = N^{-1}(N-n)n^{-1}S^2$ and $\mathrm{V}\hat{Y}_\bullet = N(N-n)n^{-1}S^2$, respectively, where $S^2 = (N-1)^{-1}\sum_i (Y_i - \bar{Y})^2$.

Result 1.8.3 $\hat{\mathrm{V}}\hat{\bar{Y}} = N^{-1}(N-n)n^{-1}\hat{S}^2$ and $\hat{\mathrm{V}}\hat{Y}_\bullet = N(N-n)n^{-1}\hat{S}^2$, where $\hat{S}^2 = (n-1)^{-1}\sum_i \delta_i(Y_i - \hat{\bar{Y}})^2$ is the *sample variance*, are design-unbiased estimators of $\mathrm{V}\hat{\bar{Y}}$ and $\mathrm{V}\hat{Y}_\bullet$, respectively.

Simple Random Sampling with Replacement

1.9 To examine the differences between simple random sampling with and without replacement, we now pretend that when the 24th elephant (Linda) came up a second time in the selection process, we chose to use *srswr* instead of *srswor*. Consequently we did not select Combo, but Linda a second time. Our selection numbers were 11, 24 (twice), 31 and 36. We did not bother to weigh Linda twice, because the few kilograms difference there might have been between the two readings would not really have conveyed any useful information, and weighing an elephant is (as we have now seen for ourselves) a cumbersome process. Our sample observations were Flimbo 3032, Linda 3328 (twice), Pamela 3427 and Sara 2910. The sample take was 16 025 and the sample mean was 3205. The sample estimate of the population total was $50 \times 3205 = 160\,250$ kg, a little over 160 tonnes. However, rather than estimate the variance and standard error of this 160 tonnes estimate in the intuitive fashion we used earlier, we shall now present the theory and substitute in the resulting formulae.

It will no longer be possible to use the zero–one indicator δ_i as our random variable. For *srswr* the relevant variable is the number of times selected or *inclusion counter*, which we shall denote by ν_i. (The Greek letter ν – transliterated as 'nu' and pronounced the same way as the English word 'new' – corresponds to n in the Roman alphabet. It is therefore an appropriate symbol for variables that take whole-number values and must not be confused with lower case v or, in italics, v.) In *srswr* the value of each individual ν_i can range from zero right up to n, though large values are rare and, of course, the total of the ν_i is itself n. For our sample, the values of ν_i are $\nu_{11} = 1$, $\nu_{24} = 2$, $\nu_{31} = 1$, $\nu_{36} = 1$ and zero for the 46 remaining values of i. The number of ν_i that are non-zero will be denoted by ν, and could also be written $\sum_i \delta_i$. For our sample, $\nu = 4$.

Under *srswr*, the sample mean is defined by $\hat{\bar{Y}} = n^{-1}\sum_i \nu_i Y_i = n^{-1} \times \sum_s \nu_i y_i = n^{-1}\sum_i^n y_i$ where there are only ν non-zero terms in the first two summations, but a full n in the third. Following the standard design-oriented paradigm, we will first show that $\hat{\bar{Y}}$ is an unbiased estimator of $\bar{Y}$ and hence that $\hat{Y}_{\bullet} = N\hat{\bar{Y}}$ is an unbiased estimator of $Y_{\bullet}$.

Lemma 1.9.1 Under *srswr*, $\mathrm{E}\nu_i = N^{-1}n$ for all $i = 1, 2, \ldots, N$.

Proof. Since each of the n draws is conducted identically, independently of every other draw, and symmetrically with respect to the N population units, each of the N values ν_i has the same expectation. Further, since their sum is n for any given sample, each of the ν_i has the expectation $N^{-1}n$. ◇

Theorem 1.9.1 Under *srswr*, $\mathrm{E}\hat{\bar{Y}} = \bar{Y}$ and $\mathrm{E}\hat{Y}_{\bullet} = Y_{\bullet}$.

Proof. This follows immediately from Lemma 1.9.1. ◇

For the second step of the paradigm, we develop expressions for the variances of $\hat{\bar{Y}}$ and $\hat{Y}_{\bullet}$.

Theorem 1.9.2 Under *srswr*, $\mathrm{V}\hat{\bar{Y}} = n^{-1}S_{\infty}^2$ and $\mathrm{V}\hat{Y}_{\bullet} = N^2 n^{-1} S_{\infty}^2$. (Note that $S^2/S_{\infty}^2 \to 1$ as $N \to \infty$; compare Theorem 1.7.2.)

Proof. From Corollary 1.7.1, when $n = 1$, $\mathrm{V}\hat{\bar{Y}} = N^{-1}(N-1)S^2 = S_{\infty}^2$ and $\mathrm{V}\hat{Y}_{\bullet} = N(N-1)S^2 = N^2 S_{\infty}^2$. (This is true regardless of whether selection is with or without replacement, because when $n = 1$ the two procedures are identical.) Under *srswr*, the sample draws are independent and the variances are therefore proportional to n^{-1}. Hence, for a sample of size n, $\mathrm{V}\hat{\bar{Y}} = n^{-1}S_{\infty}^2$ and $\mathrm{V}\hat{Y}_{\bullet} = N^2 n^{-1} S_{\infty}^2$. ◇

For the third and final step of the paradigm, we find a design-unbiased estimator for S_{∞}^2 and use it to construct design-unbiased estimators for $\mathrm{V}\hat{\bar{Y}}$ and $\mathrm{V}\hat{Y}_{\bullet}$.

Lemma 1.9.2 Under *srswr*, $\hat{S}^2_\infty = (n-1)^{-1} \sum_i \nu_i (Y_i - \hat{\bar{Y}})^2$ is a design-unbiased estimator of S^2_∞.

Proof.

$$\begin{aligned}
\mathrm{E}\hat{S}^2_\infty &= (n-1)^{-1}\mathrm{E}\left\{\sum_i \nu_i (Y_i - \hat{\bar{Y}})^2\right\} \\
&= (n-1)^{-1}\mathrm{E}\left\{\sum_i \nu_i [(Y_i - \bar{Y}) - (\hat{\bar{Y}} - \bar{Y})]^2\right\} \\
&= (n-1)^{-1}\mathrm{E}\left\{\sum_i \nu_i (Y_i - \bar{Y})^2 - 2(\hat{\bar{Y}} - \bar{Y})\sum_i \nu_i (Y_i - \bar{Y}) \right. \\
&\qquad \left. + (\hat{\bar{Y}} - \bar{Y})^2 \sum_i \nu_i \right\} \\
&= (n-1)^{-1}\mathrm{E}\left\{\sum_i \nu_i (Y_i - \bar{Y})^2 - n(\hat{\bar{Y}} - \bar{Y})^2\right\} \\
&= (n-1)^{-1}\left\{N^{-1} n \sum_i (Y_i - \bar{Y})^2 - n\mathrm{V}\hat{\bar{Y}}\right\} \\
&= (n-1)^{-1}\left\{N^{-1} nNS^2_\infty - nn^{-1}S^2_\infty\right\} \\
&= S^2_\infty.
\end{aligned}$$

◇

Theorem 1.9.3 Under *srswr*, design-unbiased estimators of $\mathrm{V}\hat{\bar{Y}}$ and $\mathrm{V}\hat{Y}_\bullet$ are $\hat{\mathrm{V}}\hat{\bar{Y}} = n^{-1}\hat{S}^2_\infty$ and $\hat{\mathrm{V}}\hat{Y}_\bullet = N^2 n^{-1}\hat{S}^2_\infty$, respectively.

Proof. This follows immediately from Theorem 1.9.2 and Lemma 1.9.2. ◇

Substituting our numerical values of Y_i in the relevant formulae, we find:

$$\begin{aligned}
\hat{S}^2_\infty &= \frac{196\,496}{4} = 49\,124, \\
\hat{\mathrm{V}}\hat{Y}_\bullet &= \frac{50^2}{5} \times 49\,124 = 24\,562\,000\,\mathrm{kg}^2,
\end{aligned}$$

and the *estimated standard error* of $\hat{Y}_\bullet$ to the nearest whole kilogram is

$$\widehat{\mathrm{SE}}\hat{Y}_\bullet = 4956\,\mathrm{kg}.$$

Rounding as before, we write our estimate of the total weight of the herd as 160 ± 5 tonnes, lower and apparently far more accurate than the *srswor*-based estimate which was 174 ± 15 tonnes. The apparently greater accuracy may cause surprise, because the theory indicates that the variance should increase rather than decrease when we move from *srswor* to *srswr*. The truth is that the variance has indeed increased, and that it is only our estimate of the variance that has decreased.

It is not difficult to see why this should be so. Looking back at the calculations for the estimate of *srswor* variance in **1.4**, we see there that Combo's contribution dominated it. But Combo was not selected for the *srswr* sample, Linda being selected a second time instead. The elephants corresponding to the five *srswr* selections all happened to be approximately the same size; consequently the *estimated* standard error was smaller than for the *srswor* sample, even though (as the theory indicates) the *actual* standard error was necessarily higher. Such paradoxical results (estimates of variance going in one direction and the variances themselves in the other) occur not infrequently in survey sampling, especially when the samples are small. Further, estimates of variance and standard error are noticeably more sensitive to sampling variability than estimates of total and mean are. We conclude, therefore, that we still need to achieve greater accuracy in the estimation process, either by increasing the sample size, or by sharpening up the methodology, or by doing both at the same time.

It is worth noting, however, that if exactly the same samples had been selected using *srswor* and *srswr*, the differences between the two sets of inferences would have been far more modest. Suppose, for instance, that when the sample was being selected, '55' had been the fifth pair of random digits, instead of the sixth. Then the *srswr* sample, just like the *srswor* sample, would have consisted of Combo, Flimbo, Linda, Pamela and Sara. The two samples would then have had the same estimates of population total and of population mean, but their estimates of the variance would have been different.

It may be seen from **1.5** that the rounded estimate of population total from *srswor* was 174 ± 15 tonnes, and from the end of **1.4** that the corresponding estimate from *srswr* would have been 174 ± 16 tonnes. So the large differences between the *srswor* and *srswr* inferences that we observed earlier were *almost* (but not quite) entirely due to differences between the samples selected. Differences between the relevant formulae were affecting only the standard errors and their estimates and, even then, only to a relatively minor extent.

1.10 It is convenient now to summarize the mathematical results that we have obtained in this section for *srswr*. They correspond directly to the three we obtained for *srswor* in **1.8**.

Result 1.10.1 If our estimators of the population mean, $\bar{Y} = N^{-1} \sum_i Y_i$, and the population total, $Y_{\bullet} = \sum_i Y_i$, are $\hat{\bar{Y}} = n^{-1} \sum_i \nu_i Y_i$ and $\hat{Y}_{\bullet} = N\hat{\bar{Y}} = Nn^{-1} \sum_i \nu_i Y_i$, respectively, then $\mathrm{E}\hat{\bar{Y}} = \bar{Y}$ and $\mathrm{E}\hat{Y}_{\bullet} = Y_{\bullet}$; so $\hat{\bar{Y}}$ and $\hat{Y}_{\bullet}$ are design-unbiased.

Result 1.10.2 The design variances of $\hat{\bar{Y}}$ and $\hat{Y}_{\bullet}$ are $\mathrm{V}\hat{\bar{Y}} = n^{-1}S^2_{\infty}$ and $\mathrm{V}\hat{Y}_{\bullet} = N^2n^{-1}S^2_{\infty}$, respectively, where $S^2_{\infty} = N^{-1} \sum_i (Y_i - \bar{Y})^2$.

Result 1.10.3 $\hat{V}\hat{\hat{Y}} = n^{-1}\hat{S}^2_\infty$ and $\hat{V}\hat{Y}_\bullet = N^2 n^{-1}\hat{S}^2_\infty$, where $\hat{S}^2_\infty = (n-1)^{-1} \times \sum_i \nu_i(Y_i - \hat{\hat{Y}})^2$ is the *sample variance*, are design-unbiased estimators of $V\hat{\hat{Y}}$ and $V\hat{Y}_\bullet$, respectively.

We may summarize the differences between the *srswor* and *srswr* formulae as follows. Result 1.10.1 differs from Result 1.8.1 only in that δ_i is replaced by ν_i. Result 1.10.2 differs from Result 1.8.2 only by the disappearance of a factor $(N-1)^{-1}(N-n)$. Result 1.10.3 differs from Result 1.8.3 in both these respects: δ_i (in the formula for $\hat{S}^2$) is replaced by ν_i (in the formula for $\hat{S}^2_\infty$), and the factor $N^{-1}(N-n)$ no longer appears (explicitly for $\hat{V}\hat{\hat{Y}}$ or implicitly for $\hat{V}\hat{Y}_\bullet$).

Remark 1.10.1 In these first ten sections we have given the same prominence to the estimation of the population mean as to that of the population total. Since the two analyses are so similar, we shall not continue to do so. From this point on, we shall concentrate on the estimation of the population total and leave it to the reader to make the necessary changes required to estimate the mean, to find an expression for the variance of that estimate, and to construct a sample estimator of that variance. ◇

Simple Random Sampling: the Prediction-Based Theory

1.11 The design-based results established in **1.6–1.10** have long histories of success behind them when applied to relatively large samples (say, 500 sample units or larger). We now know, however, that they can produce much less impressive results when applied to very small samples. We shall next see whether prediction-based sampling inference can do any better in that context.

The design-based and prediction-based (or model-based) approaches use entirely different sets of assumptions. Sometimes the two lead to identical formulae and sometimes to quite different ones. As this book proceeds, we will find that each approach has its own advantages and limitations. Using the two together, it is often possible to have the advantages of both without the limitations of either. (It is rather like a game of football, where it is a help to be able to kick both with the right foot and with the left.) For the time being, however, we will concentrate on what the prediction-based approach can do by itself, first with *srswor* and then with *srswr*.

When we approach the only genuine prediction-oriented statistician we happen to know, she begins by asking why we decided to select our samples randomly at all. She is prepared to allow a limited role for randomization, just so long as statistical inferences are not based on it, but of course ours were based on it, right up to the end of **1.10**. We therefore acknowledge the fact that prediction-oriented statisticians generally prefer to use other procedures for sample selection, and ask her if she would please overlook that point and just tell us how she would have estimated the herd weight, first using the sample that we selected earlier using *srswor* and then using the one that we pretended to select using *srswr*.

She is still reluctant to accede to our request, and we are at a loss to know why. But we know that design-oriented and model-oriented statisticians often have great difficulty in understanding each other's thought processes and even each other's language, so we just keep on asking what we hope will be helpful questions and listening very hard until we do finally grasp her point. Her two points actually, for she has two misgivings and each feeds on the other.

The first is that she is objecting in principle to analysing any sample data where it is taken for granted from the start that she has to take into account the number of times any sample unit has been selected, and give these numbers a part to play in the analysis. The second is that she objects even more strongly in principle to having to take into account the possibility that a unit or units *could have been* selected more than once, even if none of them actually was.

This comes as something of a revelation to us, because we had been taught from the beginning that both these features of the sample were highly relevant. We remember in particular one eminent sampling statistician who, when brought data to analyse, always started by grumbling that he had not been consulted about how the sample *was to be* selected and followed up by asking how it *had been* selected. Then if you told him it had been selected using *srswor* he would analyse it one way (**1.2–1.8**), but if you said it had been selected using *srswr* he would analyse that identical sample a different way (**1.9** and **1.10**) and give you different (and always slightly larger) variance estimates.

We saw nothing wrong in that at the time. I don't think we were ever asked what the relevance was of something that could have happened but didn't actually happen, but if we had been, we would have replied, 'Well, you just don't know how it should be analysed unless you know that!' But now we are being shown how to analyse sample data without that knowledge, and are left without any adequate answer to the question. We have to admit that, on the face of it, it doesn't make much sense to analyse the same data in different ways just because they were gathered differently; or at least, it would only make sense if the choice of which units were to be included in the sample depended directly on the data themselves. In that case the sampling would be informative, and we are well aware that informative samples need very careful analysis if any conclusion is to be drawn from them at all.

We acknowledge all this, and our mentor brightens up visibly. We are learning how to use her language and the communication proceeds apace. It turns out that she has yet a third misgiving. It is this. We are giving her two samples to analyse that are genuinely different. Combo is in one of them and not in the other. Of course she would arrive at different estimates from these two samples, but she needs to be reassured that we won't take the difference between those answers as reflecting the difference between the way a prediction-oriented statistician would analyse an *srswor* and an *srswr* sample, because in fact there would be no difference at all if the two samples provided the same relevant information – the manner of selecting the sample and the number of times each sample unit was selected being most definitely *ir*relevant.

At this point we are in something of an ethical dilemma, because our curiosity is such that, once we know how to go about it, we are not going to be deterred from attempting to analyse an *srswr* sample using the model-based approach. Just to see what happens. On impulse, my colleague confesses this intention. 'That's torn it,' I think privately, 'she'll never show us now.' But in fact our mentor just shrugs her shoulders and implies that if we want to waste our time that's none of her business.

One last hurdle. We want her to make absolutely minimal assumptions regarding the weights of the non-sample elephants (ignoring, for instance, such clues as we have already picked up about bulls tending to be heavier than cows). She is not altogether happy about this last request, because her natural inclination is to use models that are as realistic as possible. However, knowing that it is good teaching practice to start with the simplest situation, she agrees to proceed along those lines.

1.12 First, she writes down a linear regression model which could be taken as generating the weight of the ith elephant:

$$\xi: \quad Y_i = \mu + U_i; \quad \mathrm{E}_\xi U_i = 0; \quad \mathrm{E}_\xi U_i^2 = \sigma^2; \quad \mathrm{E}_\xi(U_iU_j) = 0, \\ j \neq i; \quad i,j = 1,2,\ldots,N.$$

There is some new notation here. ξ is the name of the model. (The Greek letter ξ – transliterated as 'xi' and pronounced the same way as in the English word 'anxiety' – corresponds to x in the Roman alphabet.) E_ξ, like E, is an expectation operator, but instead of the expectation being taken over all possible samples, it is now taken over all realizations of the model ξ, holding the sample constant. (Our mentor reminds us again that there is only one real sample, the selected one, and that it is pointless to consider any other.)

Y_i is, as before, the weight of the ith elephant on the population list, but it is no longer regarded as a fixed number but as a random variable drawn from a continuous distribution. The N distributions (in our case, $N = 50$) each have the same mean μ and the same variance σ^2.

The 'residual' random variable, U_i, describes the extent to which Y_i differs from μ. Its logical status differs from that of Y_i in that, while it is possible to know a realized value of a Y_i (by weighing an elephant), it is never possible to know the realized value of any U_i. That realized value can be estimated, but the relevant estimator is still a random variable (and we denote it by $\hat{U}_i$).

The condition $\mathrm{E}_\xi(U_iU_j) = 0, j \neq i$, would usually be interpreted as implying that if the ith elephant in a particular finite population of size N generated by model ξ happened to be larger than μ, there would be no tendency for the jth elephant in that finite population to be either larger or smaller than μ. Because of this, some authors have felt the need to generalize the model by setting $\mathrm{E}_\xi(U_iU_j) = \rho\sigma^2$ where ρ is a constant correlation coefficient, but against this practice Brewer and Tam (1990) have shown that, in the absence of relevant and recognizable subsets, the condition $\mathrm{E}_\xi(U_iU_j) = 0$ involves no loss of generality.

Given the model ξ, it is easy to proceed to the next step. Our mentor explains that since we already know the weights of the five sample elephants, there is no prediction problem so far as they are concerned. (She calls it 'a prediction problem' rather than 'an estimation problem' because in regression analysis it is only model parameters that are 'estimated'. Potential observations that have not actually been observed are 'predicted'.) It is only necessary, therefore, to predict the weights of the 45 non-sample elephants. She writes such a predictor as $\hat{Y}_i$, and the predictor of the total herd weight as

$$\hat{Y}_{\bullet} = \sum_i \delta_i Y_i + \sum_i (1 - \delta_i)\hat{Y}_i.$$

Here the δ_i are the same as the zero–one sample indicators that were introduced in **1.6**, but their logical status is different. For design-based inference they were random variables, but for prediction-based inference they are fixed numbers: 1 for each unit in the selected sample and 0 for each of the rest; still numerically identical with the realized values that the random variables δ_i took in *srswor*. It is well known that the *least squares* or *best linear unbiased estimator* (BLUE) of the parameter μ in the model ξ is the sample mean, $\hat{\mu} = n^{-1} \sum_i \delta_i Y_i$. This $\hat{\mu}$ is also the *best linear unbiased predictor* (BLUP) of each of the non-sample Y_i. Substituting $\hat{\mu}$ for $\hat{Y}_i$ in the formula for $\hat{Y}_{\bullet}$, our mentor shows that the BLUP of $Y_{\bullet}$ is

$$\begin{aligned}
\hat{Y}_{\bullet} &= \sum_i \delta_i Y_i + \sum_i (1 - \delta_i)\hat{\mu} \\
&= \sum_i \delta_i Y_i + \left\{ \sum_i (1 - \delta_i) \right\} n^{-1} \sum_i \delta_i Y_i \\
&= \sum_i \delta_i Y_i + (N - n)n^{-1} \sum_i \delta_i Y_i \\
&= Nn^{-1} \sum_i \delta_i Y_i \\
&= N\hat{\mu}.
\end{aligned}$$

This being the formula for the best linear unbiased predictor, the *best linear unbiased prediction* is obtained simply by substituting realized values for random variables, the notation being the same, but Y_i now having a different logical status.

Remark 1.12.1 If the need ever arises to distinguish between the best linear unbiased predictor and the best linear unbiased prediction, both of which have the same acronym, BLUP, the latter could be described instead as the *best predicted value* (BPV) of $Y_{\bullet}$. The BPV is also identical with the design-based expansion estimate of the same quantity obtained using *srswor* (see **1.6**). Such identical results occur fairly frequently, and in this instance the identity arises because the same strong symmetry appears in the two very different treatments of the population units.

An Excursus on Independence, Exchangeability and Non-informative Sampling

1.13 In the design-based approach, the symmetry described in Remark 1.12.1 is purely a property of the manner in which the units are selected for the sample. It relates to the sample values (that is, those of the population units that happened to be selected at the first, second, . . . , nth sample draw) rather than to the values associated with particular and uniquely identifiable population units. The precise nature of the symmetry differs slightly between *srswor* and *srswr*.

Under *srswr*, where the procedures for the n sample draws are identical in specification and carried out independently, it is immediately obvious that the values observed at these draws must be identically and independently distributed (i.i.d.) random variables, each equally likely to take on any of the N permissible values Y_i.

In *srswor* the symmetry stems not from independence, but from the property of exchangeability that was described when leading up to Lemma 1.7.3, namely that each moment of the joint probability distribution of the n sample values is symmetrical in the N population units. (For instance, the covariances between pairs of sample values are all equal, even though they are not zero.) The sample distribution is then said to be *exchangeable* among the N population units. (Independence implies exchangeability, but exchangeable distributions are not necessarily independent.)

In prediction-based sampling the nature of the symmetry is different again. The Y_i all share the same mean and variance, and each of them is perfectly uncorrelated with every other, not only within the real (or observable) population, but also over all possible realizations of the model ξ. This is sufficient to ensure that the least-squares estimates and predictors are symmetrical in the sample values, but it is not enough to ensure exchangeability. For that, it would be necessary to assume that the distributions of the individual Y_i were identical in all their moments, not just in their means and variances. Even then, they would not necessarily be independent of each other. It would, for instance, be possible for all pairs of Y_i within an exchangeable set to have identical non-zero correlations, a property incompatible with independence.

It would of course have been possible, and perhaps simpler, to make the stronger assumption that the Y_i were exchangeable or even i.i.d., but it is always best to keep one's options open. It might happen one day that a situation arises where this stronger assumption does not hold, but the weaker ones needed to obtain the symmetric predictors still do. The prediction-based theory is to that extent more general than the design-based, which both requires and ensures exchangeability.

Prediction-based theory is, moreover, applicable even when the sample is not selected randomly, for no use is made of the selection process when arriving at the estimators or predictors.

There are penalties of course. Suppose someone went around deliberately selecting all the units that looked as though they would have the largest values of Y_i. (It is often possible to do this sort of thing, even before the Y_i are actually measured. One could, for example, select all the tallest elephants, and be fairly sure that one had selected most of the heaviest.) Then the model ξ would provide a very misleading description of the *sample* Y_i, even if they had all actually been generated by that model. This kind of sampling, where the method of selection is either explicitly or implicitly dependent on the survey values themselves, is called *informative*, because the very fact that a unit is in sample provides some information about its survey value, even before that value is measured. It requires very subtle methods to analyse an informative sample. Such methods have no place in an introductory text. It is best for the beginner to become familiar with the theory of non-informative sampling first, and in the meantime to avoid informative sampling very carefully. The use of random sampling is a simple way of doing just that.

Prediction-Based Theory (Continued)

1.14 Our mentor next derives the model variance of $\hat{\mu} = n^{-1}\sum_i \delta_i Y_i$. This is simply $V_\xi \hat{\mu} = V_\xi(n^{-1}\sum_i \delta_i Y_i) = n^{-2}\sum_i \delta_i V_\xi Y_i = n^{-1}\sigma^2$. It follows that the model variances of $\hat{\bar{Y}} = \hat{\mu}$ and $\hat{Y}_{\bullet} = N\hat{\mu}$ are $V_\xi \hat{\bar{Y}} = n^{-1}\sigma^2$ and $V_\xi \hat{Y}_{\bullet} = N^2 n^{-1}\sigma^2$, respectively.

How can these variances be estimated? She first needs to find an unbiased estimator of σ^2. An obvious candidate is the sample variance, $\hat{S}^2 = (n-1)^{-1} \times \sum_i \delta_i (Y_i - \hat{\bar{Y}})^2$. (In Lemma 1.7.4 this quantity was shown to be design-unbiased for the adjusted population variance $S^2 = (N-1)^{-1}\sum_i (Y_i - \bar{Y})^2$.) Since the model ξ requires $E_\xi(Y_i - \hat{\bar{Y}})^2$ to be independent of i, the model expectation of $\hat{S}^2$ is $E_\xi \hat{S}^2 = (n-1)^{-1}\sum_i \delta_i E_\xi(Y_i - \hat{\bar{Y}})^2 = (n-1)^{-1} n E_\xi(Y_i - \hat{\bar{Y}})^2$. But for all $i \in s$ (and using C_ξ as the prediction-based covariance operator),

$$
\begin{aligned}
E_\xi(Y_i - \hat{\bar{Y}})^2 &= V_\xi(Y_i - \hat{\bar{Y}}) + \{E_\xi(Y_i - \hat{\bar{Y}})\}^2 \\
&= V_\xi Y_i + V_\xi \hat{\bar{Y}} - 2C_\xi(Y_i, \hat{\bar{Y}}) + 0^2, \qquad \text{since } E_\xi(Y_i - \hat{\bar{Y}}) = 0, \\
&= \sigma^2 + n^{-1}\sigma^2 - 2C_\xi(Y_i, n^{-1}Y_i), \qquad \text{since } C_\xi(Y_i, Y_j) = 0, \forall j \neq i, \\
&= \sigma^2 + n^{-1}\sigma^2 - 2n^{-1}\sigma^2 \\
&= \sigma^2(1 - n^{-1}).
\end{aligned}
$$

So $E_\xi \hat{S}^2 = (n-1)^{-1}\sum_i \delta_i \sigma^2(1 - n^{-1}) = \sigma^2$; that is, $\hat{S}^2$ is a model-unbiased estimator of σ^2. Hence model-unbiased estimators of $V_\xi \hat{\mu} = V_\xi \hat{\bar{Y}}$ and of $V_\xi \hat{Y}_{\bullet}$ are $\hat{V}_\xi \hat{\mu} = \hat{V}_\xi \hat{\bar{Y}} = n^{-1}\hat{S}^2$, and $\hat{V}_\xi \hat{Y}_{\bullet} = N^2 n^{-1}\hat{S}^2$, respectively.

Another important characteristic of an estimator is its *mean squared error* (MSE). This provides a measure of how far the estimate is likely to be from the estimated quantity *itself*, as opposed to from the estimator's expected value, which is what the variance provides. This implies, however, that the MSE of an unbiased estimator is equal to its variance, so for instance the model

MSE of $\hat{\mu}$, which is written $\text{MSE}_\xi \hat{\mu}$, is the same as $\text{V}_\xi \hat{\mu}$. In full, $\text{MSE}_\xi \hat{\mu} = \text{E}_\xi(\hat{\mu} - \mu)^2 = \text{V}_\xi \hat{\mu} = n^{-1}\sigma^2$.

The model MSE of $\hat{\bar{Y}}$, however, is not the same as the model MSE of $\hat{\mu}$, because $\hat{\bar{Y}}$ is then regarded as an estimator of $\bar{Y}$ and not of μ. We therefore have instead

$$\begin{aligned}
\text{MSE}_\xi \hat{\bar{Y}} &= \text{E}_\xi(\hat{\bar{Y}} - \bar{Y})^2 \\
&= \text{V}_\xi(\hat{\bar{Y}} - \bar{Y}) + \{\text{E}_\xi(\hat{\bar{Y}} - \bar{Y})\}^2 \\
&= \text{V}_\xi(\hat{\bar{Y}} - \bar{Y})^2 + 0^2 \qquad \text{since } \text{E}_\xi \hat{\bar{Y}} = \text{E}_\xi \bar{Y} = \mu, \\
&= \text{V}_\xi \hat{\bar{Y}} + \text{V}_\xi \bar{Y} - 2\text{C}_\xi(\hat{\bar{Y}}, \bar{Y}) \\
&= n^{-1}\sigma^2 + N^{-1}\sigma^2 - 2\text{C}_\xi\left(n^{-1}\sum_i \delta_i Y_i,\ N^{-1}\sum_i Y_i\right) \\
&= n^{-1}\sigma^2 + N^{-1}\sigma^2 - 2n^{-1}N^{-1}\sum_i \delta_i \sigma^2 \\
&= (n^{-1} - N^{-1})\sigma^2;
\end{aligned}$$

and, since $Y_{\bullet} = N\bar{Y}$ and $\hat{Y}_{\bullet} = N\hat{\bar{Y}}$ (note that $\hat{Y}_{\bullet}$ is an estimator of $Y_{\bullet}$), the MSE of $\hat{Y}_{\bullet}$, is

$$\text{MSE}_\xi \hat{Y}_{\bullet} = \text{V}_\xi(\hat{Y}_{\bullet} - Y_{\bullet}) = N^2(n^{-1} - N^{-1})\sigma^2 = N(N - n)n^{-1}\sigma^2.$$

Strangely, the MSEs of $\hat{\bar{Y}}$ and $\hat{Y}_{\bullet}$ are smaller than their variances! This is impossible when the estimand (meaning 'whatever is being estimated') is a constant, because then the MSE is the sum of the variance and the squared bias, but the estimands in this case are $\bar{Y}$ and $Y_{\bullet}$ and, under the model ξ, each of these is a random variable positively correlated with its estimator.

To put the same point another way, $\hat{\bar{Y}}$ is typically closer to $\bar{Y}$ than to μ, and $\hat{Y}_{\bullet} = N\hat{\mu}$ is typically closer to $Y_{\bullet}$ than to $N\mu$. To see why, first note that the sample is selected exclusively from the actual or observable finite population. That observable (finite) population is notionally a realization (or sample of one population) from a hypothetical infinity of populations. Each population contains N units, and each unit has the expected value μ. Because the sample is selected exclusively from the actual or observable population, it reflects the properties of that particular population more closely than it reflects the properties of the hypothetical infinity of populations. In particular, the sample mean, $\hat{\bar{Y}} = n^{-1}\sum_i \delta_i Y_i$, will, on average, be closer to the observable population mean, $\bar{Y}$, than to the superpopulation mean, which is the model parameter, μ.

Finally, recall that $\hat{S}^2$ is both design-unbiased (under *srswor*) for S^2, and model-unbiased for σ^2. Thus a design-unbiased estimator of $\text{MSE}\hat{\bar{Y}}$ is $(n^{-1} - N^{-1})\hat{S}^2$ and a model-unbiased estimator of $\text{MSE}_\xi \hat{\bar{Y}}$ is also $(n^{-1} - N^{-1})\hat{S}^2$. Similarly the design-unbiased and model-unbiased estimators of $\mathrm{MSE}\hat{Y}_{\bullet}$ and $\mathrm{MSE}_{\xi}\hat{Y}_{\bullet}$ are equal at $\widehat{\mathrm{MSE}}\hat{Y}_{\bullet} = \widehat{\mathrm{MSE}}_{\xi}\hat{Y}_{\bullet} = N(N-n)n^{-1}\hat{S}^2$. However, we intend to use the symbol MSE_{ξ} sparingly from now on, preferring (for instance) to write $\mathrm{V}_{\xi}(\hat{Y}_{\bullet} - Y_{\bullet})$ rather than $\mathrm{MSE}_{\xi}\hat{Y}_{\bullet}$.

The remarkable closeness of the two analyses, the one design-based and the other prediction-based, has led to some confusion in the past. It is important to recognize their closeness, but it is even more important to keep them conceptually separate. When we move away from *srswor* on the one hand and from the simple model ξ on the other, the differences become more important than the similarities.

1.15 In summary, the four important prediction-based results for equally weighted samples are:

Result 1.15.1 Under the model ξ, the BLUE of the model parameter and superpopulation mean, μ, is $\hat{\mu} = n^{-1}\sum_i \delta_i Y_i$. The BLUPs of the actual population mean, $\bar{Y}$, and of the corresponding population total, $Y_{\bullet} = N\bar{Y}$, and the BRPVs of each individual non-sample value, Y_i, are $\hat{\bar{Y}} = \hat{\mu}$, $\hat{Y}_{\bullet} = N\hat{\mu}$ and $\hat{Y}_i = \hat{\mu}$, respectively.

Result 1.15.2 The model variances of $\hat{\mu}$, $\hat{\bar{Y}}$ and $\hat{Y}_{\bullet}$ are $\mathrm{V}_{\xi}\hat{\mu} = n^{-1}\sigma^2, \mathrm{V}_{\xi}\hat{\bar{Y}} = n^{-1}\sigma^2$ and $\mathrm{V}_{\xi}\hat{Y}_{\bullet} = N^2 n^{-1}\sigma^2$, respectively.

Result 1.15.3 The model MSEs of $\hat{\mu}$, $\hat{\bar{Y}}$ and $\hat{Y}_{\bullet}$ are $\mathrm{MSE}_{\xi}\hat{\mu} = n^{-1}\sigma^2, \mathrm{MSE}_{\xi}\hat{\bar{Y}} = \mathrm{E}_{\xi}(\hat{\bar{Y}} - \bar{Y})^2 = (n^{-1} - N^{-1})\sigma^2$ and $\mathrm{MSE}_{\xi}\hat{Y}_{\bullet} = \mathrm{V}_{\xi}(\hat{Y}_{\bullet} - Y_{\bullet}) = N(N-n)n^{-1}\sigma^2$, respectively.

Result 1.15.4 The sample variance $\hat{S}^2 = (n-1)^{-1}\sum_i \delta_i(Y_i - \hat{\bar{Y}})^2$ is a model-unbiased estimator of the variance parameter σ^2 in model ξ. It may therefore equally be represented by $\hat{\sigma}^2$. To obtain an unbiased estimator of any of the variances or MSEs of $\hat{\mu}$, $\hat{\bar{Y}}$ or $\hat{Y}_{\bullet}$, substitute $\hat{\sigma}^2$ (or equivalently $\hat{S}^2$) for σ^2 in the formula for the variance or MSE itself. For example, a model-unbiased estimator of $\mathrm{MSE}_{\xi}\hat{\mu} = n^{-1}\sigma^2$ is $\widehat{\mathrm{MSE}}_{\xi}\hat{\mu} = n^{-1}\hat{\sigma}^2 \equiv n^{-1}\hat{S}^2$.

1.16 Is there anything at all that corresponds to *srswr* in terms of model-based inference? A model-oriented survey statistician would probably be inclined to say there was not, because she would have no incentive to select a sample that contained the same observation more than once. For her, the meaning of the word 'sample' is the set of population units from which survey information is meant to be collected, and who would deliberately collect the same information twice?

It is, however, possible to ask what would the model variance be if we chose to select a 'sample' (with possible repeats) using *srswr*, and then used the design-unbiased estimator as a predictor of the population total. That predictor would be $\hat{Y}_{\bullet} = Nn^{-1}\sum_i \nu_i Y_i$, where ν_i, while retaining its original meaning as the number of appearances in the *srswr* sample, would no longer have the logical status of a random variable, but would simply be a fixed weight. The model variance of $\hat{Y}_{\bullet}$ under ξ would therefore be $V_{\xi}\hat{Y}_{\bullet} = N^2 n^{-2}(\sum_i \nu_i^2)\sigma^2$. Bearing in mind that the ν_i are all integers and that their sum is n, $\sum_i \nu_i^2$ takes its minimum value of n when the ν_i are all either zero or one. One way to ensure that they are all either zero or one is to use *srswor* rather than *srswr*. Moreover, when estimating σ^2, our model-oriented mentor would use only the distinct sample values, with the result that any repeats would reduce the degrees of freedom available for estimation. Finally, her analysis is not simplified by the use of *srswr* but actually made slightly more complicated. In short, if the sampling *has* to be random (for instance, to ensure non-informativeness) she has everything to gain and nothing to lose by using *srswor*.

Result 1.16.1 If intending to use model-based inference, it is best to avoid *srswr*.

Summary

1.17 Estimators that assign the same weight to each sample are most frequently used in combination with simple random sampling. There are two forms of this: simple random sampling without replacement (*srswor*) and simple random sampling with replacement (*srswr*).

In the context of design-based inference, *srswor* is more efficient and is therefore used more frequently, even though *srswr* is simpler analytically and – for small enough sample fractions – only marginally less efficient.

It has, however, been objected (by model-oriented sampling statisticians) that the way in which a sample is selected should have no bearing on the manner in which the mean or the total is estimated. Equally weighted estimators only make sense if the population is adequately described by the model ξ. When inference is based directly on that model, *srswr* is clearly seen to be inappropriate. It is both less efficient and more complicated to handle than *srswor*.

Further, if prediction-based inference is to be used on its own, there is no requirement for the sampling to be random at all. Any subset of the population can serve as a sample, just so long as the model ξ provides an adequate description of that sample as well as of the population. However, even if the model ξ is an adequate descriptor of the population, it cannot be trusted to describe the sample well when the sampling is informative; and simple random sampling does provide a convenient way to ensure that the sample is non-informative. In addition, ξ can never be trusted to describe the sample well in any absolute sense, for when the sample is chosen randomly there is always the possibility that it will contain some quite atypical population units.

Since both design-based and prediction-based sampling have quite different shortcomings and therefore complementary virtues, there are benefits in using both at the same time. A sample selected using *srswor* is then the obvious choice. To appreciate the full benefits of combining design-based and prediction-based inference, however, it will be necessary to consider estimators that are not restricted to assigning equal weights to all units. For that we will need to wait until Chapter 3. In the meantime, however, there is a simple and ubiquitous technique called stratification that must be considered first.

Exercises

1.1 Consider the following hypothetical sample survey. It is based on a simple random sample of n individuals selected without replacment from a population of size N, where N is large enough for the distinction between N and $N-1$ to be of no importance. Each of the n sample individuals was recorded as being either 'fit' or 'unfit'. There was no failure to contact, and no incidence of any other kind of non-response.

In order to estimate variances quickly, the n sample individuals were divided into ten exactly equal and mutually exclusive subsamples, and the percentages of those 'fit' and 'unfit' in each of those ten subsamples were as follows:

Subsample	1	2	3	4	5	6	7	8	9	10
'Fit'	36	41	34	46	39	45	37	44	40	38
'Unfit'	64	59	66	54	61	55	63	56	60	62

(a) From these data, estimate the population mean of the zero–one variable 'Fit'. Then, *using that estimate only*, derive estimates of that variable's population variance and population standard deviation.

(b) Compare your derived estimate of population variance for the variable 'Fit' with the observed variance of the ten subsample estimates of that variable. From that comparison, estimate the number of respondents in the entire sample.

Hint. It is often useful in such problems to start by converting the percentages to proportions.

1.2 In financial auditing, the population units are transactions. Transactions can either be 'in error' or 'correct'. It is convenient for some purposes to regard the 'error' and the 'correct' transactions as being two separate subpopulations.

The remainder of this question refers to these two subpopulations themselves, rather than to any sample drawn from them. It relates primarily to three of the basic kinds of population statistics that can be estimated from audit sample surveys, namely:

(i) the proportions of all transactions, P_1 and $P_0 = 1 - P_1$, that are in the 'Error' subpopulation and in the 'Correct' subpopulation, respectively;

(ii) the net sum of the errors, $Y_{\bullet} = \sum_{i=1}^{N} Y_i$, measured in dollars, over the entire population; and

(iii) the population variances of the individual Y_i, and of the indicator variable Δ_i (which takes the value 1 when the transaction is in error and the value 0 otherwise).

In estimating the 'net sum of the errors', those Y_i that are to the organization's disadvantage (deficit errors) are given a positive sign, and those that are in the organization's favour (surplus errors) are given a negative sign. So the Y_i in the 'error' subpopulation can be of either sign, but $Y_i \neq 0$ for all $i = 1, 2, \ldots, N_1$. In the 'correct' subpopulation, however, Y_i takes the value 0 for all $i = N_1 + 1, N_1 + 2, \ldots, N$.

The relevant statistics being estimated by the sample survey, are $N_1, P_1 = N_1/N$, $Y_{\bullet} = \sum_{i=1}^{N} Y_i$, $\bar{Y} = Y_{\bullet}/N$, and the population variances of the individual Y_i and of the Δ_i. The population variance of the Y_i is $S_Y^2 = N^{-1} \sum_{i=1}^{N} (Y_i - \bar{Y})^2 = N^{-1} \sum_{i=1}^{N} Y_i^2 - \bar{Y}^2$. The population variance of the Δ_i is $S_\Delta^2 = N^{-1} \sum_{i=1}^{N} (\Delta_i - P_1)^2$.

Since the great majority of transactions are almost always found to be 'correct', it is convenient to make sample estimates, in the first instance, only of the mean and variance of the Y_i within the 'error' subpopulation, that is to say, of $\bar{Y}_1 = Y_{\bullet}/N_1$ and $S_{Y_1}^2 = N_1^{-1} \sum_{i=1}^{N_1} (Y_i - \bar{Y}_1)^2 = N_1^{-1} \sum_{i=1}^{N_1} Y_i^2 - \bar{Y}_1^2$ respectively. Also, N and P_1 are unknown.

The sample estimates of subpopulation mean and variance can then be used to form corresponding estimates for the entire population. Demonstrate this by finding expressions for $\bar{Y}, S_\Delta^2$ and S_Y^2 in terms of $N, P_1, \bar{Y}_1$ and $S_{Y_1}^2$.

Hint. It is not necessary to consider any sample estimates in order to answer this question. Concentrate entirely on the population and subpopulation statistics.

2

Stratification and Poststratification

Stratifying the Population 29
Poststratified Estimation 29
Designing a Stratified Sample 34
Summary 37
Exercises 38

Stratifying the Population

2.1 In the course of Chapter 1 we found that our sample of five elephants was not telling the circus owner anything that he did not know already. Either the sample size needed to be increased or the information gathered had to be used more efficiently.

The second option is clearly preferable, but how can it be achieved? It is no use concentrating only on the sample data. Both the design-oriented and prediction-oriented statistician have used all the information in the sample data in accordance with their own theories of *srswor*, and each has come up with the same pair of numerical estimates: 174 tonnes for the population total itself and 15 tonnes for the standard deviation of that estimate.

There is, however, additional information about the population that has not yet been used. In the alphabetical list that we used to select the sample there were two kinds of names; 25 ended with -a and most of them looked like women's names, while the other 25 ended with -mbo. We check with the elephant trainer and he confirms our guess that the first group are cow elephants and the second group bull elephants. Perhaps if we estimate the average weights of bulls and cows separately we will be better off.

Statisticians call this division of the population into groups of similar units (or, as they put it, 'groups that are homogeneous within and heterogeneous between') *stratification*. Each group is called a *stratum* (plural *strata*) and the entire process of designing and analysing a sample this way is *stratified sampling*. Usually more than two strata are formed, but our case is a very simple one and requires two only.

Poststratified Estimation

2.2 Had we been starting from scratch, we would probably have decided that, since there were equal numbers of elephants in the two strata, we should select equal numbers in each sample, either two or three, by *srswor*. In fact though, we have two bulls and three cows from the sample we actually selected. If we are prepared to settle for this as our sample, we have a *poststratified* sampling strategy – 'post-' because we introduced the stratification after the sample was selected.

Once we have made that decision, however, everything is straightforward. We treat the two strata as though they were completely separate populations and apply the *srswor* formulae as before. The only additional notation required is a subscript, traditionally taking the value 1 for males and 2 for females. However, to avoid confusion with notation such as Y_{11} – which could then mean either the weight of the first elephant in the bulls' stratum (Anembo) or the weight of the 11th elephant in the entire herd (Flimbo) – we will here use the subscripts B for bulls and C for cows.

For the bulls' stratum we then have $N_B = 25, n_B = 2, \delta_{Bi} = 1$ for $i = 3$ (Combo) and 5 (Flimbo), otherwise $\delta_{Bi} = 0$. The sample observations are $Y_{B3} = 4675$ and $Y_{B5} = 3032$, so the estimated stratum mean is $\hat{\bar{Y}}_B = (4675 + 3032)/2 = 3853.5$ and the estimated stratum total is $\hat{Y}_{B\bullet} = 25 \times 3853.5 = 96\,337.5$.

We will of course be interested in estimating the variance of this estimate. Introducing the subscript B into Result 1.8.3, we obtain $\hat{V}\hat{Y}_{B\bullet} = N_B(N_B - n_B)n_B^{-1}\hat{S}_B^2$, where $\hat{S}_B^2 = (n_B - 1)^{-1}\sum_i \delta_{Bi}(Y_{Bi} - \hat{\bar{Y}}_B)^2$. Substituting our known values, we have

$$\begin{aligned}
\hat{V}\hat{Y}_{B\bullet} &= 25 \times \frac{23}{2}\left\{(4675 - 3853.5)^2 + (3032 - 3853.5)^2\right\} \\
&= 287.5\left\{821.5^2 + (-821.5)^2\right\} \\
&= 388\,045\,793.75 \\
&\cong 19\,699^2.
\end{aligned}$$

For the cows' stratum we have $N_C = 25$, $n_C = 3$, $\delta_{Ci} = 1$ for $i = 12$ (Linda), 16 (Pamela) and 18 (Sara), otherwise $\delta_{Ci} = 0$. The sample observations are $Y_{C12} = 3328$, $Y_{C16} = 3427$ and $Y_{C18} = 2910$, so the estimated stratum mean is $\hat{\bar{Y}}_C = (3328 + 3427 + 2910)/3 \cong 3221.67$ and the estimated stratum total is $\hat{Y}_{C\bullet} \cong 25 \times 3221.67 \cong 80\,541.67$.

Correspondingly, we obtain $\hat{V}\hat{Y}_{C\bullet} = N_C(N_C - n_C)n_C^{-1}\hat{S}_C^2$, where $\hat{S}_C^2 = (n_C - 1)^{-1}\sum_i \delta_{Ci}(Y_{Ci} - \hat{\bar{Y}}_C)^2$. Substituting our known values, we have

$$\begin{aligned}
\hat{S}_C^2 &\cong \frac{1}{2}\left\{(3328 - 3221.67)^2 + (3427 - 3221.67)^2 + (2910 - 3221.67)^2\right\} \\
&= 0.5\left\{106.33^2 + 205.33^2 + (-311.67)^2\right\} \\
&\cong 75\,302.33 \\
&\cong 274.4^2
\end{aligned}$$

and

$$\begin{aligned}
\hat{V}\hat{Y}_{C\bullet} &\cong 25 \times \frac{22}{3} \times 75\,302.33 \\
&\cong 13\,805\,428 \\
&\cong 3716^2.
\end{aligned}$$

The selections within the two poststrata were not independent, for the total number of elephants to be selected was fixed at 5, so the larger the number of bulls selected, the smaller the number of cows, and vice versa. We had agreed, however, to proceed with the analysis as though the selections had been carried out independently, and realistically the magnitudes of the estimates within the poststrata are determined not so much by the number of bulls or cows selected as by the weights of the sample animals. It therefore makes sense, even within the design-based approach, to estimate conditionally on the numbers of bulls and the numbers of cows selected and ignore any correlation between the two poststratum estimates.

It makes even more sense within the model-based approach, because the two strata clearly require separate models, and the information obtained regarding bulls' weights should clearly be ignored when estimating cows' weights (and again vice versa). So regardless of the approach used, it is reasonable to treat the two estimates of stratum total, $\hat{Y}_{B\bullet}$ and $\hat{Y}_{C\bullet}$ as independent.

The overwhelming concern of our client, the circus owner, is the total weight of the herd, $Y_{\bullet} = Y_{B\bullet} + Y_{C\bullet}$. The obvious estimator to use is $\hat{Y}_{\bullet} = \hat{Y}_{B\bullet} + \hat{Y}_{C\bullet}$. The estimates in this case are 96 337.5 kg and 80 541.7 kg respectively, a total of 176 879.2 kg, or about 177 tonnes, very similar to the 174 tonnes obtained in Chapter 1.

The estimation of the variance of this estimate is, however, somewhat less straightforward. Superficially it seems simple enough. Since $\hat{Y}_{B\bullet}$ and $\hat{Y}_{C\bullet}$ are independent of each other in both the design-based and the model-based approach, the variance of their sum is the sum of their variances. The same argument regarding independence also makes it reasonable to use the sum of the two estimated variances as the estimated variance of their sum. We may therefore write

$$\hat{V}\hat{Y}_{\bullet} = \hat{V}\hat{Y}_{B\bullet} + \hat{V}\hat{Y}_{C\bullet} \cong 388\,045\,794 + 13\,805\,428 = 401\,851\,222 \cong 20\,046^2.$$

There are, however, two serious matters of concern here. The immediately obvious one is the extent to which the estimated variance for the bulls' stratum swamps that for the cows'. Even more problematical, from our point of view as consultants, is the fact that the estimated variance of the stratified sampling estimate exceeds that for plain *srswor*. Something is seriously amiss, and we need to see what has happened to bring this counter-intuitive answer about.

One thing is obvious: the problem lies with the bulls rather than the cows. If the bulls' stratum were as 'well behaved' as the cows', we would have very little problem. We cannot even blame the fact that we selected fewer bulls than cows, for the ratio of bulls to cows in our sample was 2 : 3, so the ratio of the estimated variances should have been about 3 : 2. Our ratio is about 28 : 1.

The problem clearly lies with the very large difference in the weights of the two sample bulls. The question we must ask is whether there is an intrinsically greater variability among the weights of bulls than there is among the weights of cows, or whether perhaps is there something odd about the sample. We ask the elephant trainer. His answer is 'Yes' to both questions. Bulls are generally heavier than cows (which means for us that a 20% variability in the weights of bulls is more important in absolute terms than a 20% variability in the weights of cows).

Beyond that, he suspects that there is a further variability among bulls, over and above what could be explained by their generally larger size.

And that brings him to our second question, whether there is something odd about our sample. The answer to this turns out to be embarrassing! The elephant trainer hadn't liked to mention it earlier, seeing as we were supposed to know all about statistical sampling and that, but now that we had asked, hadn't we noticed something unusual about Flimbo? Flimbo is a strange one, Flimbo is. The clown of the elephant herd. Sometimes people only have to look at him to start laughing. Hadn't we noticed that he was a bit scrawny, like? Some of the big ones must be nearly twice his weight. Jumbo, for instance, he would have to be for one. And perhaps some of the others too, though he wouldn't be so sure about them. Flimbo, though, he was quite the other way. Funny we should have ever thought a sample with Flimbo in it would give any sensible idea about the total weight of the herd. 'Though of course you'll have your own ways of handling things like that', he adds, diplomatically.

Making a mental note to consult with the subject-matter experts sooner and in greater depth in our next consultation, we return to our sample design problem. Unusual population units like Flimbo need to be put into a completely enumerated (or 'take all') stratum. We should obviously do this with Flimbo himself, but are there any others? It did sound as though Jumbo might be in that category, but it might not be politic to ask the elephant trainer questions like that just now. In any case, how could we frame the question without asking him to make a decision that we should really be making ourselves? We decide to carry out a quick visual inspection of the entire herd instead.

One bull elephant is noticeably larger than the others, but not so much larger as to justify taking him out of the bulls' stratum. We feel reasonably safe in recasting the existing sample as made up of Flimbo, who now represents himself only, a sample of one reasonably typical bull out of the remaining 24, and finally a reasonably typical sample of three cows out of the 25.

We already have for the cows an estimated stratum total $\hat{Y}_{C\bullet} \cong 80\,566.67$. We can also estimate the total of the (ordinary) bulls' stratum as 24 times Combo's weight, $24 \times 4675 = 112\,200$. We can add to that 3032 for Flimbo. The estimate of the total herd weight is therefore $\hat{Y}_{\bullet} \cong 112\,200 + 3032 + 80\,566.67 = 195\,798.67$, or about 196 tonnes.

Now we come to the estimated variance. For the cows' stratum it is 13 805 428. We need add nothing to the variance for Flimbo, since his stratum is completely enumerated and, whenever $n = N$, both the *srswor* variance and its estimator are identically zero. We have a problem, however with the bulls' stratum, for with $N > n$ and $n = 1$ the estimator of variance is zero divided by zero, which is indeterminate.

We can nevertheless make an educated guess ('guestimate' or imputation). The estimated population variance for the cows' stratum is 75 302.33 or 274.4^2. We first multiply this 274.4 by the estimated ratio of a bull's weight to a cow's weight. Our sample estimate of this ratio is now $4675 \div 3221.67 \cong 1.45$, and 1.45 times 274.4 is about 398, or 400 after rounding. The imputed population variance is at that stage 160 000.

We have, however, been informed by the elephant trainer that there is a further variability among bulls, over and above what could be explained by their generally larger size. We therefore need to multiply this 160 000 by an additional factor to allow for that 'further variability'. We must be careful about this additional factor. An appropriate choice or imputation for our immediate purpose – estimating the standard error of our stratified estimate of total – needs to be fairly generous, to be on the safe side. But if we use this generous imputation later for design purposes (specifically, to decide what proportion of our sample should be bulls) it will lead us to include too large a proportion of bulls in our sample. We therefore need two imputations, first a generous one and then another that is as realistic as possible.

For the generous imputation we might multiply the population variance by a factor of 2, arriving at $\tilde{S}_B^2 = 320\,000 \cong 566^2$. Using that factor, our imputation of the variance for the bulls' stratum can be written as

$$
\begin{aligned}
\hat{V}\hat{Y}_{B\bullet} &= N_B(N_B - n_B)n_B^{-1}\tilde{S}_B^2 \\
&= 24 \times \frac{23}{1} \times 320\,000 \\
&= 176\,640\,000 \\
&\cong 13\,291^2.
\end{aligned}
$$

The imputed variance of $\hat{Y}_\bullet$ is therefore

$$
\begin{aligned}
\tilde{V}\hat{Y}_\bullet &= 176\,640\,000 + 13\,805\,000 \\
&= 190\,445\,000 \\
&\cong 13\,800^2.
\end{aligned}
$$

This is appreciably smaller than the $401\,851\,222 \cong 20\,046^2$ that we had for $\hat{V}\hat{Y}_{B\bullet}$ before we took Flimbo out of the sampled bulls' stratum and selected him with certainty. This is despite the generous doubling of the population variance of the bulls' stratum. A further point worth noting is that because the estimate of total is now a little larger, the reduction in the *coefficient of variation* (or *relative standard deviation*) is slightly greater than that in the absolute standard deviation. In another situation, that difference might be more important than it is here. The coefficient of variation can move in the opposite direction to the absolute standard deviation.

Before leaving this section we summarize the results so far:

Result 2.2.1 Even after the sample has been selected, it may be useful to treat a population as made up of a set of distinct subpopulations called *poststrata*; but only if the numbers of units in each poststratum are known from non-sample sources and if inspection of the sample indicates that such a partition appears worthwhile.

Result 2.2.2 When analysing poststrata using design-based inference, it is both possible and desirable to ignore the dependence of the sample configuration within any poststratum on the outcomes of sampling in the other strata. This is known as 'making inferences conditional on the numbers of units selected within each poststratum'.

Result 2.2.3 If prediction-based inference is being used, this conditioning is done automatically and there is no need to provide any special justification for it.

Result 2.2.4 In some circumstances it may be necessary to single out a particularly unusual unit for special treatment. Provided it can be checked that there are no other such unusual units in the population, it is permissible to treat it as being in a poststratum all of its own, and within that poststratum selected with certainty.

Designing a Stratified Sample

2.3 We still have one more use for the sample information. That is for future design purposes. We had decided from the beginning to take only a small pilot sample in order to 'feel the water'. We now know enough to be able to design a properly stratified sample and, in particular, to estimate the optimum distribution of the sample between bulls and cows.

Suppose that for the hth stratum, $h = 1, \ldots, H$, there are N_h units in total and that its population variance, $S_h^2 = (N_h - 1)^{-1} \sum_i (Y_{hi} - \bar{Y}_h)^2$, is known. There are n sample units to be drawn from the H strata combined. We provisionally define the optimum allocation as the one which results in a minimum variance for the estimated population total, $\hat{Y}_{\bullet} = \sum_{h=1}^{H} \{(N_h/n_h) \sum_{i=1}^{n_h} Y_{hi}\}$.

Theorem 2.3.1 The optimum allocation of the n sample units over the H strata occurs when the individual stratum sample sizes n_h are chosen to be as nearly proportional as possible to the corresponding $N_h S_h$.

Proof. Since the selection processes within each of the strata are carried out independently, the variance of $\hat{Y}_{\bullet}$ is the sum of the individual stratum variances, that is, $V\hat{Y}_{\bullet} = \sum_{h=1}^{H} V\hat{Y}_{h\bullet} = \sum_{h=1}^{H} N_h(N_h - n_h)n_h^{-1}S_h^2$. At the optimum, $\sum_{h=1}^{H} N_h(N_h - n_h)n_h^{-1}S_h^2$ is minimized subject to $\sum_{h=1}^{H} n_h = n$. Setting $L = \sum_{h=1}^{H} (N_h^2 n_h^{-1} - N_h)S_h^2 + \lambda\left(\sum_{h=1}^{H} n_h - n\right)$, the condition for the optimum is $\partial L/\partial n_h = 0$, that is, $-N_h^2 n_h^{-2} S_h^2 + \lambda = 0$ for all h. This condition holds only when $n_h \propto N_h S_h$ for all h, and so $n_h = n\left(N_h S_h / \sum_k N_k S_k\right)$. ◇

Corollary 2.3.1 Substituting this expression for n_h, the variance of the estimator $\hat{Y}_{\bullet}$ at the optimum becomes $V\hat{Y}_{\bullet} = n^{-1}\left(\sum_{h=1}^{H} N_h S_h\right)^2 - \sum_{h=1}^{H} N_h S_h^2$, where both the summations and the value of the total sample size, n, are calculated over the sampled strata only.

Remark 2.3.1 This is a very useful equation, as people are always wanting to know how large a sample size they 'need'. We may interpret this as meaning 'How large a sample is required to yield a given but as yet unstated level of accuracy?' If we change the subject of the formula from $\mathrm{V}\hat{Y}_{\bullet}$ to n, it can be used to tell us the required sample sizes for a range of required variances. The equation then reads

$$n = \frac{\left(\sum_{h=1}^{H} N_h S_h\right)^2}{\mathrm{V}\hat{Y}_{\bullet} + \sum_{h=1}^{H} N_h S_h^2}.$$

Remark 2.3.2 A very similar formula, with σ_h taking the place of S_h, can be obtained by minimizing the prediction-based variance instead of the design-based variance.

Remark 2.3.3 The application of the condition derived from Theorem 2.3.1 frequently leads in practice to 'optimal' values of n_h that exceed N_h. Since it is not possible to draw such a sample without replacement, what is done in practice is to set these n_h equal to their maximum feasible values, N_h. The sum of the n_h then falls short of the required n, and it is necessary to recalculate the optimal allocation of the remaining n_h (that is, excluding those that have been set to equal N_h). Their required sum in that case is the value of n originally chosen, minus the sum of the N_h in the completely enumerated strata.

Remark 2.3.4 Here we have chosen a value of n and optimized the sample allocation by minimizing the variance of the sample estimate. Choosing a value for the sample variance and minimizing the required sample size leads to the same allocation rule, namely, $n_h \propto N_h S_h$ for all h.

Remark 2.3.5 This allocation rule is usually attributed to Neyman (1934), a classical paper that led to the establishment of design-based inference as a virtually unchallenged paradigm from the 1940s through to the 1970s. The rule was in fact given earlier in Tschuprow (1923), but that paper is highly mathematical and so difficult to read that even to find this famous allocation rule within it is itself a task of some magnitude!

Remark 2.3.6 In our case, there is no difference in cost between the weighing of a bull and of a cow elephant, but if there were, it would be the total cost rather than the sample number which would need to be minimized. The more general allocation rule (derivable in exactly the same way as the simpler version) would then be $n_h \propto N_h S_h c_h^{-1/2}$, where c_h is the cost of obtaining the relevant information regarding a unit in stratum h.

We now need to substitute numerical values in the formula for n in Remark 2.3.1. We already know that $N_B = 24$, $N_C = 25$ and $S_C \cong 275$. We will also need to make as realistic an estimate as possible for S_B. Being somewhat unwilling to ask the elephant trainer for his opinion (partly at least because of the difficulty of explaining what a population standard deviation is and why we need to impute it) we make our own stab at a factor of 1.2 for the standard deviation or 1.44 for the variance. That gives us an imputed population standard deviation of $400 \times 1.2 = 480$ for S_B, in which case

$$\begin{aligned}\tilde{\mathrm{V}}\hat{Y}_{\bullet} &= n^{-1}(24 \times 480 + 25 \times 275)^2 - (24 \times 480^2 + 25 \times 275^2)\\ &\cong 338\,376\,025n^{-1} - 7\,420\,225.\end{aligned}$$

All that remains is to decide what value of $\mathrm{V}\hat{Y}_{\bullet}$ to aim for. You will remember that in Chapter 1 we worked out that if we aimed for the standard error to be a little more than 2% of the sample estimate of total, we should be just about right.

Now $\hat{Y}_{\bullet}$ is nearly 200 000, so that 2% of $\hat{Y}_{\bullet}$ is a little less than 4000. The required variance is the square of that; say 16 000 000. Substituting this figure for $\tilde{\mathrm{V}}\hat{Y}_{\bullet}$ we obtain $n \cong (24 \times 480 + 25 \times 275)^2/(16\,000\,000 + 24 \times 480^2 + 25 \times 275^2) \cong 14.45$. Using Neyman (or Tschuprow) allocation we divide this 14.45 in the ratio $(24 \times 480):(25 \times 275)$ or $11\,520:6875$ to obtain the required sample of 9.05 bulls and 5.40 cows, or more realistically 9 bulls and 6 cows.

To this we must add Flimbo, so that the required sample size will actually be $n = 16$ if we follow the above assumptions consistently. However, to be on the safe side we should use the generous factor 2 rather than the more realistic 1.44 when guessing $\tilde{\mathrm{V}}\hat{Y}_{\bullet}$ (only for the variance calculations though, not for the allocation ratio which remains at $11\,520:6875$). So this time we have

$$n \cong \frac{(24 \times 566 + 25 \times 275)^2}{16\,000\,000 + 24 \times 566^2 + 25 \times 275^2} \cong 16.36.$$

This 16.36 is allocated 10.25 to the bulls and 6.11 to the cows. We might risk it and still say 10 bulls and 6 cows (bearing in mind the rather cavalier assumptions we have been making) but we decide to be on the safe side and say 11 bulls and 6 cows, or, with Flimbo, a total sample of 18.

The more generous estimate of variance for the bulls has made comparatively little difference to the required sample size, but how does either of them compare with the required size for simple random sampling without replacement? When we used *srswor* in Chapter 1 we found $\hat{S}^2$ to be 494 846.3 or $\hat{S}$ to be 703.5. We can now use these figures with $N = 50$ to work out the required sample size for *srswor*. We use the same level of accuracy as before ($\tilde{\mathrm{V}}\hat{Y}_{\bullet} = 16\,000\,000$) and we now have only a single stratum, so

$$n = \frac{(N\hat{S})^2}{\tilde{\mathrm{V}}\hat{Y}_{\bullet} + N\hat{S}^2} \cong \frac{(50 \times 703.5)^2}{16\,000\,000 + 50 \times 703.5^2} \cong 30.37,$$

or, in practice, 31. Our 16 or 18 for poststratified sampling is considerably smaller, but we must also remember that the circus owner originally wanted to weigh only one elephant. Clearly poststratification, or even stratification if we could use it, though helpful, would not be enough. We must find some other sampling strategy that will be quite substantially more efficient again if we are going to satisfy this client.

Result 2.3.1 The rule for optimally allocating a sample among strata is $n_h \propto N_h S_h$ when the cost of obtaining information from a sampling unit does not differ from stratum to stratum, and $n_h \propto N_h S_h c_h^{-1/2}$ when it does.

Result 2.3.2 If the sample unit costs do not vary among strata, then, given optimal allocation, the variance of the estimator $\hat{Y}_{\bullet}$ is $\mathrm{V}\hat{Y}_{\bullet} = n^{-1}\left(\sum_h N_h S_h\right)^2 - \sum_h N_h S_h^2$, where both the summations and the value of the total sample size, n, are calculated over the sampled strata only.

Result 2.3.3 Changing the subject of the above formula from $\tilde{\mathrm{V}}\hat{Y}_{\bullet}$ to n allows the required sample size to be calculated for any given level of precision.

Summary

2.4 If, after the sample has been selected, inspection of it indicates that the population consists of two or more subpopulations with recognizably different characteristics, and if the numbers of units in these subpopulations are known from non-sample sources, it will usually pay to analyse the samples from these two subpopulations separately. This technique is known as *poststratification* and the subpopulations are called *poststrata*. In this instance, the sample was poststratified into bull and cow elephants, because they tended to differ markedly in their average weights.

In the circumstances described in this chapter, it was also found necessary to single out a particularly unusual unit (Flimbo) for special treatment. Since it could be checked that there was no other such unusual unit in the population, it was treated as being in a poststratum all of its own and as having been selected with certainty. (The situation where no such check is possible will be considered in Chapter 14.) It was necessary to impute one of the stratum variances but, even with a generous imputation, the variance of the estimated total was substantially reduced as compared with the situation where the unusual unit was kept in its original poststratum.

The poststratified sample was used to design a properly stratified sample, including an optimum allocation of the required sample between the bulls' stratum and the cows' stratum.

Stratification and poststratification can be very powerful techniques where the units in each stratum are more like each other than they are like the units in other strata. Even in situations such as the elephant weighing problem considered here, where there is a considerable overlap of characteristics from stratum to stratum, stratification (and even poststratification) roughly halves the required sample size. Where the units within a stratum or poststratum are relatively more like each other than the cows and the bulls are in this example ('groups even more homogeneous within and heterogeneous between'), stratification and poststratification will be even more effective in reducing the sample size required to deliver a given level of precision.

Remark 2.4.1 Very little has been said in this chapter concerning prediction-based inference. It has only been mentioned that the latter provides a stronger argument for ignoring the interdependence of poststratified estimates than the former does. Indeed, from the standpoint of prediction-based inference, there is no interdependence. Other than that, the two inferential approaches behave very similarly in the case of poststratification, and still more similarly in that of stratification proper. Prediction-based inference requires a separate model for each (post)stratum. Other than that, its treatment of stratified sampling is virtually the same as its treatment of simple random sampling (described in **1.11–1.14**).

Exercises

2.1 A sample of 1500 is selected (supposedly using *srswor*) from a population of 30 000 adult persons. The sample is found to consist of 300 male smokers, 500 male non-smokers, 200 female smokers and 500 female non-smokers. Initially, the proportion of smokers in the population is estimated using only the information already given. Subsequently, it is found that the population actually consisted of 14 600 males and 15 400 females.

(a) Use the above information to compare the proportion of males in the sample with the subsequently known proportion of males in the population. Is the proportion of males in the sample sufficiently in excess of that in the population to cast serious doubt on the claim that the selection was *srswor*? (You may use the normal approximation for the distribution of the proportion of males in the sample. You may also use the critical two-sided limits of 1.96, 2.58 and 3.09 standard deviations for the 95%, 99% and 99.9% confidence intervals, respectively.)

(b) Again using the information given above, calculate:

(i) the estimate of the number of smokers in the population arrived at using the simple expansion estimator, $Nn^{-1}\sum_i \delta_i Y_i$; and

(ii) a poststratification estimate that takes into account the fact that the numbers of males and females in the population were 14 600 and 15 400, respectively.

(c) Estimate the variances of the simple expansion estimate and the poststratification estimate described in (b) above. Calculate the 95% confidence intervals around these two estimates, once again using the assumption that the sample size is large enough to use the normal approximation to do so. Comment on the relative sizes of the two variance estimates, and the overlap or lack of overlap between the two confidence intervals. What, if anything, has been gained by poststratification?

2.2 A population of businesses stratified by numbers of employees consists of H strata. Within the hth stratum there are N_h units, their population standard deviation is S_h, and the cost of collecting information from any one of them is c_h. The population total (value of sales) is $Y_{\bullet} = \sum_{h=1}^{H}\sum_{i=1}^{N_h} Y_{hi}$, the sample estimator of that population total is $\hat{Y}_{\bullet} = \sum_{h=1}^{H} N_h n_h^{-1} \sum_{i=1}^{N_h} \delta_{hi} Y_{hi}$, where δ_{hi} is the sample inclusion indicator (taking the value 1 when the ith population unit within the hth stratum is included in the sample and 0 otherwise), and the variance of $\hat{Y}_{\bullet}$ is $V\hat{Y}_{\bullet} = \sum_{h=1}^{H} (N_h^2 n_h^{-1} - N_h) S_h^2$.

(a) Show, using an undetermined multiplier, that the allocation of n sample units over the H strata has minimum cost when the individual stratum sample sizes n_h are chosen to be as nearly proportional as possible to the corresponding $N_h S_h c_h^{-1/2}$.

(b) Suppose that $H = 3$, $N_1 = 120$, $N_2 = 800$, $N_3 = 2000$, $S_1 = 5000$, $S_2 = 750$, $S_3 = 100$, $c_1 = \$25$, $c_2 = \$25$ and $c_3 = \$100$ (it usually being more difficult to collect statistics from small businesses than from larger ones). Find the feasible sample, with collection cost no greater than $C = \$15\,000$, that has minimum variance for $\hat{Y}_{\bullet}$.

Hints. (i) A sample having any $n_h > N_h$ is not feasible. (ii) If stratum h is completely enumerated, the cost of collecting information for the survey includes that of collecting from each of the N_h population units in that stratum.

3

Ratio Estimation (Design-Based)

Finding a Supplementary Variable 40
The Classical Ratio Estimator under Design-Based Inference 41
Exact Bias of Ratio Estimator 43
Asymptotic Approximations to the Relative Design Bias and Relative Design Variance of the Ratio Estimator 44
Asymptotic Approximations to the Actual Design Bias and Actual Design Variance of the Ratio Estimator 46
Numerical Results 48
Across-Stratum (or Combined) Ratio Estimation 52
Exercises 57

Finding a Supplementary Variable

3.1 Since we need to improve substantially on the stratified sampling design of Chapter 2, we will need to find yet more relevant information about the individual population units (elephants). Ideally, we would like to find the values of some *supplementary variable*, x, already known for each population unit, that happened to be exactly proportional to the value of the variable (weight) for which we want to estimate the total. If we had such information, we would only need to weigh a single elephant to know exactly what the constant of proportionality was, and then we would be able to calculate the total weight of the herd without error. (This, of course, would also have fulfilled the circus owner's original wish to weigh just a single elephant!) In practice, however, it is almost always necessary to settle for a far less ideal variable, and estimate the proportionality relationship from a sample of several units.

The usual source of such information is some kind of historical record. 'Have the elephants ever been weighed before,' we ask, 'or have any other measurements been taken of them?' If they have, no one seems to know about it. We consider the possibility of taking some relevant measurements now. They would need to be cheap, compared with the cost of weighing, or there would be no point in using them.

Measuring heights is one possibility, but it fails on at least two counts. First, it is not all that easy to measure the height of an elephant. Also the relationship between height and weight is certainly not going to be linear, and it is not clear what transformation of the heights would be most nearly proportional to the weights. (The obvious choice, the cube of the height, fails miserably for human beings.)

However, the elephant trainer is probably in a good position to come up with a set of predictions as to what the weights would be. Unfortunately, he does not seem to hold statisticians in very high esteem. (The previous circus statistician, whom Basu informs us was dismissed on account of his rather strange views on estimation, would not have endeared him to the profession. Our own initial acceptance of Flimbo as 'representative' has not exactly advanced our cause either.)

We decide to talk with the circus owner and put our cards on the table. He understands the nature of our intended solution and is sympathetic with our problem. He undertakes to get the information we need from the elephant trainer. The elephant trainer does not attempt to supply estimates in kilograms, but he does compare all the bull elephants with Sambo and all the cow elephants with Kara, and provides multiplicative factors that he believes to be nearly proportional to the weights. (Fortunately, the elephant trainer was not present at the time of the sample weighing and has never bothered to enquire what the weights were. Had he known them, they would almost certainly have influenced his estimates for the sample elephants and made the standard estimators of variance completely useless!)

[The narrator did not know at the time that the elephant trainer had boycotted the weighing because he was upset at having no input into the selection process; nor did he know that the trainer had washed his hands of the whole project once he learned that Flimbo had been selected. The circus owner had to bear quite heavily on him to obtain the eye estimates, and even took the trouble to check each one of them himself for credibility, in order to ensure that they had been arrived at carefully. The consultants were most fortunate in having had such a versatile and conscientious client. (Appendix B contains all the relevant numerical information, including the actual weight in kilograms of each elephant in the herd, of which only the five in sample were at that stage known to the narrator.) K.B.]

The Classical Ratio Estimator under Design-Based Inference

3.2 So now we are able to compare the actual weighings, $Y_{B3}, Y_{B5}, Y_{C12}, Y_{C16}$ and Y_{C18}, for our five original sample elephants with the elephant trainer's factors $X_{B3}, X_{B5}, X_{C12}, X_{C16}$ and X_{C18}. For the bulls we have $Y_{B3} = 4675$, $X_{B3} = 0.95$ (Combo); and $Y_{B5} = 3032$, $X_{B5} = 0.6$ (Flimbo). Since to the nearest kilogram $4675 \div 0.95 = 4921$ and $3032 \div 0.6 = 5053$, there is some hope that the X_{Bi} will prove useful. For the cows we have $Y_{C12} = 3328$, $X_{C12} = 1.1$ (Linda); $Y_{C16} = 3427$, $X_{C16} = 1.1$ (Pamela); and $Y_{C18} = 2910$, $X_{C18} = 1.0$ (Sara). Now $3328 \div 1.1 = 3025$, $3427 \div 1.1 = 3115$ and $2910 \div 1.0 = 2910$, so once again it seems as though the elephant trainer is a good judge of weights and that his estimates will be useful. We also have confirmation that the bulls are heavier than the cows, because the two estimates of 'kilograms per Sambo' are about 5000 and the three of 'kilograms per Kara' are all about 3000. This is in accordance with our informal observations and adds to our confidence that this line of attack is worth pursuing.

3.3 It might be supposed that we would proceed (at least for the cows) by averaging the three 'kilograms per Kara' ratios and applying that average to the total of Kara equivalents for the 25 cows, which is available to us and is in fact 25.3. This would give us (again to the nearest kilogram for each elephant)

$$\frac{3025 + 3115 + 2910}{3} \times 25.3 = 3016.67 \times 25.3 = 76\,322.$$

The *classical ratio estimator* of total for the cows' stratum is, however,

$$\hat{Y}_{C.R} = \frac{\hat{Y}_{C.}}{\hat{X}_{C.}} X_{C.} \tag{3.1}$$

where $\hat{Y}_{C.}$ is the *expansion* estimator or *number-raising estimator* of $Y_{C.}$, as defined in Chapter 1, and $\hat{X}_{C.}$ is the corresponding expansion estimator of $X_{C.}$, which in turn is the population sum of the X-variable values for the cows' stratum. Substituting the relevant numerical values, we obtain the corresponding estimate

$$\hat{Y}_{C.R} = \frac{25(3328 + 3427 + 2910)/3}{25(1.1 + 1.1 + 1.0)/3} 25.3 = \frac{80\,542}{26.667} 25.3 = 76\,414.$$

This is very close to our 'average of ratios' estimate of 76 322 (both being about 4 tonnes lower than the 80 542 kg estimate of Chapter 2). It is in fact seldom that they differ sharply, but it is as well to explain why the classical ratio estimator is used far more often. That is not a straightforward matter and will take a little time.

3.4 From the 1940s until at least the 1970s, design-based inference went almost unchallenged. For design-based inference, $\hat{Y}_{C.}$ and $\hat{X}_{C.}$ are unbiased estimators (as proved for the single-stratum $\hat{Y}_{.}$ in Chapter 1). The classical ratio estimator is not design-unbiased, but it is in one sense of the word 'consistent', and in a way that the 'average of ratios' is not. This statement itself requires explanation.

In statistics generally, the notion of consistency is inextricably bound up with the possibility of increasing the sample size indefinitely. A *consistent estimator* is one which converges in probability to the true value as the sample size tends to infinity. In *srswr*, of course, one can keep on sampling indefinitely, but in survey sampling we usually prefer to sample without replacement, so the maximum size of our sample is that of the entire population, which in our present case is N_C. That fact led Cochran (1953, p. 12; 1963, p. 20; 1977, p. 21) to write: 'In this book, a method of estimation is called *consistent* if the estimate becomes equal to the population value when $n = N$, that is, when the sample consists of the whole population.' In some instances, however, we will wish to use the more usual definition involving the possibility of the sample size increasing indefinitely, so we will call consistency according to Cochran's definition *Cochran consistency*.

3.5 We shall be proving the following theorem generally (not just for the cows' stratum), so we shall temporarily drop the suffix C.

Theorem 3.5.1 The classical ratio estimator is Cochran consistent for *srswor*, but the 'averages of ratios' estimator, in general, is not.

Proof. The classical ratio estimator is $\hat{Y}_{\cdot R} = \hat{R}X_{\cdot}$, where $\hat{R} = \hat{Y}_{\cdot}/\hat{X}_{\cdot}$. When the sample consists of the whole population, $\hat{Y}_{\cdot} = Y_{\cdot}$ and $\hat{X}_{\cdot} = X_{\cdot}$, so $\hat{R}$ is a Cochran-consistent estimator of $R = Y_{\cdot}/X_{\cdot}$ and $\hat{Y}_{\cdot R}$ of $Y_{\cdot}$.

The average of ratios estimator is

$$\hat{Y}_{\cdot AR} = \left\{ n^{-1} \sum_{i} \delta_i \left(\frac{Y_i}{X_i} \right) \right\} X_{\cdot}. \tag{3.2}$$

When the sample consists of the whole population, $\hat{Y}_{\cdot AR} = \left\{ N^{-1} \sum_i (Y_i/X_i) \right\} X_{\cdot}$. This is not the same as $Y_{\cdot}$. To take a simple counterexample, let $N = n = 2$, $Y_1 = 1$, $X_1 = 2$, $Y_2 = 1$, $X_2 = 4$. Then $\bar{X} = N^{-1}X_{\cdot} = 3$, $Y_1/X_1 = 1/2$ and $Y_2/X_2 = 1/4$, so $\hat{Y}_{\cdot AR} = 3/2 + 3/4 = 9/4$, whereas $Y_{\cdot} = 1 + 1 = 2$. So in general $\hat{Y}_{\cdot AR} \neq Y_{\cdot}$, even when the sample consists of the whole population, and $\hat{Y}_{\cdot AR}$ is not Cochran consistent. ◇

Remark 3.5.1 This theorem applies only to *srswor*. While that is an important special case, there are other important circumstances in which Cochran consistency is meaningless, even for a finite population. In such circumstances, it may be possible for the average of ratios estimator to be consistent (according to another rather special definition of the word) and the classical ratio estimator inconsistent. Design consistency in general is not a particularly straightforward concept, and is always heavily dependent on the manner in which the sample has been selected. Nevertheless the ascendancy of design-based inference over the period from the 1940s to at least the 1970s was such that no estimator was regarded as statistically acceptable unless it was either design-unbiased or at least (in some sense) design-consistent.

The acceptance of the classical ratio estimator over all its rivals within the context of *srswor* is almost certainly due to these two properties: that it was a function of estimators that were design-unbiased and that it was itself Cochran consistent. To appreciate the potentialities of other possible estimators, and in particular the average of ratios estimator, it is necessary to consider the prediction-based approach, and this will be done in Chapter 5. In the meantime, however, we return to the problem of weighing circus elephants, to see whether the classical ratio estimator can indeed satisfy the circus owner's current objective, which is to know the total weight of his herd within 10% with 99% confidence without having to weigh any more elephants. To do this within the design-based approach we will need to be able to estimate the design-based mean squared error of our ratio estimator. The MSE is the sum of the squared bias and the variance.

Exact Bias of Ratio Estimator

3.6 We consider the bias first.

Theorem 3.6.1 The bias in $\hat{Y}_{\bullet}$ is $-\mathrm{C}(\hat{R}, \hat{X}_{\bullet})$, that is, minus the covariance between $\hat{R}$ and $\hat{X}_{\bullet}$.

Proof (Hartley and Ross, 1954; Cochran, 1963, p. 162).

$$\begin{aligned} \mathrm{C}(\hat{R}, \hat{X}_{\bullet}) &= \mathrm{E}(\hat{R}\hat{X}_{\bullet}) - (\mathrm{E}\hat{R})\mathrm{E}\hat{X}_{\bullet} \\ &= Y_{\bullet} - X_{\bullet}\mathrm{E}\hat{R}. \end{aligned}$$

Hence,

$$\begin{aligned} \mathrm{E}\hat{R} &= \frac{Y_{\bullet}}{X_{\bullet}} - \frac{\mathrm{C}(\hat{R}, \hat{X}_{\bullet})}{X_{\bullet}} \\ &= R - \frac{\mathrm{C}(\hat{R}, \hat{X}_{\bullet})}{X_{\bullet}} \end{aligned}$$

so that

$$\mathrm{E}\hat{Y}_{\bullet R} = X_{\bullet}\mathrm{E}\hat{R} = Y_{\bullet} - \mathrm{C}(\hat{R}, \hat{X}_{\bullet});$$

and the bias in $\hat{Y}_{\bullet R}$ is

$$\mathrm{E}\hat{Y}_{\bullet R} - Y_{\bullet} = -\mathrm{C}(\hat{R}, \hat{X}_{\bullet}). \tag{3.3}$$

◇

An important consequence of this result is the following:

Theorem 3.6.2 The ratio of the absolute value of the bias in $\hat{Y}_{\bullet R}$ to its standard error cannot be greater than the coefficient of variation of $\hat{X}_{\bullet}$ (that is, the ratio of the standard error of $\hat{X}_{\bullet}$ to the expectation of $\hat{X}_{\bullet}$).

Proof (Hartley and Ross, 1954; Cochran, 1963, p. 162). $|\mathrm{E}\hat{Y}_{\bullet R} - Y_{\bullet}| = |\mathrm{C}(\hat{R}, \hat{X}_{\bullet})| \leq (\mathrm{SE}\hat{R})\mathrm{SE}\hat{X}_{\bullet}$, where $\mathrm{SE}(\cdot)$ denotes standard error. Dividing both sides by $\mathrm{SE}\hat{Y}_{\bullet R} = X_{\bullet}\mathrm{SE}\hat{R}$, $|\mathrm{E}\hat{Y}_{\bullet R} - Y_{\bullet}|/\mathrm{SE}\hat{Y}_{\bullet R} \leq \mathrm{SE}\hat{X}_{\bullet}/X_{\bullet}$. ◇

Cochran draws from this the conclusion that if the coefficient of variation of $\hat{X}_{\bullet}$ is less than 0.1, the bias of $\hat{Y}_{\bullet R}$ may safely be regarded as negligible in relation to its standard error.

Asymptotic Approximations to the Relative Design Bias and Relative Design Variance of the Ratio Estimator

3.7 The exact results of **3.6** are useful as far as they go, but (3.3) is not a convenient formula for estimating the bias and, even more importantly, no similar approach to an exact formula for the variance of $\hat{Y}_{\bullet R}$ has yet been found. Approximate expressions for both the bias and the variance of $\hat{Y}_{\bullet R}$ can, however, be found using a Taylor expansion, and both lend themselves easily to the formation of sample estimators.

It will be convenient for this section to work in terms of the mean rather than of the total. Define $\Delta\hat{\bar{Y}}$ and $\Delta\hat{\bar{X}}$ by $\Delta\hat{\bar{Y}} = (\hat{\bar{Y}} - \bar{Y})/\bar{Y}$ and $\Delta\hat{\bar{X}} = (\hat{\bar{X}} - \bar{X})/\bar{X}$, respectively. (Note that the design expectations of $\Delta\hat{\bar{Y}}$ and $\Delta\hat{\bar{X}}$ are both zero.) In order to obtain a large-sample approximation that is as meaningful as possible for our actually rather small population and even smaller sample, we will imagine that the population itself is replicated many times, that the large population we are considering is the sum of all such replicates, and that the relevant sample is obtained by applying the same *srswor* procedure independently within each replicate of the population (Brewer, 1979). We will also, for convenience, be working in terms of the *relative bias* (the ratio of the bias to the value of the quantity estimated) and the *relative variance* (the ratio of the variance to the square of the quantity estimated) rather than in terms of the bias and variance themselves.

Theorem 3.7.1 Under the asymptotics set out in the immediately preceding paragraph, the relative design bias of $\hat{\bar{Y}}_R = (\hat{\bar{Y}}/\hat{\bar{X}})\bar{X}$, the ratio estimator of the population mean, is asymptotically equal to $\mathrm{V}\hat{\bar{X}}/\bar{X}^2 - \mathrm{C}(\hat{\bar{Y}},\hat{\bar{X}})/\bar{Y}\bar{X}$, $\mathrm{C}(\hat{\bar{Y}},\hat{\bar{X}})$ being the design covariance between $\hat{\bar{Y}}$ and $\hat{\bar{X}}$.

Proof. Regardless of the composition of the original population, as the number of replicates increases, a point will eventually be reached where $\Delta\hat{\bar{Y}}$ and $\Delta\hat{\bar{X}}$ are both less than unity. From that point onwards we are able to write:

$$\begin{aligned}\hat{\bar{Y}}_R - \bar{Y} = \left(\frac{\hat{\bar{Y}}}{\hat{\bar{X}}}\right)\bar{X} - \bar{Y} &= \left\{\frac{\bar{Y}(1+\Delta\hat{\bar{Y}})}{\bar{X}(1+\Delta\hat{\bar{X}})}\right\}\bar{X} - \bar{Y} \\ &= \frac{\bar{Y}}{\bar{X}}\left\{(1+\Delta\hat{\bar{Y}})(1+\Delta\hat{\bar{X}})^{-1} - 1\right\}\bar{X} \\ &= \left[(1+\Delta\hat{\bar{Y}})\left\{1 - \Delta\hat{\bar{X}} + (\Delta\hat{\bar{X}})^2 - \cdots\right\} - 1\right]\bar{Y} \\ &= \left\{\Delta\hat{\bar{Y}} - \Delta\hat{\bar{X}} - (\Delta\hat{\bar{Y}})(\Delta\hat{\bar{X}}) + (\Delta\hat{\bar{X}})^2 + \cdots\right\}\bar{Y}.\end{aligned}$$

Hence the relative design bias in $\hat{\bar{Y}}_R$, defined as $\mathrm{E}(\hat{\bar{Y}}_R - \bar{Y})/\bar{Y}$, is asymptotically equal to

$$\begin{aligned}\mathrm{E}\left\{\Delta\hat{\bar{Y}} - \Delta\hat{\bar{X}} - (\Delta\hat{\bar{Y}})(\Delta\hat{\bar{X}}) + (\Delta\hat{\bar{X}})^2\right\} &= \mathrm{E}\left\{(\Delta\hat{\bar{X}})^2 - (\Delta\hat{\bar{Y}})(\Delta\hat{\bar{X}})\right\} \\ &= \frac{\mathrm{V}\hat{\bar{X}}}{\bar{X}^2} - \frac{\mathrm{C}(\hat{\bar{Y}},\hat{\bar{X}})}{\bar{Y}\bar{X}}. \qquad (3.4)\end{aligned}$$

◇

In this asymptotic expression for the relative bias, $\mathrm{V}\hat{\bar{X}}/\bar{X}^2$ is the *relative variance* of $\hat{\bar{X}}$ and $\mathrm{C}(\hat{\bar{Y}},\hat{\bar{X}})/\bar{Y}\bar{X}$ is the *relative covariance* of $\hat{\bar{Y}}$ and $\hat{\bar{X}}$. Ignoring for the moment the finite-sample correction, both $\mathrm{V}\hat{\bar{X}}/\bar{X}^2$ and $\mathrm{C}(\hat{\bar{Y}},\hat{\bar{X}})/\bar{Y}\bar{X}$ are inversely proportional to the sample size, so asymptotically the design bias of $\hat{\bar{Y}}_R$ is also inversely proportional to the sample size.

Remark 3.7.1 If the least-squares linear regression of the Y_i on the X_i passes through the origin, $\mathrm{C}(\hat{\bar{Y}},\hat{\bar{X}})/\bar{Y}\bar{X} = \mathrm{V}\hat{\bar{X}}/\bar{X}^2$ and there is no design bias in the ratio estimator.

Theorem 3.7.2 Given the same assumptions as used for Theorem 3.7.1, the relative design MSE of $\hat{\bar{Y}}_R = (\hat{\bar{Y}}/\hat{\bar{X}})\bar{X}$, the ratio estimator of the population mean, is asymptotically equal to $\mathrm{V}\hat{\bar{Y}}/\bar{Y}^2 - 2\mathrm{C}(\hat{\bar{Y}},\hat{\bar{X}})/\bar{Y}\bar{X} + \mathrm{V}\hat{\bar{X}}/\bar{X}^2$.

Proof. Proceeding as in the proof of Theorem 3.7.1, the relative design MSE of $\hat{\bar{Y}}_R$, defined as $\mathrm{E}\{(\hat{\bar{Y}}_R - \bar{Y})/\bar{Y}\}^2$, is asymptotically equal to

$$\begin{aligned}\mathrm{E}\{\Delta\hat{\bar{Y}} - \Delta\hat{\bar{X}} - (\Delta\hat{\bar{Y}})(\Delta\hat{\bar{X}}) + (\Delta\hat{\bar{X}})^2\}^2 &\cong \mathrm{E}(\Delta\hat{\bar{Y}} - \Delta\hat{\bar{X}})^2 \\ &= \mathrm{E}\{(\Delta\hat{\bar{Y}})^2 - 2(\Delta\hat{\bar{Y}})(\Delta\hat{\bar{X}}) + (\Delta\hat{\bar{X}})^2\} \\ &= \frac{\mathrm{V}\hat{\bar{Y}}}{\bar{Y}^2} - \frac{2\mathrm{C}(\hat{\bar{Y}},\hat{\bar{X}})}{\bar{Y}\bar{X}} + \frac{\mathrm{V}\hat{\bar{X}}}{\bar{X}^2}. \qquad (3.5)\end{aligned}$$

◇

Once again ignoring the finite-sample correction, each of these three expressions is asymptotically inversely proportional to the sample size. This is in accordance with the earlier result, deriving from Theorem 3.6.2, that the square of the bias is asymptotically negligible compared within the variance. Hence both the design variance and the design MSE of $\hat{\bar{Y}}_R$ are themselves asymptotically inversely proportional to the sample size.

Asymptotic Approximations to the Actual Design Bias and Actual Design Variance of the Ratio Estimator

3.8 It is commonly allowed that since $\hat{Y}_{\bullet R} = N\hat{\bar{Y}}_R$ and N is a constant, $\hat{Y}_{\bullet R}$ may itself be described as asymptotically design unbiased. However, among the assumptions used to establish the asymptotic design unbiasedness of $\hat{\bar{Y}}_R$ there was one that N should be allowed to increase indefinitely. Provided this caveat is kept in mind, the common usage should not give rise to any confusion.

We shall next obtain convenient expressions for the design bias and design variance of $\hat{Y}_{\bullet R}$ that take advantage of some cancellation within the formulae obtained in **3.6.**

The design bias of $\hat{Y}_{\bullet R}$ is $Y_{\bullet}$ times its relative design bias; that is,

$$\begin{aligned}\mathrm{E}(\hat{Y}_{\bullet R} - Y_{\bullet}) &\cong Y_{\bullet}\left\{\frac{\mathrm{V}\hat{\bar{X}}}{\bar{X}^2} - \frac{\mathrm{C}(\hat{\bar{Y}},\hat{\bar{X}})}{\bar{Y}\bar{X}}\right\} \\ &= Y_{\bullet}\left\{\frac{\mathrm{V}\hat{X}_{\bullet}}{X_{\bullet}^2} - \frac{\mathrm{C}(\hat{Y}_{\bullet},\hat{X}_{\bullet})}{Y_{\bullet}X_{\bullet}}\right\}\end{aligned}$$

$$= N(N-n)n^{-1}Y_{\bullet}\left(\frac{S_X^2}{X_{\bullet}^2} - \frac{S_{Y,X}}{Y_{\bullet}X_{\bullet}}\right),$$

where $S_X^2 = (N-1)^{-1}\sum_i (X_i - \bar{X})^2$ and $S_{Y,X} = (N-1)^{-1}\sum_i (Y_i - \bar{Y})(X_i - \bar{X})$. Hence

$$\mathrm{E}(\hat{Y}_{\bullet R} - Y_{\bullet}) \cong N(N-n)n^{-1}Y_{\bullet}(N-1)^{-1} \times \left\{\frac{\sum_i (X_i - \bar{X})^2}{X_{\bullet}^2} - \frac{\sum_i (Y_i - \bar{Y})(X_i - \bar{X})}{Y_{\bullet}X_{\bullet}}\right\}$$

Writing $\bar{R} = Y_{\bullet}/X_{\bullet} = \bar{Y}/\bar{X}$, $Y_{\bullet}\sum_i (X_i - \bar{X})^2 - X_{\bullet}\sum_i (Y_i - \bar{Y})(X_i - \bar{X}) \equiv X_{\bullet}\sum_i \{X_i(\bar{R}X_i - Y_i)\}$. So

$$\mathrm{E}(\hat{Y}_{\bullet R} - Y_{\bullet}) \cong N(N-n)n^{-1}X_{\bullet}^{-1}(N-1)^{-1}\sum_i \{X_i(\bar{R}X_i - Y_i)\}. \tag{3.6}$$

Two Cochran-consistent estimators of this approximation to $\mathrm{E}(\hat{Y}_{\bullet R} - Y_{\bullet})$ are $N(N-n)n^{-1}X_{\bullet}^{-1}(n-1)^{-1}\sum_i \delta_i\{X_i(\hat{\bar{R}}X_i - Y_i)\}$ and $N(N-n)n^{-1}\hat{X}_{\bullet}^{-1}(n-1)^{-1}\sum_i \delta_i\{X_i(\hat{\bar{R}}X_i - Y_i)\}$. While the former might seem the more obvious, there is an argument for using the latter. This is that given the kind of estimates that the elephant trainer was asked to make, the standard deviations of the $\hat{\bar{R}}X_i - Y_i$ could reasonably be expected to increase proportionally with the X_i. A natural estimator of the relative design bias would therefore use $\hat{\bar{X}}$ and $\hat{\bar{Y}}$ in the denominators rather than $\bar{X}$ and $\hat{\bar{Y}}_R$, so that the extent to which the numerators were overestimates or underestimates (as a result of selecting large or small sample units by chance) would be balanced by corresponding overestimates or underestimates in the denominators. This would correspond to using the multiplier $\hat{X}_{\bullet}^{-1}$ rather than $X_{\bullet}^{-1}$. The latter expression will be used for that reason.

The design variance of $\hat{Y}_{\bullet R}$ is $Y_{\bullet}^2$ times its relative design variance; that is,

$$\begin{aligned}
\mathrm{V}\hat{Y}_{\bullet R} &\cong Y_{\bullet}^2\left\{\frac{\mathrm{V}\hat{\bar{Y}}}{\bar{Y}^2} - \frac{2\mathrm{C}(\hat{\bar{Y}},\hat{\bar{X}})}{\bar{Y}\bar{X}} + \frac{\mathrm{V}\hat{\bar{X}}}{\bar{X}^2}\right\} \\
&= Y_{\bullet}^2\left\{\frac{\mathrm{V}\hat{Y}_{\bullet}}{Y_{\bullet}^2} - \frac{2\mathrm{C}(\hat{Y}_{\bullet},\hat{X}_{\bullet})}{Y_{\bullet}X_{\bullet}} + \frac{\mathrm{V}\hat{X}_{\bullet}}{X_{\bullet}^2}\right\} \\
&= \mathrm{V}\hat{Y}_{\bullet} - 2\bar{R}\mathrm{C}(\hat{Y}_{\bullet},\hat{X}_{\bullet}) + \bar{R}^2\mathrm{V}\hat{X}_{\bullet} \\
&= N(N-n)n^{-1}\left(S_Y^2 - 2\bar{R}S_{Y,X} + \bar{R}^2S_X^2\right) \\
&= N(N-n)n^{-1}(N-1)^{-1}\sum_i \left(Y_i^2 - 2\bar{R}X_iY_i + \bar{R}^2X_i^2\right)
\end{aligned}$$

$$= N(N-n)n^{-1}(N-1)^{-1}\left\{\sum_i (Y_i-\bar{Y})^2 - 2\bar{R}\sum_i (Y_i-\bar{Y})(X_i-\bar{X}) + \bar{R}^2\sum_i (X_i-\bar{X})^2\right\}. \tag{3.7}$$

As with the approximate expression for the bias of $\hat{Y}_{\cdot R}$, this formula readily simplifies down, and (3.7) may also be written as

$$\mathrm{V}\hat{Y}_{\cdot R} \cong N(N-n)n^{-1}S^2_{(Y-\bar{R}X)} \tag{3.8}$$

where

$$S^2_{(Y-\bar{R}X)} = (N-1)^{-1}\sum_i (Y_i - \bar{R}X_i)^2. \tag{3.9}$$

This expression for the approximate variance, (3.8) with (3.9), is more convenient to use than (3.7), which involves three large terms which can nearly cancel out. When computers are used such calculations can end up losing a great deal of accuracy through rounding error, and when they are not used it is easy to make gross mistakes without realizing it.

As with the approximate design bias, there are two Cochran-consistent estimators of the approximate design variance worth considering. $N(N-n)n^{-1}(n-1)^{-1}\sum_i \delta_i(Y_i-\bar{R}X_i)^2$ is attractively simple, but again $N(N-n)n^{-1}X_{\cdot}^2\hat{X}_{\cdot}^{-2}(n-1)^{-1}\sum_i \delta_i(Y_i-\bar{R}X_i)^2$ contains a natural compensating factor to counter the effects of selecting relatively large or small sample units and is therefore preferable.

The expression $X_{\cdot}^2\hat{X}_{\cdot}^{-2}(n-1)^{-1}\sum_i \delta_i(Y_i-\bar{R}X_i)^2$ is the corresponding Cochran-consistent estimator of $S^2_{(Y-\bar{R}X)}$ and will therefore be denoted by $\hat{S}^2_{(Y-\bar{R}X)}$.

Numerical Results

3.9 We can now not only calculate the classical ratio estimates (for bulls and cows separately) in the context of our elephant weighing problem, but also estimate their biases and variances. It is true that we will be using asymptotic expressions in a situation where our sample sizes are unambiguously small, but even if the asymptotic formulae are considerably in error we will still be able to obtain some idea of the reduction in design variances (as compared with the designs used in Chapters 1 and 2). We will consider first the likely behaviour of the design variance and the design bias in relation to our own problem.

We again start with the cows' stratum, because there is no complication there with any atypical observation. Our estimate of the total weight of the cows is

76 414 kg, for which the estimated design variance is

$$
\begin{aligned}
\hat{V}\hat{Y}_{C.R} &= N_C(N_C - n_C)n_C^{-1}\hat{S}^2_{C(Y-\bar{R}X)} \\
&= N_C(N_C - n_C)n_C^{-1}X_{C.}^2\hat{X}_{C.}^{-2}(n_C - 1)^{-1}\sum_i \delta_{Ci}(Y_{Ci} - \bar{R}_C X_{Ci})^2 \\
&\cong 25\frac{22}{3}\left(\frac{25.3}{26.667}\right)^2\frac{1}{3-1}\big[(3328 - 3020.3125 \times 1.1)^2 \\
&\quad + (3427 - 3020.3125 \times 1.1)^2 + (2910 - 3020.3125 \times 1.0)^2\big] \\
&\cong 183.333 \times 0.900\,13 \times 0.5 \times [31.99 + 10\,952.94 + 12\,168.85] \\
&\cong 183.333 \times 0.900\,13 \times 11\,576.89 \\
&\cong 183.333 \times 10\,420.66 \\
&\cong 1\,910\,451 \\
&\cong 1382^2.
\end{aligned}
$$

This is a big reduction on the 3716^2 we had in Chapter 2 using the unbiased estimator $\hat{V}\hat{Y}_{C.} = N_C(N_C - n_C)n_C^{-1}\hat{S}_C^2$. Things are looking distinctly hopeful.

Now we must consider the bulls' stratum. In Chapter 2 we had to treat Flimbo as an extreme outlier and put him in a stratum all by himself, but under ratio estimation the relevant stratification variable is not the elephant's weight, but the ratio of the elephant's weight to the elephant trainer's estimate of his weight. We have only two sample bull elephants, but we can see that if the variability between these two ratios is of the same order of magnitude as the variability among the three corresponding ratios for the sample cows, there will be no need to treat Flimbo any longer as in a stratum all by himself. The two ratios are for Combo $4675/0.95 = 4921$ and for Flimbo $3032/0.6 = 5053$. The difference is clearly of the same order of magnitude as was found among the cows (3025, 3115 and 2910). We therefore put Flimbo back in the bulls' stratum and form the ratio estimator of the total weight for that stratum as $\{24.35/(0.95 + 0.6)\}\{4675 + 3032\} = 121\,074$ kg or about 121 tonnes. (This is considerably larger than the 96 338 kg originally obtained in Chapter 2, before Flimbo was separated off as an outlier, but not so much in excess of the 115 tonnes – including Flimbo – finally arrived at in that chapter.) The corresponding estimator of variance is

$$
\begin{aligned}
\hat{V}\hat{Y}_{B.R} &= N_B(N_B - n_B)n_B^{-1}\hat{S}^2_{B(Y-\bar{R}X)} \\
&= N_B(N_B - n_B)n_B^{-1}X_{B.}^2\hat{X}_{B.}^{-2}(n_B - 1)^{-1}\sum_i \delta_{Bi}(Y_{Bi} - \bar{R}_B X_{Bi})^2 \\
&\cong 25\frac{25-2}{2}\left(\frac{24.35}{19.375}\right)^2\big[(4675 - 4972.258 \times 0.95)^2 \\
&\quad + (3032 - 4972.258 \times 0.6)^2\big] \\
&\cong 287.5 \times 1.579\,48 \times (2366.35 + 2366.35)
\end{aligned}
$$

$$\cong 287.5 \times 7475.21$$
$$\cong 2\,149\,123$$
$$\cong 1466^2.$$

This is quite a remarkable reduction on the $19\,699^2$ we obtained in Chapter 2, but of course the main reason for the reduction is that Flimbo need no longer be regarded as an outlying observation. For the two strata combined, the estimate of total is $121 + 76 = 197$ tonnes with a standard error of $(2\,149\,123 + 1\,910\,451)^{1/2} = 2015$ kg or almost exactly 2 tonnes.

So we now have a standard error of only 1.0%, which is well below the 2% for which we were aiming! But we need to be triply careful. Cochran (1977, p. 153) suggests that: 'As a working rule, the large sample results [for a ratio estimate] may be used if the sample size exceeds 30 and is also large enough so that the coefficients of variation of [$\hat{\hat{X}}$ and $\hat{\hat{Y}}$] are both less than 10%.' We can meet none of these three conditions. Our only hope is to investigate our situation more closely. First, we can and must estimate the bias. Next, we must examine the higher-order terms in the Taylor series expansion for the variance. Finally, even if there is no appreciable bias and the variance is about right, the sample is so small that the distribution of the estimate of total may be far from normal. Before we inform the circus owner that all is well, we will need to check on all these three points.

3.10 First, then, the bias. It is not usual for sampling statisticians to worry about estimating bias, but our sample is very small and has been split between two strata, so we need to be particularly careful. For the cows, our estimate of design bias is

$$N_C(N_C - n_C)n_C^{-1}\hat{X}_C^{-1}(n_C - 1)^{-1}\sum_i \delta_{Ci}\{X_{Ci}(\hat{\hat{R}}_C X_{Ci} - Y_{Ci})\}$$
$$\cong 183.333\left(\frac{25.3}{26.667^2}\right)\frac{1}{3-1}[1.1(3020.3125 \times 1.1 - 3328)$$
$$+ 1.1(3020.3125 \times 1.1 - 3427) + (3020.3125 - 2910)]$$
$$\cong 183.333 \times 0.0375 \times 0.5 \times [-6.221\,875 - 115.121\,875 + 110.3125]$$
$$\cong 183.333 \times 0.0375 \times 0.5 \times [-11.031\,25]$$
$$\cong -183.333 \times 0.206\,84$$
$$\cong -37.920$$
$$\cong -37.9.$$

For the bulls, it is

$$N_B(N_B - n_B)n_B^{-1}\hat{X}_B^{-1}(n_B - 1)^{-1}\sum_i \delta_{Bi}\{X_{Bi}(\hat{\hat{R}}_B X_{Bi} - Y_{Bi})\}$$
$$\cong 287.5(19.375)^{-1}\frac{1}{2-1}[0.95(4972.258 \times 0.95 - 4675)$$
$$+ 0.6(4972.258 \times 0.6 - 3032)]$$

$$\begin{aligned}
&\cong 287.5 \times 0.051\,612\,9 \times 1 \times [46.212\,93 - 29.187\,09] \\
&\cong 287.5 \times 0.051\,612\,9 \times 17.025\,84 \\
&\cong 287.5 \times 0.878\,753 \\
&\cong 252.641\,5 \\
&\cong 252.6.
\end{aligned}$$

The estimated bias for bulls and cows together is therefore about 214.7 kg and the squared bias is only 46 096, compared with the 4 059 574 estimated for the variance. This appears to be promising, but the bias-corrected estimator obtained by subtracting this estimate of bias from $\hat{Y}_{\bullet R}$ is the Hartley and Ross (1954) estimator, and this has a dubious reputation. Cochran (1977, p. 177) notes that some studies of natural populations have shown relatively high variances for that estimator for samples of size 2. Moreover, we have no idea how precise our particular estimate of bias is, and in fact we can never know its precision because we would need to use fourth-order sample moments to estimate that precision, and that is impossible when we only have one sample of two units and one sample of three. The fact that our estimate of the squared bias is only one-fiftieth of the corresponding estimated variance does tend to reassure us, but the other signals are all unfavourable.

We turn to something less perplexing: the Taylor series approximation for the variance. Our fundamental assumption was that

$$\mathrm{E}\{\Delta\hat{\bar{Y}} - \Delta\hat{\bar{X}} - \Delta\hat{\bar{Y}}\Delta\hat{\bar{X}} + (\Delta\hat{\bar{X}})^2\}^2 \cong \mathrm{E}(\Delta\hat{\bar{Y}} - \Delta\hat{\bar{X}})^2.$$

If we take the next higher-order terms into account, we have

$$\mathrm{E}\{\Delta\hat{\bar{Y}} - \Delta\hat{\bar{X}} - \Delta\hat{\bar{Y}}\Delta\hat{\bar{X}} + (\Delta\hat{\bar{X}})^2\}^2 \cong \mathrm{E}\{(\Delta\hat{\bar{Y}} - \Delta\hat{\bar{X}})^2(1 - \Delta\hat{\bar{X}})\}.$$

The extra terms are of third order and are zero when the distributions of $\Delta\hat{\bar{Y}}$ and $\Delta\hat{\bar{X}}$ are both symmetrical. We use the elephant trainer's estimates, X_i, to see whether the sizes of bulls and of cows are reasonably symmetrical. There is an appreciable bimodality among the bulls, of the type that produces a slight skewness, but nothing like the extent of skewness typically found in populations of businesses, so we feel confident that the third-order quantities will all be negligible. That pushes the problem into the fourth-order terms, which we are unable to estimate.

We therefore resort to common sense. It is true that we fail to meet Cochran's requirement that the coefficients of variation of $\Delta\hat{\bar{Y}}$ and $\Delta\hat{\bar{X}}$ both be less than 10%, but that is primarily because we selected Flimbo, and he is unusual only on account of his low weight. In terms of the relationship between weight and eye estimate of weight, Flimbo is a reasonably average bull. Cochran's criterion only puts a ceiling on the bias in any case. To apply it in this situation does not seem appropriate.

Finally the question of normality. We are dealing with a natural population and would expect the distributions of bull sizes and cow sizes to be approximately normal. Despite the bimodality previously noted in the bulls' sizes, neither the distribution for bulls nor that for cows is too far from normal. We would also expect the distributions of $\hat{X}$ and $\hat{Y}$ to be slightly closer to normal than those of the X_i and Y_i themselves. Realistically, we should have nothing to worry about in this regard.

Across-Stratum (or Combined) Ratio Estimation

3.11 We are therefore morally convinced that we have already more than fulfilled the requirements of the circus owner. But to our fellow sampling statisticians, all the considerations above are going to look suspiciously like 'hand-waving' or like Huff's (1954) 'statisticulation'. We are going to have to do much more work to convince them!

We consider our possible strategies. My Australian colleague, who once worked in the Australian Bureau of Statistics sampling area (the one started by Ken Foreman shortly after World War II), remembers the rule of thumb used there that a sample of size six was regarded as sufficient to use *stratum-by-stratum* (or *separate*) *ratio estimators*. Where the sample was smaller, the Australians used the *across-stratum* (or *combined*) *ratio estimator*. The formula for this was

$$\hat{Y}_{.RA} = \hat{\hat{R}}X_{.} = \frac{\sum_h \hat{Y}_{h.}}{\sum_h \hat{X}_{h.}} \sum_h X_{h.} \tag{3.10}$$

and it had a smaller bias than $\hat{Y}_{.R}$. We decide to try that. The estimate itself is

$$\begin{aligned}
\hat{Y}_{.RA} &= \frac{\hat{Y}_{B.} + \hat{Y}_{C.}}{\hat{X}_{B.} + \hat{X}_{C.}}(X_{B.} + X_{C.}) \\
&\cong \frac{96\,337.5 + 80\,541.667}{19.375 + 26.667}(24.35 + 25.3) \\
&\cong \frac{176\,879.167}{46.042}49.65 \\
&\cong 3841.7 \times 49.65 \\
&\cong 190\,740,
\end{aligned}$$

or about 191 tonnes, 6 tonnes less than $\hat{Y}_{.R}$.

This result is a little disappointing. The estimated standard error of $\hat{Y}_{.R}$ was only 2 tonnes and its estimated bias less than one-quarter of a tonne. We would have hoped for $\hat{Y}_{.R}$ and $\hat{Y}_{.RA}$ to be substantially closer.

We nevertheless press on with estimating the variance of $\hat{Y}_{\bullet RA}$. The Taylor expansion approximation for $\mathrm{V}\hat{Y}_{\bullet RA}$ is

$$
\begin{aligned}
\mathrm{V}\hat{Y}_{\bullet RA} &\cong Y_{\bullet}^{2}\left\{\frac{\mathrm{V}\hat{\bar{Y}}}{\bar{Y}^{2}}-\frac{2\mathrm{C}(\hat{\bar{Y}},\hat{\bar{X}})}{\bar{Y}\bar{X}}+\frac{\mathrm{V}\hat{\bar{X}}}{\bar{X}^{2}}\right\} \\
&= Y_{\bullet}^{2}\left\{\frac{\mathrm{V}\hat{Y}_{\bullet}}{Y_{\bullet}^{2}}-\frac{2\mathrm{C}(\hat{Y}_{\bullet},\hat{X}_{\bullet})}{Y_{\bullet}X_{\bullet}}+\frac{\mathrm{V}\hat{X}_{\bullet}}{X_{\bullet}^{2}}\right\} \\
&= \mathrm{V}\hat{Y}_{\bullet}-2\bar{R}\mathrm{C}(\hat{Y}_{\bullet},\hat{X}_{\bullet})+\bar{R}^{2}\mathrm{V}\hat{X}_{\bullet}, \qquad \text{where} \quad \bar{R}=Y_{\bullet}/X_{\bullet}, \\
&= \sum_{h} N_{h}(N_{h}-n_{h})n_{h}^{-1}\left(S_{hy}^{2}-2\bar{R}S_{hy,x}+\bar{R}^{2}S_{hx}^{2}\right) \qquad (3.11) \\
&= \sum_{h} N_{h}(N_{h}-n_{h})n_{h}^{-1}(N_{h}-1)^{-1}\left\{\sum_{i}(Y_{hi}-\bar{Y}_{h})^{2}\right. \\
&\qquad \left. -2\bar{R}\sum_{i}(Y_{hi}-\bar{Y}_{h})(X_{hi}-\bar{X}_{h})+\bar{R}^{2}\sum_{i}(X_{hi}-\bar{X}_{h})^{2}\right\} \\
&= \sum_{h} N_{h}(N_{h}-n_{h})n_{h}^{-1}(N_{h}-1)^{-1}\sum_{i}\{Y_{hi}-\bar{Y}_{h}-\bar{R}(X_{hi}-\bar{X}_{h})\}^{2}. \qquad (3.12)
\end{aligned}
$$

Two Cochran-consistent estimators of this approximation to $\mathrm{V}\hat{Y}_{\bullet RA}$ are

$$\sum_{h} N_{h}(N_{h}-n_{h})n_{h}^{-1}(n_{h}-1)^{-1}\sum_{i}\delta_{hi}\left\{(Y_{hi}-\hat{\bar{Y}}_{h})-\hat{\bar{R}}(X_{hi}-\hat{\bar{X}}_{h})\right\}^{2}$$

and

$$\sum_{h} N_{h}(N_{h}-n_{h})n_{h}^{-1}(n_{h}-1)^{-1}\sum_{i}\delta_{hi}\left\{(Y_{hi}-\hat{\bar{Y}}_{h})-\hat{\bar{R}}(X_{hi}-\hat{\bar{X}}_{h})\right\}^{2}X_{\bullet}^{2}\hat{X}_{\bullet}^{-2}.$$

For the reason given earlier we prefer the second. In our case, we then have

$$
\begin{aligned}
\hat{\mathrm{V}}\hat{Y}_{\bullet RA} &= N_{B}(N_{B}-n_{B})n_{B}^{-1}(n_{B}-1)^{-1} \\
&\quad \times \sum_{i}\delta_{Bi}\left\{(Y_{Bi}-\hat{\bar{Y}}_{B})-\hat{\bar{R}}(X_{Bi}-\hat{\bar{X}}_{B})\right\}^{2}X_{\bullet}^{2}\hat{X}_{\bullet}^{-2} \\
&\quad + N_{C}(N_{C}-n_{C})n_{C}^{-1}(n_{C}-1)^{-1}\sum_{i}\delta_{Ci}\left\{(Y_{Ci}-\hat{\bar{Y}}_{C})\right. \\
&\quad \left. -\hat{\bar{R}}(X_{Ci}-\hat{\bar{X}}_{C})\right\}^{2}X_{\bullet}^{2}\hat{X}_{\bullet}^{-2}
\end{aligned}
$$

$$\begin{aligned}
&\cong 287.5[\{(4675 - 3853.5) - 3841.72(0.95 - 0.775)\}^2 \\
&\quad + \{(3032 - 3853.5) - 3841.72(0.60 - 0.775)\}^2] \\
&\quad \times 49.65^2 \left\{\frac{25}{2}(0.95 + 0.60) + \frac{25}{3}(1.1 + 1.1 + 1.0)\right\}^{-2} \\
&\quad + 183.333 \times 0.5[\{(3328 - 3221.667) - 3841.72(1.1 - 1.066\,67)\}^2 \\
&\quad + \{(3427 - 3221.667) - 3841.72(1.1 - 1.066\,67)\}^2 \\
&\quad + \{(2910 - 3221.667) - 3841.72(1.0 - 1.066\,67)\}^2] \\
&\quad \times 49.65^2 \left\{\frac{25}{2}(0.95 + 0.60) + \frac{25}{3}(1.1 + 1.1 + 1.0)\right\}^{-2} \\
&\cong [287.5\{(821.5 - 672.301)^2 + (-821.5 + 672.301)^2\} \\
&\quad + 91.6667\{(106.333\,33 - 128.057\,33)^2 \\
&\quad + (205.333\,33 - 128.057\,33)^2 + (-311.666\,67 + 256.114\,67)^2\}] \\
&\quad \times 49.65^2\{19.375 + 26.6667\}^{-2} \\
&\cong [287.5\{22\,260.342 + 22\,260.342\} \\
&\quad + 91.6667\{471.932\,18 + 5971.5802 + 3086.0247\}] \\
&\quad \times (2465.1225/2119.8351) \\
&= (12\,799\,697 + 873\,541)1.162\,884\,1 \\
&= 15\,900\,391 \\
&\cong 3988^2,
\end{aligned}$$

so the standard deviation is about 4 tonnes.

This is a more considerable disappointment. We would not have expected a doubling of the standard error just by changing from stratum-by-stratum to across-stratum ratio estimation. Still, 4 tonnes is not that much more than 2% of 191 tonnes, and we know that the circus owner is most averse to weighing any more elephants. So we might still get away with it, especially if the bias is reduced considerably. That is our next concern.

The Taylor expansion approximation for the bias of $\hat{Y}_{\cdot RA}$ is

$$\begin{aligned}
\mathrm{E}(\hat{Y}_{\cdot RA} - Y_{\cdot}) &= \mathrm{E}\left(\sum_h \hat{Y}_{h\cdot} \Big/ \sum_h \hat{X}_{h\cdot}\right) X_{\cdot} - Y_{\cdot} \\
&= \mathrm{E}\left\{\left(1 + \Delta \sum_h \hat{Y}_{h\cdot}\right) Y_{\cdot} \left(1 + \Delta \sum_h \hat{X}_{h\cdot}\right)^{-1} X_{\cdot}^{-1}\right\} X_{\cdot} - Y_{\cdot}
\end{aligned}$$

$$= \mathrm{E}\left[\left\{1 + \Delta \sum_h \hat{Y}_{h\bullet}\right\}\left\{1 - \Delta \sum_h \hat{X}_{h\bullet} + \left(\Delta \sum_h \hat{X}_{h\bullet}\right)^2 - \cdots\right\}\right] Y_\bullet - Y_\bullet$$

$$\cong \mathrm{E}\left\{\left(\Delta \sum_h \hat{X}_{h\bullet}\right)^2 - \left(\Delta \sum_h \hat{Y}_{h\bullet}\right)\left(\Delta \sum_h \hat{X}_{h\bullet}\right)\right\} Y_\bullet$$

$$\cong \left\{X_\bullet^{-2}\mathrm{V}\left(\sum_h \hat{X}_{h\bullet}\right) - Y_\bullet^{-1}X_\bullet^{-1}\mathrm{C}\left(\sum_h \hat{Y}_{h\bullet}, \sum_h \hat{X}_{h\bullet}\right)\right\} Y_\bullet$$

$$= \left\{\bar{R}\mathrm{V}\left(\sum_h \hat{X}_{h\bullet}\right) - \mathrm{C}\left(\sum_h \hat{Y}_{h\bullet}, \sum_h \hat{X}_{h\bullet}\right)\right\} X_\bullet^{-1}$$

$$= \sum_h N_h(N_h - n_h)\big[(N_h - 1)^{-1} \sum_i (X_{hi} - \bar{X}_h) \times \left\{\bar{R}(X_{hi} - \bar{X}_h) - (Y_{hi} - \bar{Y}_h)\right\}\big] X_\bullet^{-1}.$$

Two Cochran-consistent estimators of this approximation to $\mathrm{E}(\hat{Y}_{\bullet RA} - Y_\bullet)$ are

$$\sum_h N_h(N_h - n_h)\left[(n_h - 1)^{-1} \sum_i \delta_{hi}(X_{hi} - \hat{\bar{X}}_h)\left\{\hat{\bar{R}}(X_{hi} - \hat{\bar{X}}_h) - (Y_{hi} - \hat{\bar{Y}}_h)\right\}\right] X_\bullet^{-1}$$

and

$$\sum_h N_h(N_h - n_h)\left[(n_h - 1)^{-1} \sum_i \delta_{hi}(X_{hi} - \hat{\bar{X}}_h) \times \left\{\hat{\bar{R}}(X_{hi} - \hat{\bar{X}}_h) - (Y_{hi} - \hat{\bar{Y}}_h)\right\}\right] \hat{X}_\bullet^{-1};$$

and, as usual, we prefer the latter.

This gives us the estimated bias of $\hat{Y}_{\bullet RA}$ as

$$N_B(N_B - n_B)n_B^{-1}\left[(n_B - 1)^{-1} \sum_i \delta_{Bi}(X_{Bi} - \hat{\bar{X}}_B) \times \left\{\hat{\bar{R}}(X_{Bi} - \hat{\bar{X}}_B) - (Y_{Bi} - \hat{\bar{Y}}_B)\right\}\right] \hat{X}_\bullet^{-1} + N_C(N_C - n_C)n_C^{-1} \times \left[(n_C - 1)^{-1} \sum_i \delta_{Ci}(X_{Ci} - \hat{\bar{X}}_C)\left\{\hat{\bar{R}}(X_{Ci} - \hat{\bar{X}}_C) - (Y_{Ci} - \hat{\bar{Y}}_C)\right\}\right] \hat{X}_\bullet^{-1}$$

$$\begin{aligned}
&\cong 287.5[(0.95 - 0.775)\{3841.72(0.95 - 0.775) - (4675 - 3853.5)\} \\
&\quad + (0.60 - 0.775)\{3841.72(0.60 - 0.775) - (3032 - 3853.5)\}]0.021\,719\,3 \\
&\quad + 183.333 \times 0.5[(1.1 - 1.066\,67)\{3841.72(1.1 - 1.066\,67) \\
&\quad - (3328 - 3221.667)\} + (1.1 - 1.066\,67)\{3841.72(1.1 - 1.066\,67) \\
&\quad - (3427 - 3221.667)\} + (1.0 - 1.066\,67)\{3841.72(1.0 - 1.066\,67) \\
&\quad - (2910 - 3221.667)\}]0.021\,719\,3 \\
&\cong 287.5[0.175\{672.3 - 821.5\} - 0.175\{-672.3 + 821.5\}]0.023\,421\,6 \\
&\quad + 183.333 \times 0.5\left[\frac{1}{30}\{128.057 - 106.333\} + \frac{1}{30}\{128.057 - 205.333\}\right. \\
&\quad \left. + \frac{-1}{15}\left\{3841.72 \times \frac{-1}{15} - (-311.667)\right\}\right]0.021\,719\,3 \\
&\cong 287.5[-26.11 - 26.11]0.021\,719\,3 \\
&\quad + 183.333 \times 0.5(0.724\,133 - 2.575\,867 - 3.703\,489)0.021\,719\,3 \\
&\cong 287.5(-52.22)0.021\,719\,3 + 91.667(-8.815\,562)0.021\,719\,3 \\
&\cong -326.1 - 17.6 \\
&\cong -343.7,
\end{aligned}$$

opposite in sign and larger in absolute terms than the estimated bias of $\hat{Y}_{\bullet R}$.

This is our fourth disappointment in four calculations, and that is quite disturbing. There is nothing in our sample to indicate that it might yield a totally misleading estimate, yet the across-stratum ratio estimator was specifically designed to make stratified ratio estimation more acceptable for small samples. The extent of the observed difference between $\hat{Y}_{\bullet RA}$ and $\hat{Y}_{\bullet R}$ and the size of the estimated standard error for $\hat{Y}_{\bullet RA}$ are particularly disturbing. Even the relatively small direct estimate of bias is suspect, because the Hartley–Ross unbiased estimator obtained by subtracting it is known to perform poorly. So just why is this across-stratum ratio estimator not performing as expected?

My colleague draws attention to the form of $\hat{Y}_{\bullet RA}$ itself. It involves three sums, $\hat{Y}_{B\bullet} + \hat{Y}_{C\bullet}$, $\hat{X}_{B\bullet} + \hat{X}_{C\bullet}$ and $X_{B\bullet} + X_{c\bullet}$. The first sum is meaningful, because $\hat{Y}_{B\bullet}$ and $\hat{Y}_{C\bullet}$ are both expressed in the same units (whether kilograms or tonnes), but what are we to make of the other two? There we are adding so many 'Sambos' to so many 'Karas', and the two have quite different weights. Although we haven't weighed them, $\hat{\hat{Y}}_{BR} = 4972$ kg is an implicit estimate of Sambo's weight, just as $\hat{\hat{Y}}_{CR} = 3020$ kg is an implicit estimate of Kara's. We might as well (my colleague suggests) be adding apples and oranges.

So we agree that across-stratum ratio estimation seems not to be appropriate when the supplementary variable values are not comparable, but why is this warning missing from the sampling textbooks? My colleague argues that the supplementary variables used in statistical offices are invariably comparable, usually in dollars, but always the same units, so they have no need to worry about this in practice. I am not so sure. 'Would you', I ask, 'use across-stratum ratio estimation over two industries if the supplementary variable was "numbers employed" and if in industry A they were all full-time permanent staff but in industry B they were predominantly part time casuals?' 'Well,' she admits, 'not now.'

We are obviously scraping the bottom of the barrel so far as the classical ratio estimator is concerned. However, the elephant trainer's supplementary information is definitely useful, and that points to ratio estimation of some kind. What we need is a form of ratio estimation that is free (or at least virtually free) from bias. Could unequal selection probabilities help? That is our next question.

Exercises

3.1 (a) Using the figures given in Appendix B, calculate the least-squares regressions of the weights Y_i on the eye estimates X_i for bulls and for cows separately, and then for all elephants.

(b) How large are the intercepts on the two axes? What does this imply for the use of ratio estimation?

3.2 Generalize Theorems 3.7.1 and 3.7.2 so as to obtain asymptotically valid approximations for the relative bias and relative variance of the ratio of any two random variables U and W.

3.3 Cochran (1977, p. 167) states that the asymptotic difference between the variances of the across-stratum and stratum-by-stratum ratio estimators 'vanishes if within each stratum the relation between Y_{hi} and X_{hi} is a straight line through the origin'.

(a) Examine Cochran's mathematical proof of this proposition and explain why it does not seem to work in **3.11**.

(b) Even without that explanation, could Cochran's proposition still fail for samples as small as two or three?

(c) What might Cochran have said instead, had he been aware of this counterexample?

3.4 One way of fixing the problem the consultants faced with across-stratum ratio estimation would be to turn the X_{Bi} into the same units as the X_{Ci} are already in, namely 'Karas'. A sample estimate of the number of 'Sambos' in a 'Kara' is the ratio (or quotient)

$$\frac{Y_5 + Y_{11}}{X_5 + X_{11}} \div \frac{Y_{24} + Y_{31} + Y_{36}}{X_{24} + X_{31} + X_{36}},$$

the first expression (or dividend) being a sample estimate of Sambo's weight and the second expression (or divisor) a sample estimate of Kara's.

(a) Use this expression to recalculate the across-stratum ratio estimate with comparable units in the auxiliary variable. Compare it with the sum of the stratum-by-stratum estimates (197 tonnes).

(b) Estimate its variance and standard error using the formula

$$\hat{V}\hat{Y}_{\bullet RA} = N_B(N_B - n_B)n_B^{-1}\left[(n_B - 1)^{-1}\sum_i \delta_{Bi} \times \left\{(Y_{Bi} - \hat{\hat{Y}}_B) - \hat{\hat{R}}(X_{Bi} - \hat{\hat{X}}_B)\right\}^2\right] X_{\bullet}^2\hat{X}_{\bullet}^{-2} + N_C(N_C - n_C)n_C^{-1} \times \left[(n_C - 1)^{-1}\sum_i \delta_{Ci}\left\{(Y_{Ci} - \hat{\hat{Y}}_C) - \hat{\hat{R}}(X_{Ci} - \hat{\hat{X}}_C)\right\}^2\right] X_{\bullet}^2\hat{X}_{\bullet}^{-2}$$

and its bias using the formula

$$N_B(N_B - n_B)n_B^{-1}\left[(n_B - 1)^{-1}\sum_i \delta_{Bi}(X_{Bi} - \hat{\hat{X}}_B) \times \left\{\hat{\hat{R}}(X_{Bi} - \hat{\hat{X}}_B) - (Y_{Bi} - \hat{\hat{Y}}_B)\right\}\right]\hat{X}_{\bullet}^{-1} + N_C(N_C - n_C)n_C^{-1} \times \left[(n_C - 1)^{-1}\sum_i \delta_{Ci}(X_{Ci} - \hat{\hat{X}}_C)\left\{\hat{\hat{R}}(X_{Ci} - \hat{\hat{X}}_C) - (Y_{Ci} - \hat{\hat{Y}}_C)\right\}\right]\hat{X}_{\bullet}^{-1}.$$

(c) Compared with the unadjusted across-stratum ratio estimator described in **3.11**, what is encouraging and/or discouraging about the performance of this adjusted estimate?

3.5 A certain mixed forest is known from an aerial photograph to contain H different species of timber-yielding tree. The number of trees belonging to each of these species, N_h $(h = 1, 2, \ldots, H)$, is also determined from the photograph, but no sample of trees is selected from the photograph, as it is known it would be very difficult to identify, on the ground, which of the trees in the forest were the ones selected in the sample.

Instead, a random sample of n trees is selected on the ground, and the species to which each of the sample trees belongs is recorded. The ith sample tree, $i = 1, 2, \ldots, n$, is thereby assigned H indicator variables, Δ_{hi}, where $\Delta_{hi} = 1$ if that tree belongs to species h but $\Delta_{hi} = 0$ otherwise. A timber expert also makes an assessment of the quantity of usable timber, T_i, measured in cubic metres, that would be available from that ith sample tree. The sample data thus consist of n records of observations, and each of these records in turn consists of the identifier i, the H indicator variables Δ_{hi}, and T_i.

(a) Write down a formula for $\hat{T}_{h\bullet}$, the poststratified estimator of $T_{h\bullet}$ (the total available timber from species h) based on the knowledge of N_h, the n values of Δ_{hi}, and the n values of T_i.

(b) Show that this poststratified estimator, for species h, has the same form as the classical ratio estimator, $\hat{Y}_{\bullet R} = \left(\sum_{i=1}^{N} \delta_i X_i\right)^{-1}\left(\sum_{i=1}^{N} \delta_i Y_i\right)X_{\bullet}$.

What symbols, in this particular application, correspond to $\hat{Y}_{\bullet R}$, Y_i, $\sum_{i=1}^{N} \delta_i Y_i$, X_i, $\sum_{i=1}^{N} \delta_i X_i$ and $X_{\bullet}$?

(c) Use the standard randomization-based variance approximation for the classical ratio estimator $\mathrm{V}\hat{Y}_{\bullet R} \cong N(N-n)n^{-1}(N-1)^{-1}\sum_i (Y_i - \bar{R}X_i)^2$, where $\bar{R} = Y_{\bullet}/X_{\bullet}$, to construct an expression for an approximation to the randomization-based variance of the poststratification estimator arrived at in (a). Also, use the randomization-based variance estimator for the classical ratio estimator, $N(N-n)n^{-1}X_{\bullet}^2\hat{X}_{\bullet}^{-2}(n-1)^{-1}\sum_i \delta_i(Y_i - \bar{R}X_i)^2$, to construct an estimator of that poststratification estimator's variance.

4

Ratio Estimators for Unequal Probability Samples

Facing the Dilemma 60
The Lahiri–Midzuno Unbiased Ratio Estimator 60
The Horvitz–Thompson and Hansen–Hurwitz Estimators of Total 63
Poisson Sampling 74
Exercises 79

Facing the Dilemma

4.1 As a result of the events described in Chapter 3, we are faced with a difficult choice. On the one hand, the separate stratum ratio estimates, $\hat{Y}_{B\bullet R}$ and $\hat{Y}_{C\bullet R}$, look very convincing; their sum, $\hat{Y}_{\bullet R}$, has an estimated variance well within the limit of accuracy specified by the circus owner, and its estimated bias is small compared with its estimated variance. The only reason for not using it is that it violates generally recognized canons of acceptability. It is based on one sample of size 2 and one of size 3 (neither of which is anywhere near the minimum of 30 suggested by Cochran or even the minimum of 6 long used, but even then only in the context of a highly stratified sample, by the Australian Bureau of Statistics). It also fails to meet Cochran's other criterion, that the coefficients of variation of $\hat{\hat{X}}_B$ and $\hat{\hat{Y}}_B$ should be less than 0.1. (For the record, those of $\hat{\hat{X}}_C$ and $\hat{\hat{Y}}_C$ *do* meet that criterion, but partial fulfilment is not *ful*filment.)

On the other hand, the point estimate of total obtained from the across-stratum ratio estimator, $\hat{Y}_{\bullet RA}$, which was specially devised for use with small samples, is three estimated standard deviations of $\hat{Y}_{\bullet R}$ below $\hat{Y}_{\bullet R}$ itself, its estimated variance is four times as large as that of $\hat{Y}_{\bullet R}$, and its estimated bias, which we had reason to expect to be substantially smaller than that of $\hat{Y}_{\bullet R}$, actually exceeds it slightly. We do not trust $\hat{Y}_{\bullet RA}$ and would be unwilling to foist it on our client (even if we thought we could get away with it), but we are even more reluctant to face the criticism of our fellow survey statisticians if we base our report on $\hat{Y}_{\bullet R}$. Can we find a way through this dilemma?

The Lahiri–Midzuno Unbiased Ratio Estimator

4.2 We examine our armoury. The eye estimates supplied by the elephant trainer are clearly useful, and their nature strongly implies that we should use some kind of ratio estimation. Is there some third estimator that could rid us of our worry about bias? My colleague remembers reading about the Lahiri–Midzuno unbiased ratio estimator (Lahiri, 1951; Midzuno, 1952; Cochran, 1977, pp. 175–178). If our whole sample had been selected with probability proportional to the *sample sum* or *sample take* of the supplementary variable, that is $\sum_i \delta_{Bi} X_{Bi}$ for the bulls and $\sum_i \delta_{Ci} X_{Ci}$ for the cows, then our separate stratum ratio estimates would have been design-unbiased. We can see this by considering a single stratum. Denoting by $s \in S$ the sample s within the complete set of samples S,

$$
\begin{aligned}
\mathrm{E}\left\{\frac{\hat{Y}_{\bullet}}{\hat{X}_{\bullet}}\right\} X_{\bullet} &= \sum_{s \in S}\left[\Pr(s)\left\{\frac{\hat{Y}_{\bullet}(s)}{\hat{X}_{\bullet}(s)}\right\}\right] X_{\bullet} \\
&= \sum_{s \in S}\left[\frac{\sum_{i \in s} \delta_i X_i}{\sum_{t \in S}\sum_{i \in t} \delta_i X_i} \frac{(N/n)\sum_{i \in s} \delta_i Y_i}{(N/n)\sum_{i \in s} \delta_i X_i} X_{\bullet}\right] \\
&= \frac{\sum_{s \in S}\sum_{i \in s} \delta_i Y_i}{\sum_{s \in S}\sum_{i \in s} \delta_i X_i} X_{\bullet} \\
&= \frac{Y_{\bullet}}{X_{\bullet}} X_{\bullet} = Y_{\bullet}.
\end{aligned} \tag{4.1}
$$

So if only we had selected our sample that way, our estimator $\hat{Y}_{\bullet R}$ would actually have been unbiased! My reaction is 'What a pity we didn't select it that way', but my colleague is way ahead of me. 'Wait, we might very well be able to,' she says. 'Have you forgotten the Keyfitz technique?'

'Remind me', I say, not exactly lying, for the name does ring a faint bell somewhere.

'All in good time,' she promises. 'First let me tell you what Midzuno did with Lahiri's idea.'

Midzuno's (1952) contribution was this. A sample can be selected with probability proportional to the sum of the sample x_i if the first draw is made with probabilities proportional to the x_i and all the others with equal probabilities without replacement. The probability of selecting the entire sample is equal to the probability of selecting the sample unit with the smallest value of i first (and the remainder with equal probabilities), plus the probability of selecting the unit with the next smallest value of i first (and the remainder with equal probabilities), and so on. Each of these n possible ways of selecting the achieved sample has a probability proportional to the x_i of the first selected unit, so the total probability of selection of that sample is proportional to the sample sum of those x_i.

'Neat', I admit, but doubtfully, not quite sure how this will actually help.

My colleague, however, continues in full swing with her description of the Keyfitz technique (Keyfitz, 1951). Consider the cows' stratum first. Using Midzuno's specification of the problem, the probability of selecting Linda, Pamela and Sara required for $\hat{Y}_{\bullet R}$ to be design-unbiased must be

$$
\frac{1.1 + 1.1 + 1.0}{25.3} \times \frac{2}{24} \times \frac{1}{23} = \frac{1}{2182.125}.
$$

The original probability of selection of that sample is simply the prior probability that any sample of five selected from 50 elephants would include a specified three. This is

$$\binom{3}{3}\binom{47}{2}\binom{50}{5}^{-1} = \frac{1}{1960}.$$

So we have a sample chosen with probability 1/1960, and we need that same sample, but chosen with probability 1/2182.125. We therefore need to choose a random number from 0 and to 2182.125, and if it lies in the range 0 to 1960, then we retain our sample.

This is almost equivalent to drawing an integer between 1 and 10 000, and accepting the sample if it lies in the range between 1 and 8982. Holding our breath, we make our random selection. The four-digit random number is 0236, very safely within our required range, so the original sample of cows is retained.

We now turn to the bulls' stratum. The required inclusion probability of Combo and Flimbo together is

$$\frac{0.95 + 0.60}{24.35} \times \frac{1}{24} = \frac{1}{377.032\,26}.$$

The original selection probability of any two specified elephants was

$$\binom{2}{2}\binom{48}{3}\binom{50}{5}^{-1} = \frac{2}{245} = \frac{1}{122.5}.$$

This time we prepare to make a random choice of an integer between 1 and 10 000 and hope that it will lie in the range between 1 and 3249. This is a much riskier proposition. My colleague suggests that we switch the random numbers and apply the 0236 to the bulls' stratum, but I can remember what the next random number was going to be, so I can afford to be scrupulous without fear as to the outcome. No, I insist, that would be cheating. And, of course, the next random number is 3015, just within our range. We have made the necessary reselection, but I wonder uncomfortably what I would have done if I had not noticed what the next four-digit number in the table had been. Would I really have been so fastidious, and, if not, what was the real probability with which we had reselected Combo and Flimbo?

But at this juncture, it is easy to put my misgivings to one side. The next random number was in fact 3015 and I did not in fact cheat, so what is wrong with the proposition that Combo and Flimbo have been selected with the required probability? Result: we now have our original ratio estimate of $121 + 76 = 197$ tonnes in total, and it is without bias. So far, so good.

Next question: how do we estimate the variance? At this point my colleague looks rather embarrassed. It turns out that while for large samples the Lahiri ratio estimator has the same approximate variance as the classical ratio estimator, Cochran (1963, p. 178) indicates that no exact expression for its variance had then been found, and Cochran (1977) says nothing about it at all. And, of course, our samples of bulls and cows are both extremely small. We now have a biased estimator with a small estimated variance that is identical in form with an unbiased estimator of unknown variance. We also have a strong intuition that the two have very similar variances, but nothing conclusive.

A literature search is evidently called for, and we find that the definitive paper on this is Rao and Vijayan (1977). Alas, both their variance estimators involve complex calculations, and both are capable of producing negative estimates of variance, the simpler one more often than the more complicated alternative. We decide to put these options on the back-burner and return to them only if we have no other alternative.

So where do we turn next? We have already considered and rejected the Hartley–Ross estimator. Mickey's (1959) estimator is very similar to it, and identical for samples of size 2. We do not have large enough samples to use a meaningful jackknife for the estimation of variance (Quenouille, 1956; Tukey, 1958; Shao and Tu, 1995). Perhaps we should consider the circumstances in which the average of ratios estimator, $\hat{Y}_{\bullet AR}$, is unbiased?

The Horvitz–Thompson and Hansen–Hurwitz Estimators of Total

4.3 Early in Chapter 3 we found that the average of ratios estimator was initially plausible; however, it was design-biased under *srswor* and not even Cochran consistent. We can, however, eliminate the design bias if we give each unit an inclusion probability proportional to its supplementary variable value x_j and select without replacement. When used with this selection scheme the average of ratios estimator is also the famous Horvitz–Thompson (or HT) estimator of total (Horvitz and Thompson, 1952). It is easily seen to be design-unbiased, for

$$\begin{aligned}
\mathrm{E}\hat{Y}_{\bullet HT} &= \left\{ n^{-1}\mathrm{E}\sum_i \delta_i \left(\frac{Y_i}{X_i}\right)\right\} X_{\bullet} \\
&= n^{-1}\sum_i \left\{\frac{Y_i}{X_i}\frac{nX_i}{X_{\bullet}}\right\} X_{\bullet} \\
&= \sum_i Y_i = Y_{\bullet}. \qquad (4.2)
\end{aligned}$$

This time we apply the Keyfitz reselection technique unit by unit. Linda and Pamela are cow elephants of above average size and their new inclusion probabilities (both 3.3/25.3 or 0.1304) are greater than their old ones, so they are reselected with certainty. Sara, as it turns out, is also in this category, not because she is above average in size, but because we had only expected to select 2.5 cow elephants originally out of 50, and now we want three out of 25. Her original inclusion probability (like all the others') was 5/50 or 0.10. Since there are three cow elephants to be selected with probability proportional to size her new inclusion probability is 3 times her size measure divided by the sum of the cows' size measures, that is, $3 \times 1.0/25.3$ or 0.1186. This is greater than 0.1, so she also is reselected with certainty.

Reselecting the two sample bulls, however, is going to be a risky business. Combo is the better of the two bets. His original inclusion probability was 0.10. His new one is twice 0.95/24.35 or 0.0780. We therefore have a probability of 0.0780/0.10 or 0.78 of retaining Combo. We only need a two-digit random integer on this occasion. It is 64, which is in the range from 1 to 78, so Combo is also reselected. Flimbo, however, has a new inclusion probability that is only twice 0.6/24.35 or 0.0493. Our probability of reselecting Flimbo is therefore only 0.493. Our next three-digit random number is (oh dear!) 622. Sadly, we will have to do without Flimbo, but at least we still have Combo to represent the bulls.

The estimation of total seems easy enough. Our HT estimate for the cows' stratum is the same as the average of ratios estimate that we calculated in **3.3**: 76 322 kg. For the bulls we now have an inclusion probability for Combo of 0.078, but if we apply the standard HT formula, $\hat{Y}_{.HT} = \sum_i \delta_i (Y_i/\pi_i)$, where π_i is the inclusion probability for the ith unit, we get the estimate 4675/0.0780 or 59 936 kg. This is only about half of what it should be. What has gone wrong?

4.4 My colleague has met this kind of situation before. She tells me that by selecting unit by unit we have made our sample size a random variable with an expectation (in this case) of $0.780 + 0.493$ or 1.273 units. The effective selection probability for Combo was indeed 0.078 and the HT estimator of total 59 936 kg, but it is common in such cases to make a multiplicative adjustment which in this case would be the ratio of the expected sample size to the actual sample size, or 1.273 (divided by 1). That adjusts it up to 76 299 kg, but this is still well below the 120 tonnes or so that we know to be appropriate. We wonder about this and decide that the real factor we should be using is 2, but are at a loss to justify it until we remember that Keyfitz's retention technique required us to replace any unit that is not retained by another unit selected randomly from the rest of the stratum (in this case, the non-sample bulls). We know this is impossible; so is there anything else can we do instead?

Our first thought is that we have not applied the Keyfitz procedure in its completeness. Having failed to reselect Flimbo, we should now select another bull in his place, with probability proportional to size. Although that is impossible for us, we still have Combo. The initial selections of Flimbo and Combo were very nearly independent, so the 'event' that Combo is the only other bull that can be selected is also a very nearly independent event and it also has nearly the right probability. In our exigency, could we not reasonably say that Combo was selected to be Flimbo's replacement? It would certainly be in the spirit of the Keyfitz sample retention technique. It is true that we would then be selecting with replacement rather than without replacement, but sampling with replacement is not unusual when selecting with unequal probabilities. And frankly, what else can we do but double up on Combo in some *ad hoc* fashion? The Keyfitz technique does provide us with a rationale of some sort.

4.5 So we now proceed on the basis that we have selected with replacement and have selected Combo twice. The appropriate estimator, due to Hansen and Hurwitz (1943), has almost the same form as the HT estimator. Using some of the same notation as was introduced for *srswr* in Chapter 1, we have

$$\hat{Y}_{\bullet HH} = n^{-1} \sum_i \nu_i \left(\frac{Y_i}{P_i} \right), \tag{4.3}$$

where ν_i is the number of times the ith unit is selected and P_i is the probability of its selection at a single draw. To prove the design unbiasedness of $\hat{Y}_{\bullet HH}$ if units are selected with probability proportional to size with replacement (*ppswr*) we require the following lemma.

Lemma 4.5.1 Under *ppswr*, $\mathrm{E}\nu_i = nP_i$ for all $i = 1, 2, \ldots, N$.

Proof. Under *ppswr* the n draws are conducted independently. So the expected number of appearances of the ith population unit in sample, $\mathrm{E}\nu_i$, is the sum of the probabilities of selection of that unit in sample over the n draws. But the contribution of each draw to the expected number of appearances of that unit in sample is P_i. Hence $\mathrm{E}\nu_i = nP_i$ for all $i = 1, 2, \ldots, N$. ◇

Theorem 4.5.1 Under *ppswr*, the Hansen–Hurwitz (HH) estimator is a design-unbiased estimator of total.

Proof.

$$\begin{aligned}
\mathrm{E}\hat{Y}_{\bullet HH} &= n^{-1}\mathrm{E} \sum_i \nu_i \left(\frac{Y_i}{P_i} \right) \\
&= n^{-1} \sum_i \mathrm{E}\nu_i \left(\frac{Y_i}{P_i} \right) \\
&= n^{-1} \sum_i nP_i \left(\frac{Y_i}{P_i} \right) \\
&= \sum_i Y_i \\
&= Y_{\bullet}.
\end{aligned}$$

◇

Our HH estimate for the bulls' stratum in this situation is

$$\begin{aligned}
\hat{Y}_{\bullet BHH} &= \frac{1}{2} \times 2 \times \frac{4675}{0.0390} \\
&= 119\,872\,\mathrm{kg},
\end{aligned}$$

or nearly 120 tonnes. The sum for the two strata is once again the 197 tonnes we had already obtained three times over. And this time we are (at least arguably!) free from bias.

4.6 But variance estimation is not exactly straightforward, either for cows or bulls. The bulls were selected under *ppswr* and their totals were estimated using the HH estimator. For this situation we need the following theory.

Lemma 4.6.1 Under *ppswr*, $\mathrm{V}\nu_i = nP_i(1 - P_i)$ for all $i = 1, 2, \ldots, N$.

Proof. Under *ppswr* the n draws are identical and conducted independently. So $\mathrm{V}\nu_i$ is the sum over the n draws of the variances of the event that the ith unit is selected at a single draw. But that event has outcome unity with probability P_i and zero with probability $1 - P_i$, so its variance at every draw is $P_i(1 - P_i)$. Hence $\mathrm{V}\nu_i = nP_i(1 - P_i)$ for all $i = 1, 2, \ldots, N$. ◇

From Lemmas 4.5.1 and 4.6.1 we immediately obtain the following result:

Corollary 4.6.1 Under *ppswr*, $\mathrm{E}\nu_i^2 \equiv (\mathrm{E}\nu_i)^2 + \mathrm{V}\nu_i = n^2P_i^2 + nP_i(1 - P_i)$. ◇

From there we can proceed to:

Theorem 4.6.1 Under *ppswr*, the variance of the HH estimator, $\hat{Y}_{\bullet HH} = n^{-1}\sum_i \nu_i Y_i P_i^{-1}$, is

$$\mathrm{V}\hat{Y}_{\bullet HH} \equiv \mathrm{E}(\hat{Y}_{\bullet HH} - Y_{\bullet})^2 = n^{-1}\sum_i P_i\{Y_iP_i^{-1} - Y_{\bullet}\}^2. \tag{4.4}$$

Proof. Given a sample of a single unit, say unit i, the HH estimator is $Y_iP_i^{-1}$ and its variance is $\mathrm{E}(Y_iP_i^{-1} - Y_{\bullet})^2 = \sum_i P_i(Y_iP_i^{-1} - Y_{\bullet})^2$. But the n draws are conducted independently, so the variance of the HH estimator in general, which is the mean of the $Y_iP_i^{-1}$ over n independent draws, is n^{-1} times the variance for a single draw. Hence $\mathrm{V}\hat{Y}_{\bullet HH} \equiv \mathrm{E}(\hat{Y}_{\bullet HH} - Y_{\bullet})^2 = n^{-1}\sum_i P_i\{Y_iP_i^{-1} - Y_{\bullet}\}^2$. ◇

We next need to find a design-unbiased estimator for $\mathrm{V}\hat{Y}_{\bullet HH}$. We can do this using either the notation with which we are familiar, but which is rather awkward to use when sampling is with replacement, or another notation (described in **1.6**) in which y_i is the value for the sample unit selected at the ith draw and, correspondingly, p_i is the probability with which whatever population unit was *in fact selected* as the ith sample unit *could have been selected* at each and every draw. That makes the proof simpler, but because the notation is unfamiliar we will present the more complicated proof first. For that we will require $\mathrm{E}\nu_i = nP_i$ from Lemma 4.5.1, $\mathrm{E}\nu_i^2 = n^2P_i^2 + nP_i(1 - P_i)$ from Corollary 4.6.1, and finally an expression for $\mathrm{E}_{j\neq i}\nu_i\nu_j$ from the following lemma.

Lemma 4.6.2 $\mathrm{E}_{j\neq i}\nu_i\nu_j = n(n - 1)P_iP_j$.

Proof. $\mathrm{E}_{j \neq i}\nu_i\nu_j = \mathrm{E}\nu_i\mathrm{E}_{j \neq i}\nu_j = nP_i\mathrm{E}_{j \neq i}\nu_j$. But if the ith unit is already in sample, there are only $n-1$ draws remaining at which the jth unit can be selected. Hence $\mathrm{E}_{j \neq i}\nu_j = (n-1)P_j$ and $\mathrm{E}_{j \neq i}\nu_i\nu_j = n(n-1)P_iP_j$. ◇

(Note that more rigorous but lengthier proofs exist for all three of these expressions.) We may now proceed with

Theorem 4.6.2 The estimator

$$\hat{\mathrm{V}}\hat{Y}_{\bullet HH} = n^{-1}(n-1)^{-1}\sum_i \nu_i(Y_iP_i^{-1} - \hat{Y}_{\bullet HH})^2 \tag{4.5}$$

is design-unbiased for $\mathrm{V}\hat{Y}_{\bullet HH}$.

First proof.

$$\begin{aligned}
n(n-1)\mathrm{E}\hat{\mathrm{V}}\hat{Y}_{\bullet HH} &= \mathrm{E}\sum_i \nu_i\{Y_iP_i^{-1} - \hat{Y}_{\bullet HH}\}^2 \\
&= \mathrm{E}\sum_i \nu_i\{(Y_iP_i^{-1} - Y_\bullet) - (\hat{Y}_{\bullet HH} - Y_\bullet)\}^2 \\
&= \mathrm{E}\sum_i \nu_i\{(Y_iP_i^{-1} - Y_\bullet)^2 \\
&\quad - 2(Y_iP_i^{-1} - Y_\bullet)(\hat{Y}_{\bullet HH} - Y_\bullet) + (\hat{Y}_{\bullet HH} - Y_\bullet)^2\} \\
&= \sum_i \{(\mathrm{E}\nu_i)(Y_iP_i^{-1} - Y_\bullet)^2\} \\
&\quad - 2\sum_i \{(\mathrm{E}\nu_i^2)(Y_iP_i^{-1} - Y_\bullet)n^{-1}(Y_iP_i^{-1} - Y_\bullet)\} \\
&\quad - 2\sum_i\sum_{j \neq i} \{(\mathrm{E}_{j \neq i}\nu_i\nu_j)(Y_iP_i^{-1} - Y_\bullet)(Y_jP_j^{-1} - Y_\bullet)\} \\
&\quad + \left(\mathrm{E}\sum_i \nu_i\right)\mathrm{V}\hat{Y}_{\bullet HH}.
\end{aligned}$$

At this point we invoke the earlier results $\mathrm{E}\nu_i = nP_i$, $\mathrm{E}\nu_i^2 = n^2P_i^2 + nP_i(1-P_i)$ and $\mathrm{E}_{j \neq i}\nu_i\nu_j = n(n-1)P_iP_j$ and continue with

$$\begin{aligned}
n(n-1)\mathrm{E}\hat{\mathrm{V}}\hat{Y}_{\bullet HH} &= \sum_i \{nP_i(Y_iP_i^{-1} - Y_\bullet)^2\} \\
&\quad - 2\sum_i n^{-1}\{n(n-1)P_i^2 + nP_i\}(Y_iP_i^{-1} - Y_\bullet)^2
\end{aligned}$$

$$- 2n^{-1}\sum_i\sum_{j\neq i}\{n(n-1)P_iP_j(Y_iP_i^{-1}-Y_\bullet)(Y_jP_j^{-1}-Y_\bullet)\} + n\mathrm{V}\hat{Y}_{\bullet HH}$$

$$= n.n\mathrm{V}\hat{Y}_{\bullet HH} - 2(n-1)\sum_i P_i^2(Y_iP_i^{-1}-Y_\bullet)^2 - 2\sum_i P_i(Y_iP_i^{-1}-Y_\bullet)^2$$

$$- 2(n-1)\left\{\sum_i P_i(Y_iP_i^{-1}-Y_\bullet)\right\}\left\{\sum_j P_j(Y_jP_j^{-1}-Y_\bullet)\right\}$$

$$+ 2(n-1)\sum_i P_i^2(Y_iP_i^{-1}-Y_\bullet)^2 + n\mathrm{V}\hat{Y}_{\bullet HH}$$

$$= n^2\mathrm{V}\hat{Y}_{\bullet HH} - 2(n-1)\sum_i P_i^2(Y_iP_i^{-1}-Y_\bullet)^2 - 2n\mathrm{V}\hat{Y}_{\bullet HH} - 0$$

$$+ 2(n-1)\sum_i P_i^2(Y_iP_i^{-1}-Y_\bullet)^2 + n\mathrm{V}\hat{Y}_{\bullet HH}$$

$$= n(n-1)\mathrm{V}\hat{Y}_{\bullet HH}.$$

Hence $\mathrm{E}\hat{\mathrm{V}}\hat{Y}_{\bullet HH} = \mathrm{V}\hat{Y}_{\bullet HH}$. ◇

Second proof. This proof uses the alternative notation described in **1.6**. Note that if a particular population unit, say the kth, happens to be selected at both the ith and the jth draw, then $p_i = p_j = P_k$.

The proof itself commences with a transition from the old to the new notation:

$$n(n-1)\mathrm{E}\hat{\mathrm{V}}\hat{Y}_{\bullet HH} = \mathrm{E}\sum_i \nu_i(Y_iP_i^{-1} - \hat{Y}_{\bullet HH})^2$$

$$= \mathrm{E}\sum_{i=1}^n (y_ip_i^{-1} - \hat{Y}_{\bullet HH})^2$$

$$= \mathrm{E}\sum_{i=1}^n \left\{(y_ip_i^{-1} - Y_\bullet) - (\hat{Y}_{\bullet HH} - Y_\bullet)\right\}^2$$

$$= \sum_{i=1}^n \left[\mathrm{E}(y_ip_i^{-1} - Y_\bullet)^2 - 2\mathrm{E}\left\{(y_ip_i^{-1} - Y_\bullet)(\hat{Y}_{\bullet HH} - Y_\bullet)\right\}\right.$$

$$\left. + \mathrm{E}(\hat{Y}_{\bullet HH} - Y_\bullet)^2\right]$$

$$= n\left[\mathrm{E}(y_ip_i^{-1} - Y_\bullet)^2 - 2\mathrm{E}\left\{(y_ip_i^{-1} - Y_\bullet)(\hat{Y}_{\bullet HH} - Y_\bullet)\right\}\right.$$

$$\left. + \mathrm{E}(\hat{Y}_{\bullet HH} - Y_\bullet)^2\right]$$

$$= n^2\mathrm{V}\hat{Y}_{.HH} - 2n\mathrm{E}\sum_{i=1}^{n}\{(y_ip_i^{-1} - Y_.)n^{-1}(y_ip_i^{-1} - Y_.)\}$$

$$- 2n\mathrm{E}\left[\sum_{i=1}^{n}(y_ip_i^{-1} - Y_.)n^{-1}\left\{\sum_{j(\neq i)=1}^{n} y_jp_j^{-1} - (n-1)Y_.\right\}\right] + n\mathrm{V}\hat{Y}_{.HH}.$$

But the n draws are made independently, so $\mathrm{E}\{(y_ip_i^{-1} - Y_.)(y_jp_j^{-1} - Y_.)\} = 0$ for all $j \neq i$. Hence

$$\mathrm{E}\hat{\mathrm{V}}\hat{Y}_{.HH} = n^{-1}(n-1)^{-1}\mathrm{V}\hat{Y}_{.HH}n(n-2-0+1) = \mathrm{V}\hat{Y}_{.HH}. \qquad \diamond$$

Despite the availability of this simple estimator, we still have a problem with the bulls' stratum. Our only value of Y_{Bi}/P_{Bi} is identical with $\hat{Y}_{B\bullet HH}$, so our estimate of variance is zero. This always happens when the same population unit is selected at each draw. The variance estimator is technically unbiased, because its formula ensures that over all possible samples of n (two in this case) the expectation is precisely $\mathrm{V}\hat{Y}_{B\bullet HH}$, but what this means in practice is that the average over all the samples consisting of two *distinct* units must be *larger* than $\mathrm{V}\hat{Y}_{B\bullet HH}$, to compensate for its being zero when they are not distinct. However unbiased the estimator is, our present zero estimate understates the true variance and we had better do something about it, as we did when Combo was the only selected elephant from the then truncated bulls' stratum back in Chapter 2.

Then we based our imputation on our experience with the cows' stratum. But now the cows present their own problem. We selected them without replacement and used the HT estimator, $\hat{Y}_{.HT} = \sum_i \delta_i(Y_i/\pi_i)$. That was fine for estimating the total, but it is not easy to estimate the variance of that estimator.

Theorem 4.6.3 The variance of the HT estimator is

$$\mathrm{V}\hat{Y}_{.HT} \equiv \mathrm{E}(\hat{Y}_{.HT} - Y_.)^2 = \sum_{i=1}^{N} Y_i^2(1-\pi_i)\pi_i^{-1}$$

$$+\sum_{i=1}^{N}\sum_{j\neq i}^{N}(\pi_{ij} - \pi_i\pi_j)Y_i\pi_i^{-1}Y_j\pi_j^{-1}, \qquad (4.6)$$

where $\pi_{ij} \equiv \mathrm{E}(\delta_i\delta_j)$ (Horvitz and Thompson, 1952), regardless of whether the sample size is fixed or random.

Proof. For any selection scheme in which the units are selected without replacement and their inclusion probabilities are proportional to size ($\pi pswor$) the variance of the HT estimator is

$$\begin{aligned}
\mathrm{V}\hat{Y}_{\bullet HT} &\equiv \mathrm{E}(\hat{Y}_{\bullet HT} - Y_{\bullet})^2 \\
&= \mathrm{E}\left(\sum_i \delta_i Y_i \pi_i^{-1} - Y_{\bullet}\right)^2 \\
&= \mathrm{E}\left\{\left(\sum_i \delta_i Y_i \pi_i^{-1}\right)\left(\sum_j \delta_j Y_j \pi_j^{-1}\right)\right\} - 2Y_{\bullet}\mathrm{E}\left(\sum_i \delta_i Y_i \pi_i^{-1}\right) + Y_{\bullet}^2 \\
&= \mathrm{E}\left\{\sum_i \delta_i^2 Y_i^2 \pi_i^{-2} + \sum_i \sum_{j \neq i} \delta_i \delta_j Y_i \pi_i^{-1} Y_j \pi_j^{-1}\right\} \\
&\quad - 2Y_{\bullet}\mathrm{E}\left(\sum_i \delta_i Y_i \pi_i^{-1}\right) + Y_{\bullet}^2 \\
&= \sum_{i=1}^{N} Y_i^2 \pi_i^{-1} + \sum_{i=1}^{N} \sum_{j \neq i}^{N} \pi_{ij} Y_i \pi_i^{-1} Y_j \pi_j^{-1} - Y_{\bullet}^2, \qquad \text{since } \pi_{ij} \equiv \mathrm{E}(\delta_i \delta_j), \\
&= \sum_{i=1}^{N} Y_i^2 (1 - \pi_i) \pi_i^{-1} + \sum_{i=1}^{N} \sum_{j \neq i}^{N} (\pi_{ij} - \pi_i \pi_j) Y_i \pi_i^{-1} Y_j \pi_j^{-1}. \qquad \diamond
\end{aligned}$$

Horvitz and Thompson suggested using the obvious estimator of this, which was $\hat{\mathrm{V}}_{HT}\hat{Y}_{\bullet HT} = \sum_{i=1}^{N} \delta_i Y_i^2 (1 - \pi_i) \pi_i^{-2} + \sum_{i=1}^{N} \sum_{j(\neq i)=1}^{N} \delta_i \delta_j Y_i Y_j \pi_{ij}^{-1} (\pi_{ij} - \pi_i \pi_j) \pi_i^{-1} \pi_j^{-1}$, but for samples with fixed n this was soon found to be inefficient.

The results in the following lemma are useful for considering samples of fixed size.

Lemma 4.6.2 For a sample of fixed size n units:

$$\sum_{j(\neq i)=1}^{N} \pi_{ij} = (n-1)\pi_i; \tag{4.7a}$$

$$\sum_{i=1}^{N} \sum_{j(\neq i)=1}^{N} \pi_{ij} = n(n-1); \tag{4.7b}$$

$$\sum_{j(\neq i)=1}^{N} \pi_i \pi_j = \pi_i (n - \pi_i); \tag{4.7c}$$

$$\sum_{i=1}^{N} \sum_{j(\neq i)=1}^{N} \pi_i \pi_j = n^2 - \sum_{i=1}^{N} \pi_i^2. \tag{4.7d}$$

The proofs of these four results are straightforward.

Theorem 4.6.4 For a sample of fixed size n units, the variance of the HT estimator is (Sen, 1953; Yates and Grundy, 1953):

$$\mathrm{V}\hat{Y}_{\bullet HT} = \sum_{i=1}^{N} \sum_{j(<i)=1}^{N-1} (\pi_i \pi_j - \pi_{ij}) \left(Y_i \pi_i^{-1} - Y_j \pi_j^{-1} \right)^2 . \tag{4.8}$$

Proof. It is straightforward to show, using $\sum_{j=1}^{N} \pi_j = n$, that

$$\sum_{i=1}^{N} \sum_{j=1}^{N} \pi_i \pi_j \left(Y_i \pi_i^{-1} - Y_j \pi_j^{-1} \right)^2 = 2n \sum_{i=1}^{N} Y_i^2 \pi_i^{-1} - 2Y_{\bullet}^2, \tag{4.9}$$

and, using (4.7a), that

$$\sum_{i=1}^{N} \sum_{j(\neq i)=1}^{N} \pi_{ij} \left(Y_i \pi_i^{-1} - Y_j \pi_j^{-1} \right)^2 = 2(n-1) \sum_{i=1}^{N} Y_i^2 \pi_i^{-1}$$
$$- 2 \sum_{i=1}^{N} \sum_{j(\neq i)=1}^{N} \pi_{ij} Y_i \pi_i^{-1} Y_j \pi_j^{-1}. \tag{4.10}$$

Subtracting (4.10) from (4.9), and noting that since $\pi_{ij} = \pi_{ji}$ the sums over $j(\neq i) = 1$ to N are twice the sums over $j(<i) = 1$ to $N-1$, (4.8) follows. ◇

Corollary 4.6.2 The corresponding Sen–Yates–Grundy variance estimator,

$$\hat{\mathrm{V}}_{SYG} \hat{Y}_{\bullet HT} = \sum_{i=1}^{N} \sum_{j(<i)=1}^{N-1} \delta_i \delta_j \pi_{ij}^{-1} (\pi_i \pi_j - \pi_{ij}) \left(Y_i \pi_i^{-1} - Y_j \pi_j^{-1} \right)^2 , \tag{4.11}$$

is unbiased for $\mathrm{V}\hat{Y}_{\bullet HT}$. ◇

4.7 All these formulae, however, involve the joint inclusion probabilities π_{ij}. Our problem is, what are the π_{ij} in our case? Initially we think of assuming that the three selections were nearly enough independent and therefore that $\pi_{ij} \cong \pi_i \pi_j$. However, this is not an appropriate description of what we have used here because, given this specification, the probability of selecting the ith unit twice is $\pi_i^2 > 0$, so the selection cannot be without replacement. And once we reject that assumption, the extents of the actual differences between π_{ij} and $\pi_i \pi_j$ for every pair $\{i, j\}$ in sample for which i and j are distinct become critically important for the estimation of variance and must be known reasonably accurately.

Moreover, as soon as we try to evaluate these π_{ij}, we hit real trouble. If we had selected Linda, Pamela and Sara with probabilities proportional to size without replacement in the first instance, we might have found calculation of the π_{ij} awkward or tedious, but, given the precise method of selection used, it could be done. However, we initially selected with equal probabilities without replacement from the bulls and cows combined. In the event, we selected two bulls and three cows. Subsequently, we used the Keyfitz sample retention technique to reselect each of them with probability proportional to size. During the application of that technique we changed from using unconditional inclusion probabilities of five in 50 (or one in 10) to probabilities of 3.3/25.3, 3.3/25.3 and 3.0/25.3 respectively, which were conditional on the selection of three cows. What meaning could be ascribed to a π_{ij} calculated partly on the basis of unconditional and partly on the basis of conditional probabilities? Should we go back and repeat the application of the Keyfitz sample retention technique using conditional probabilities throughout? That is a possibility, but by this time we are very sensitive to the way in which random numbers can retain or reject elephants that we know we are going to have to retain if we are going to have any chance of meeting the circus owner's criterion of acceptable accuracy. We have the weights of those five elephants, we are going to have to use them; is there really no way in which we can justify this?

4.8 We agree to think about this independently for a while. After half an hour or so, my colleague comes up with a suggestion. First, we abandon the idea of selection with unequal probabilities without replacement. That is just too demanding when it comes to variance estimation. Selection with replacement is far easier to handle. We can treat the three sample cows as having been reselected with probabilities proportional to size with replacement and use the HH estimator. (For the bulls, she has an even more ingenious idea, but we will come to that later.) Our HH estimate is

$$\begin{aligned}
&\frac{1}{3}\left(3328 \times 3 \times \frac{25.3}{3.3} + 3427 \times 3 \times \frac{25.3}{3.3} + 2910 \times 3 \times \frac{25.3}{3.0}\right)\\
&\quad \cong \frac{1}{3}(76\,544 + 78\,821 + 73\,623)\\
&\quad \cong 76\,329\,\text{kg}.
\end{aligned}$$

This is the same (within rounding error) as the HT estimate in **4.3** and the average of ratios estimate in **3.3**. The corresponding HH estimate of variance is

$$\begin{aligned}
&\frac{1}{3}\left\{\frac{1}{3-1}\right\}\left\{(76\,544 - 76\,329)^2 + (78\,821 - 76\,329)^2 + (73\,623 - 76\,329)^2\right\}\\
&\quad \cong \frac{1}{3}\frac{1}{2}(46\,200 + 6\,210\,100 + 7\,322\,400)\\
&\quad \cong 2\,263\,100\\
&\quad \cong 1504^2.
\end{aligned}$$

This is slightly in excess of the 1382^2 we found for stratum-by-stratum ratio estimation, but still small enough for us to hope that, when added to the estimated variance for the bulls' stratum, the relative standard deviation for the entire herd will be less than 2%.

4.9 One little reservation here. When we started investigating the variance for the bulls' stratum we obtained an estimate of zero, because the same elephant had been selected twice. So we proceeded to impute one. We then noted that since the estimate of zero came from an unbiased estimator, the variance estimates from samples containing two or more distinct units must on balance be overestimates, to compensate for the obvious underestimates arising when the same population unit is selected at each draw. We have not yet allowed here for the possibility that the same cow elephant might have been selected at all three sample draws, or even only twice, which would also have reduced the estimated variance. After a short discussion we decide not to do anything about this. For one thing, any adjustment to the estimate we have just obtained would have to be downwards. For another, it would have to be comparatively small, and a downward adjustment of this magnitude is not worth the trouble of working out how large it should be. We already have an estimate for the cows' stratum that is small enough to be comfortable with. Time to move on!

4.10 My colleague explains her idea for the bulls' stratum this way. If we had applied the Keyfitz replacement technique many times, there would have been four possible outcomes and each would have occurred in a known proportion of occasions. We would have retained both Combo and Flimbo 0.780 times 0.493 or 0.385 of the time. We would have retained only Combo (and therefore have to treat him as selected twice) 0.780 times (1 – 0.493) or 0.396 of the time. We would have retained only Flimbo (and therefore have to treat him as selected twice) 0.493 times (1 – 0.780) or 0.108 of the time. Finally we would have retained neither Combo nor Flimbo (and therefore had to select each to replace the other) $(1-0.493)(1-0.0780)$ or 0.111 of the time. The expected sample size for the bulls' stratum is thus $2 \times (0.385 + 0.111) + (0.396 + 0.108) = 0.990 + 0.505 = 1.496$. That might just be enough to keep the estimated relative standard deviation below 2%!

In fact we have only two different cases to consider. With probability $0.385 + 0.111 = 0.496$ our sample consists of both Combo and Flimbo. Our HH estimate of total is then $\frac{1}{2}\{(4675/0.0390) + (3032/0.02465)\} = 121\,437$. Our HH variance estimate is $(2-1)^{-1}[0.0390\{(4675/0.0390) - 121\,437\}^2 + 0.02465\{3032/0.02465) - 121\,437\}^2] \cong 2\,449\,500 \cong 1565^2$.

With probability $0.396 + 0.108 = 0.504$ our sample consists of a single elephant. Theoretically our estimate of variance in such circumstances would be undefined (zero divided by zero), but because we have in fact access to sample information about both Combo and Flimbo we can sidestep that problem. The variance of the HH estimator is strictly inversely proportional to size, so all we need to do is double the estimate of variance we have just made for the situation where there are two elephants in sample. Twice 2 449 500 is 4 899 000 $\cong 2213^2$, so our weighted average variance estimator for the bulls' stratum is $0.496 \times 2\,449\,500 + 0.504 \times 4\,899\,000 = 3\,684\,000 \cong 1919^2$.

The two estimated variances together are $2\,263\,100 + 3\,684\,000 \cong 2439^2$. This means the estimated relative standard error is $2439/(121\,437 + 76\,329) = 2439/197\,766$ or 1.2%. It looks as though we are home and dry!

4.11 But my colleague soon has second thoughts about her own ingenious idea for the bulls' stratum. Two sets of second thoughts. The first is that it might be too ingenious by half for our statistical peers. There is so much shuffling of data that it once again smells of being able to prove anything by statistics. The second is that the actual sample size for the bulls is not 1.496, but (in accordance with the Keyfitz retention method) one and one only.

We investigate the second point first. If we play fair by the result of that random draw, the HH estimate is not 121 437 but 4675/0.0390 or 119 872. More to the point, the bulls' imputed variance should not be 3 684 000 but 4 899 000. But that turns out to be tolerable. It would make the total imputed variance $2\,263\,100 + 4\,899\,000 = 7\,162\,100 \cong 2676^2$ and the imputed relative standard error $2676/(119\,872 + 76\,329)$, but this is still only 1.4%. So the accuracy of the estimate is not a problem after all, even with only a single elephant in sample for the bulls' stratum. And if that is the case, surely we need not be worried about the double shuffling with the bulls' stratum? Is this not the end of the quest?

No, it is not. My colleague is a perfectionist. The HH estimator, she insists, was designed for use with a sample of fixed size. We have no right to use it for a sampling scheme which is clearly yielding samples for which the sample size is a random variable. We should be finding a sampling procedure, and an estimator to go with it, which allows for the sample size to be variable.

Poisson Sampling

4.12 As it happens, such a sampling strategy is readily available. It is known as *Poisson sampling* (Hájek, 1958; Grosenbaugh, 1964; 1965). For Poisson sampling, every unit in a stratum is given a particular probability of inclusion in sample, and the decision as to whether each is actually to be in sample or not is made by carrying out a *Bernoulli trial*. Bernoulli trials are what we have been carrying out already in applying the Keyfitz retention procedure, so that does look very much like Poisson sampling. My colleague reckons that we should analyse our sample as though every bull had been assigned the inclusion probability $2X_{Bi}/24.35$ (only Combo being selected) and every cow the probability $3X_{Ci}/25.3$ (Linda, Pamela and Sara being selected).

'Why do you choose 2 for the bulls and 3 for the cows instead of 2.5 for each?' I ask.

'I'm not really sure,' she replies, 'and we might get much the same answer if we did, but I feel safer using the conditional rather than the unconditional analysis.'

'And what is the appropriate estimator?'

This turns out to be a form of the HT ratio estimator with the X_{Bi} as the supplementary variable for the bulls and X_{Ci} for the cows.

So we analyse our sample that way. Our HT estimate for the cows' stratum remains the same at 77 330 kg, and there is no ratio adjustment to make because the number of cows actually selected is the same as the expected number of 3. Our HT estimator for the bulls is now $4675 \times (24.35/1.90)$ or 59 914 kg, the difference from the earlier 59 936 kg being entirely due to rounding. The ratio adjustment factor now, however (the ratio of the actual total of the X_{Bi} to the HT estimate of that total), is $24.35/12.175 = 2$, and the HT ratio estimate is therefore 119 828 kg, definitely in the right ball park.

4.13 Now comes the crunch. How do we estimate the variances? As usual, we start with the cows, because they are simpler. It turns out that foresters have several possible ways of estimating the variance of the HT ratio estimator, and at least one of them (Gregoire, 1999) is more efficient than the one in the statistical literature (Brewer *et al.*, 1984) but we choose to stay with the latter because it is easier to see how it was arrived at. First, however, we need a formula for the variance itself. Ignoring the adjustment term that takes care of the possibility that no sample is selected (usually small, although admittedly not small in this instance) the variance of the HT estimator under Poisson sampling can be obtained by using the fact that the first-order inclusion probabilities are independent of each other. Substituting $\pi_{ij} = \pi_i\pi_j$ into (4.6) and simplifying, we arrive at

$$\mathrm{V}\hat{Y}_{.HT} = \sum_{i=1}^{N} \pi_i^{-1}(1 - \pi_i)Y_i^2. \tag{4.12}$$

Analogously, $\mathrm{V}\hat{X}_{.HT} = \sum_{i=1}^{N} \pi_i^{-1}(1 - \pi_i)X_i^2$ and $\mathrm{C}(\hat{Y}_{.HT}, \hat{X}_{.HT}) = \sum_{i=1}^{N} \pi_i^{-1} \times (1 - \pi_i)Y_iX_i$.

The variance of $\hat{Y}_{.HTR} = (\hat{Y}_{.HT}/\hat{X}_{.HT})X_.$ can therefore be approximated by

$$\begin{aligned} \mathrm{V}\hat{Y}_{.HTR} &\cong \mathrm{V}\hat{X}_{.HT} + R^2\mathrm{V}\hat{Y}_{.HT} - 2R\mathrm{C}(\hat{Y}_{.HT}, \hat{X}_{.HT}), \qquad \text{where } R = Y_./X_., \\ &= \sum_{i=1}^{N} \pi_i^{-1}(1 - \pi_i)\{Y_i - RX_i\}^2. \end{aligned} \tag{4.13}$$

This may be estimated by

$$\begin{aligned} \hat{\mathrm{V}}\hat{Y}_{.HTR} &= n^{-1}\mathrm{E}n\left\{\frac{n}{n-1}\right\}\sum_{i=1}^{N} \delta_i\pi_i^{-2}(1 - \pi_i)\{Y_i - \hat{R}X_i\}^2 \\ &= \frac{\mathrm{E}n}{n-1}\sum_{i=1}^{N} \delta_i\pi_i^{-2}(1 - \pi_i)\{Y_i - \hat{R}X_i\}^2, \end{aligned} \tag{4.14}$$

where $\hat{R} = \hat{Y}_{.HT}/\hat{X}_{.HT}$ and the factor $n/(n-1)$ is an approximate allowance for the fact that $\hat{R}$ is an estimator of R based on a sample of size n. We may think of this as correcting for the loss of a degree of freedom, so long as we recognize that this is only an approximation. Finally, the factor $n^{-1}\mathrm{E}n$ corrects for the existence of n terms in the summation when there are an expected $\mathrm{E}n$ of them.

For the cows, $\hat{R}_C = 76\,329/25.3 = 3017$; so

$$
\begin{aligned}
\hat{V}\hat{Y}_{C.HTR} &\cong \frac{3}{2}[0.1304^{-2}(1-0.1304)\{(3328-3017\times 1.1)^2 \\
&\quad + (3427-3017\times 1.1)^2\} + 0.1186^{-2}(1-0.1186) \\
&\quad \times (2910-3017\times 1.0)^2] \\
&\cong \frac{3}{2}\left[51.14\{9.3^2+108.3^2\}+62.66\times(-107)^2\right] \\
&\cong \frac{3}{2}(604\,200+717\,400) \\
&= 1\,982\,400 \\
&\cong 1408^2.
\end{aligned}
$$

4.14 This is credible and encouraging. Moreover, although we again have an imputation problem for the bulls, we are not quite as short of data as we were in Chapter 2. Then, we could not count Flimbo as a regular bull, because his weight was extraordinarily low. Now, however, the ratio of his actual weight to the elephant trainer's eye estimate is within an acceptable range for the bulls, and although our failure to retain him in sample using Keyfitz's procedure forbids us from using him for direct estimation of herd weight, it does not prevent us from using his data to impute a variance, for which the rules are far less strict. So we can start to work as though Combo and Flimbo had both been retained in sample, just as long as we know where to stop! On that hypothetical basis we have that the HT estimate is

$$
\begin{aligned}
\hat{Y}_{B.HT} &= 0.5\times 24.35\times\left(\frac{4675}{0.95}+\frac{3032}{0.6}\right) \\
&= 12.175\times(4921.05+5053.33) \\
&= 121\,438.
\end{aligned}
$$

It follows that $\hat{R}_B \cong 121\,438/24.35 \cong 4987.19$, and hence also that

$$
\begin{aligned}
\sum_i \delta_i\pi_i^{-2}(1-\pi_i)\{Y_i-\hat{R}X_i\}^2 &= 0.0780^{-2}(1-0.0780) \\
&\quad \times (4675-4987.19\times 0.95)^2 \\
&\quad + 0.0493^{-2}(1-0.0493) \\
&\quad \times (3032-4987.19\times 0.60)^2 \\
&= 151.55\times 3947.67+391.16\times 1574.98 \\
&= 598\,269+616\,069 \\
&= 1\,214\,338.
\end{aligned}
$$

Once again we need the factor $n/(n-1)$ to correct for the fact that we lose a degree of freedom when we estimate R_B by $\hat{R}_B$. We used two observations to form

$\hat{R}_B$, so the appropriate value for n in this calculation is 2. Finally, the factor $n^{-1}\mathrm{E}n$ again corrects for the existence of n terms in the summation when there are an expected $\mathrm{E}n$ of them. In our case there are two terms in the summation and the expectation of n is also 2, so the $\mathrm{E}n$ cancels with the n^{-1} (so no net correction on that account) and our imputed variance for the bulls' stratum is

$$\begin{aligned}\hat{\mathrm{V}}\hat{Y}_{B.HTR} &\cong \frac{2}{1} \times 1\,214\,338 \\ &= 2\,428\,676 \\ &\cong 1558^2.\end{aligned}$$

The sum of these estimated variances over the two strata is

$$\begin{aligned}\hat{\mathrm{V}}\hat{Y}_{.HTR} &\cong 1\,982\,400 + 2\,428\,700 \\ &= 4\,411\,100 \\ &\cong 2100^2.\end{aligned}$$

4.15 I am about to remark that this time we have scored a bull's-eye and can start to relax when my colleague cuts in: 'Wait! I'm not satisfied with the imputed variance for the bulls. Do you realize that this is exactly the value that we would have regarded as the unbiased estimator of variance if we had actually had both Combo and Flimbo in sample?'

'Why, so it is, but why should we worry about that when the expected sample size of our Poisson sample is also 2?'

'Because our achieved sample size is only 1!'

'But that doesn't matter,' I protest. 'What we are estimating is the variance of the estimator over all samples, samples of size one, two, three, whatever!'

'Including size zero?' she demands.

I grit my teeth. I was hoping that issue would not be brought up. There is an answer, of course, but it will take some time to explain.

'Zero is a special case,' I begin. 'Usually it isn't worth worrying about, because the probability of selecting an empty sample is trivial.'

'But in our case?'

'Well, it's true, it isn't entirely trivial in our case, but it is small, and it didn't happen, did it?'

'That's irrelevant,' she insists. 'I thought what we were after was an estimator of variance that was genuinely over all possible samples, including the one of size zero.'

'Very well,' I concede, 'but as you and I know very well, if an empty sample is selected, it is standard practice to try again and keep on trying until one does have a sample size greater than zero. It's called *modified Poisson sampling*. The foresters do that too (see Grosenbaugh, 1965).'

The long and the short of this is that my colleague insists on going back to the beginning and treating the problem as one of modified Poisson sampling.

'First of all, then,' I say, 'we need to know the probability of selecting an empty sample at the first attempt. That is the product of the probabilities of not selecting each of the 25 bulls in the population. Let's get an order-of-magnitude estimate first. We have been working conditionally on two bulls having been selected, so the probability of selecting any one of them would be about $\{1 - (2/25)\}$, and $\{1 - (2/25)\}^{25}$ is about e^{-2} or 0.135, so then ...'

'Wait! Isn't there a contradiction there? How can we get a meaningful estimate of the probability of selecting an empty sample conditional on having selected two units?'

'It does sound a bit strange I suppose, but what we are doing is modelling a selection of two elephants as though it had been a Poisson sample with an expected sample size of 2.'

'When the expected sample size was really 2.5?'

'When there's a choice between an unconditional and a conditional analysis, it's nearly always better to use the conditional one.'

'Then let's analyse this as a Poisson sample conditionally on the selection of *two*!'

I should have been noticing the warning note in her voice, but I press on regardless. 'Wouldn't it have to be "conditional on a sample size of one"? We reckoned we couldn't retain Flimbo.'

Her answer is not one that I have been ready for. 'Frankly, I'm getting very cynical about the relevance of all this game-playing with random numbers. Can you lay your hand on your heart and swear that it mattered whether we got one random number rather than another when we ditched Flimbo?'

This touches a sensitive spot. I have never been really easy in my mind since we took the decision to retain Flimbo and Combo together for the Lahiri–Midzuno analysis. That was the time when I had known what random number was coming up next, and wondered afterwards whether I would be so ready to accept the result if I had known that it would require their rejection. On impulse, I make a full confession. Not a wise move.

'You did that and you never told me? Well, that's the last straw! I've had enough now of being at the mercy of random events. I'm also tired of pretending that something has happened when it hasn't happened. And I'm sick of torturing our data until they fairly scream at us to leave them alone to tell their own story. Most of all, I resent having to pretend that we didn't select poor old Flimbo when we did, we did, we did! As it happens, I weighed him myself! We have the weights of *five* elephants and *I* want to use them *all.* I'm going back to see that woman who reckoned we should make all our inferences using prediction models. I reckon she was talking a lot of sense; more sense than you and I have been talking recently. And I don't care whether you come with me or not!'

Was it really less than an hour ago that I was being lectured on the need for a variance estimator that allowed for the sample size to be variable? No matter. There are times when logic has to take second place to intuition. Pausing only to pick up my books, I follow her straight out. I am barely in time to prevent her from driving off without me.

Exercises

4.1 Under *srswr* with $n = 2$, the form of the unbiased estimator of variance necessarily leads to the unbiased estimate being zero for every stratum in which the same sample unit is selected twice. The probability that a single sample unit will be selected twice in any given stratum is easily calculable beforehand. Hence the estimates supplied by the unbiased estimator, whenever the two sample units are *different*, overestimate the sample variance in that stratum, on average, by that calculable factor.

Two colleagues are collaborating in the design and analysis of a survey with many small strata, and the selection of the sample units within each stratum is necessarily *ppswr*. One of them suggests to the other that the variances in the individual strata would be more accurately estimated if the unbiased estimates in those strata where the two sample units are different were adjusted downwards by that calculable factor, and the difference between the sum of the unbiased estimates and the sum of those adjusted estimates were attributed to those strata where the two sample units were the same. He further suggests that the difference be distributed among those strata proportionally to their size.

(a) If the ith population unit in a given stratum has the probability P_i of being selected at either draw, what is the total probability that a single sample unit will be selected twice to represent the stratum?

(b) Imagine you are the other colleague. How would you respond to that suggestion for spreading the total estimate of variance around?

4.2 Set out the unconditional analysis referred to in **4.15** and comment on the differences between the conditional and unconditional approaches.

5

Ratio Estimation (Prediction-Based)

Understanding the Difference 80
The Ratio Prediction Model 83
Exercises 93

Understanding the Difference

5.1 Arriving unannounced at the office of our mentor, a very busy woman, not surprisingly we have to cool our heels a little until she is ready to see us. Not a bad thing really, because it gives us time to cool our tempers too. Fortunately, my colleague is not one to stay angry for long, so the fences are soon mended and we have time to discuss dispassionately the implications of relying wholly on prediction-based inference. 'You do realize', I put to her, 'that if we go along the path you are suggesting we shall be regarded at best as eccentric and at worst as part of some lunatic fringe?'

'I think you're still living in the 1980s,' she responds. 'No doubt it was like that then, but ideas have moved on quite a bit since. Several well-respected academic statisticians favour prediction-based inference these days.'

'But there's very little use of it outside the universities. Know any government statistical bureau that uses it?'

'There are many that use synthetic estimates. They're prediction-based.'

'But only for small domains, and they don't use them unless they have to.'

'Well, precisely. And aren't we working with a very small sample? And don't we have to?'

'Are you saying that prediction-based inference is particularly good for very small samples?'

'No, it's more that design-based inference is particularly bad for very small samples. Haven't the events of the last few days convinced you of that?'

This is a new idea for me. Up till now I had taken it for granted that small samples had problems simply because they were small, not because the inference being used for them was inappropriate.

'The last few days? Would you mind explaining what you mean?'

'OK. I've been feeling more and more uncomfortable ever since we got those eye estimates of weights from the elephant trainer. Up till then, Flimbo was an exceptional elephant and we had to treat him separately from the other bulls. Now all of a sudden he became just one of the boys. What had changed?'

'His ratio of weight to eye estimate wasn't atypical.'

'Yes; before that, he hadn't fitted our model. Now he did. It was our model that changed, not Flimbo.'

'I can see that. So?'

'So suddenly the question was not just how many cows there were and how many bulls, and how many of those bulls were exceptional. It was how many elephants fitted the cows' model and how many fitted the bulls' model. And we knew that, 25 each.'

'Wasn't there just a single model with 50 then? Weight proportional to eye estimate?'

'There would have been if the elephant trainer had related them all to a single elephant. But he related the cows to Kara and the bulls to Sambo. And Sambo was much heavier than Kara. Two models.'

I feel I am beginning to understand. 'You mean, before we had the eye estimates, it was important that we had a representative sample of bulls, some heavy ones and some light ones, and the same with cows. But once we had the ratio-to-eye-estimate model, it didn't matter whether we had heavy ones or light ones, so the inclusion probabilities became irrelevant and ...'

'Hold on,' she interrupts, 'you're going a bit fast there. Yes, before we had the eye-estimate model we effectively had one where the bulls' weights were randomly distributed around an unknown mean, but the differences between the heavy bulls and the light ones were very noticeable. Without consciously or deliberately doing so, you could have found yourself picking all big ones and biasing the sample mean upwards. Random selection was a crude way of avoiding that possibility; crude because it would still have been possible to choose all big ones, just by chance. A safer way would have been to group them in fives, the five biggest, the five next biggest and so on down to the five smallest, and pick one randomly from each group.'

'Another kind of stratification?'

'Yes, stratification by size is very common and very useful, but the point is that then you would know exactly how many elephants in the herd each sample one was *resembling*. The whole idea of randomization is to be able to say, "We have this one in sample. Its inclusion probability is (or rather was) one in five, so there must be four other elephants in the non-sample part of the herd that resemble him sufficiently closely for us to pretend that they are (or model them to be) exact replicas of this one." I guess that's why the process is sometimes called *randomization modelling*.'

'And once we had the eye estimates we had a different model, prediction-based, so we didn't need the randomization!'

'Will you just wait? Once we had the eye estimates, we were not as dependent on the randomization model as we were before, but we still had at least to consider the possibility of the prediction model breaking down. Perhaps the elephant trainer has a bit of a tendency to overestimate the weights of the larger elephants relative to the smaller ones, so it is still good to be able to ensure a reasonable spread of sizes within the sample if you can. But when you only have two or three in sample, well, that's very difficult to do. With very small samples like that, all one can do is say, "Here are 25 elephants, here are the two of them we have selected in sample, is there anything we can detect, after controlling on the supplementary information if we have any, that would disqualify either of them as representative?" If there isn't, you've got the relevant data for them and you use it as best you can. Before we had the eye estimates, we disqualified Flimbo on casual observation. He just wasn't typical. But after controlling on the eye estimates, Flimbo's data turned out to be perfectly typical. All that soul-searching about whether or not we could use the data, and if so with what probability, became irrelevant – as you said yourself five minutes ago.'

'What you are saying is that you should make the best model you can, and analyse the sample data in those terms; but that you should also be prepared for some measure of prediction model breakdown, and use the randomization model as an adjunct to minimize the damage that might cause?'

'I'd go along with most of that, but I wouldn't say "minimize". Randomization is a pretty blunt instrument, especially for small samples. If you've got the time and resources, you might try to select a *balanced sample*. That would actually minimize the damage (Royall and Herson, 1973a).'

'Balanced sample?'

'A balanced sample is one where the sample moments of the supplementary variable or variables are equal to the corresponding population moments. Everyone who ever selects a random sample would be delighted if it happened to be balanced. Balancing is what randomization is aiming at. Using randomization to choose a small sample is just a quick and dirty way of arriving at an approximately balanced sample. And since all random samples are possible, some are going to be badly imbalanced.'

'Balancing on every moment of every supplementary variable sounds a tall order.'

'It is, and in practice prediction-oriented statisticians balance on the mean of the most important one, and trust to that to facilitate approximate balance on the rest.' (See Tam and Chan, 1984.)

'If prediction inference is so good for small samples, why isn't it just as good for large ones, too?'

'I've just started thinking about that. I imagine it's because the larger the sample is, the greater the chance that any breakdown in the prediction model will become detectable.'

'Isn't there something else too? The larger the sample and the larger the population it is drawn from, the more plausible that randomization model that you were describing earlier starts to sound.'

'That too, I guess. The randomization model is unlike any other I know. The larger the sample, the better it works. I think that may be because it is not actually specified until we know the sample data. All other models start to break down at some stage and require further elaboration if they are still going to be useful.'

'And that may be why government statistical bureaus are so loath to touch prediction-based inference. The other has worked so well for them for so long, and most of their samples are so large that nothing else can match it.'

At that stage the door opens and we are once again being welcomed by our mentor.

The Ratio Prediction Model

5.2 When we explain why we have come, our mentor is grimly amused; but she does not say 'I told you so' straight out. She just starts writing out the prediction model we are going to need – a linear regression which could be taken as generating the weight of the *i*th elephant in either the bulls' or the cows' stratum:

$$\xi_R\colon\quad Y_{hi} = \beta_h X_{hi} + U_{hi};\quad \mathrm{E}_{\xi_R} U_{hi} = 0;\quad \mathrm{E}_{\xi_R} U_{hi}^2 = \sigma_{hi}^2;\quad \mathrm{E}_{\xi_R}(U_{hi}U_{hj}) = 0,$$
$$j \neq i;\quad i = 1, 2, \ldots, N_h;\quad h = B, C.$$

This differs somewhat from the ξ of Chapter 1. Instead of the N distributions each having the same mean and variance, each individual elephant has his or her own individual mean $\beta_h X_{hi}$, and variance σ_{hi}^2. With this model, there is no need to worry about how the sample was selected. Every elephant for which we have survey data is a relevant sample unit. Our estimator of total for stratum h is not quite the classical ratio estimator of Chapter 3, $\hat{Y}_{h\bullet R} = \hat{R}_h X_{h\bullet}$ where $\hat{R}_h = \hat{Y}_{h\bullet}/\hat{X}_{h\bullet}$. Instead, since we already know the weights of the five sample elephants 'without error' (meaning 'without sample error' of course, not 'without measurement error'!) we need only to estimate the weights of the non-sample elephants.

Our mentor tells us next that, if we do not know the individual σ_{hi}^2 (and of course we don't) we are unable to use the best linear unbiased estimator of β_h, but that the usual thing to do in such circumstances is to use $\hat{\beta}_h = \sum_i \delta_{hi} Y_{hi} / \sum_i \delta_{hi} X_{hi}$, which is unbiased under the model ξ_R and leads to a particularly simple estimator. 'In fact,' she says, 'it's probably the one that you've been using already.' And she's right.

Theorem 5.2.1 The estimator $\hat{\beta}_h = \sum_i \delta_{hi} Y_{hi} / \sum_i \delta_{hi} X_{hi}$ is prediction-unbiased for the β in ξ_R, and the corresponding prediction estimator $\hat{Y}_{h\bullet \xi_R} = \sum_i \delta_{hi} Y_{hi} + \hat{\beta}_h \sum_i (1 - \delta_{hi}) X_{hi}$ is prediction-unbiased for $Y_{h\bullet}$.

(Remember that, under prediction inference, Y_{hi} becomes a random variable, but X_{hi} and δ_{hi} are fixed numbers.)

Proof. The proof of the first part of the theorem is trivial:

$$\mathrm{E}_{\xi_R} \hat{\beta}_h = \frac{\sum_i \delta_{hi} (\mathrm{E}_{\xi_R} Y_{hi})}{\sum_i \delta_{hi} X_{hi}} = \frac{\sum_i \delta_{hi} \beta X_{hi}}{\sum_i \delta_{hi} X_{hi}} = \beta.$$

For the second part, we note that

$$
\begin{aligned}
\mathrm{E}_{\xi_R}(\hat{Y}_{h\bullet\xi_R} - Y_{h\bullet}) &= \mathrm{E}_{\xi_R}\left\{\sum_i \delta_{hi} Y_{hi} + \hat{\beta}_h \sum_i (1-\delta_{hi}) X_{hi} - \sum_i Y_{hi}\right\} \\
&= \mathrm{E}_{\xi_R} \sum_i \delta_{hi} Y_{hi} + \frac{\mathrm{E}_{\xi_R} \sum_i \delta_{hi} Y_{hi}}{\sum_i \delta_{hi} X_{hi}} \sum_i (1-\delta_{hi}) X_{hi} \\
&\quad - \mathrm{E}_{\xi_R} \sum_i Y_{hi} \\
&= \mathrm{E}_{\xi_R}\left[\sum_i \delta_{hi}(\beta_h X_{hi} + U_{hi})\right. \\
&\quad + \frac{\mathrm{E}_{\xi_R} \sum_i \delta_{hi}(\beta_h X_{hi} + U_{hi})}{\sum_i \delta_{hi} X_{hi}} \sum_i (1-\delta_{hi}) X_{hi} \\
&\quad \left. - \mathrm{E}_{\xi_R} \sum_i (\beta_h X_{hi} + U_{hi})\right] \\
&= \beta_h \sum_i \delta_{hi} X_{hi} + \beta_h \sum_i (1-\delta_{hi}) X_{hi} - \beta_h \sum_i X_{hi} \\
&= 0. \qquad \diamond
\end{aligned}
$$

Remark 5.2.1 $\hat{\beta}_h$ is numerically equivalent to $\hat{R}_h$, but as an estimator of the model parameter β_h it carries a different meaning.

We know from Chapter 3 that with Combo and Flimbo both in sample, $\sum_i \delta_{Bi} Y_{Bi} = 7707$, $\sum_i (1-\delta_{Bi}) X_{Bi} = 24.35 - 1.55 = 22.8$ and $\hat{R}_B = 7707/1.55$. Hence for the bulls, $\hat{Y}_{B\bullet\xi_R} = 7707\{1 + (22.8/1.55)\} \cong 121\,074$ kg, and similarly, for the cows, $\hat{Y}_{C\bullet\xi_R} = 9665\{1 + (22.1/3.2)\} \cong 76\,414$ kg.

These figures look suspiciously familiar. They are in fact (and as a result of the point made in Remark 5.2.1) numerically equivalent to the classical ratio estimates of Chapter 3. We raise this point with our mentor. Yes, she agrees, in this particular case the two approaches do yield the same numerical estimates, but with other ways of estimating the parameter β_h they could be different, and it is a good habit of thought to treat the sample values as known 'without error', so estimating only for the remainder.

This sounds reasonable, and we recall that in Chapter 1 we discovered that prediction-based and design-based estimates were often the same (or, as it seemed at the time, were always going to be the same). We now begin to expect that something like that will happen also with the estimator of sample variance, but we are mistaken. When we consider the prediction variance of $\hat{Y}_{h\bullet R} - Y_{h\bullet}$ under model ξ_R, the contribution from the $\sum_i \delta_{hi} Y_{hi}$ is zero, and

$$
\mathrm{V}_{\xi_R}(\hat{Y}_{h\bullet R} - Y_{h\bullet}) = \left\{\sum_i (1-\delta_{hi}) X_{hi}\right\}^2 \mathrm{V}_{\xi_R} \hat{\beta}_h.
$$

We begin to appreciate what we were told earlier about acquiring a good habit of thought concerning the sample values; always treat them as being known without error!

Theorem 5.2.2 The prediction variance of $\hat{Y}_{h\bullet R} - Y_{h\bullet}$ under ξ_R is $w_h(w_h - 1)\times \sum_i \delta_{hi}\sigma_{hi}^2 - \left(\sum_i w_h\delta_{hi}\sigma_{hi}^2 - \sum_i \sigma_{hi}^2\right)$, where $w_h = \sum_i X_{hi}/\sum_i \delta_{hi}X_{hi}$ is the *stratum weight* applied to each sample unit in the stratum.

Proof.

$$
\begin{aligned}
\mathrm{V}_{\xi_R}(\hat{Y}_{h\bullet R} - Y_{h\bullet}) &= \mathrm{V}_{\xi_R}\left\{\hat{\beta}_h \sum_i (1-\delta_{hi})X_{hi} - \sum_i (1-\delta_{hi})Y_{hi}\right\} \\
&= \mathrm{V}_{\xi_R}\left\{\frac{\sum_i \delta_{hi}Y_{hi}}{\sum_i \delta_{hi}X_{hi}} \sum_i (1-\delta_{hi})X_{hi} - \sum_i (1-\delta_{hi})Y_{hi}\right\} \\
&= \mathrm{V}_{\xi_R}\left\{\frac{\sum_i (1-\delta_{hi})X_{hi}}{\sum_i \delta_{hi}X_{hi}} \sum_i \delta_{hi}Y_{hi} - \sum_i (1-\delta_{hi})Y_{hi}\right\} \\
&= \left\{\frac{\sum_i (1-\delta_{hi})X_{hi}}{\sum_i \delta_{hi}X_{hi}}\right\}^2 \sum_i \delta_{hi}\sigma_{hi}^2 + \sum_i (1-\delta_{hi})^2\sigma_{hi}^2
\end{aligned}
$$

Since δ_{hi} is always either 0 or 1, $(1-\delta_{hi})^2 = 1 - \delta_{hi}$, so

$$
\begin{aligned}
\mathrm{V}_{\xi_R}(\hat{Y}_{h\bullet R} - Y_{h\bullet}) &= (w_h - 1)^2 \sum_i \delta_{hi}\sigma_{hi}^2 + \sum_i (1-\delta_{hi})\sigma_{hi}^2 \\
&= (w_h^2 - 2w_h) \sum_i \delta_{hi}\sigma_{hi}^2 + \sum_i \sigma_{hi}^2 \\
&= w_h(w_h - 1) \sum_i \delta_{hi}\sigma_{hi}^2 + \sum_i \sigma_{hi}^2 - w_h \sum_i \delta_{hi}\sigma_{hi}^2. \qquad (5.1)
\end{aligned}
$$

$\diamond$

The first term here is the leading term and will be estimable provided we can estimate the individual sample σ_{hi}^2. The second term is the population sum of the σ_{hi}^2, and the third is a sample estimator of that sum.

The third term is actually the classical ratio estimator of the second. This may be seen as follows. The third term may be written as

$$
\begin{aligned}
w_h \sum_i \delta_{hi}\sigma_{hi}^2 &= \frac{\sum_i X_{hi}}{\sum_i \delta_{hi}X_{hi}} \sum_i \delta_{hi}\sigma_{hi}^2 \\
&= \frac{(N_h/n_h)\sum_i \delta_{hi}\sigma_{hi}^2}{(N_h/n_h)\sum_i \delta_{hi}X_{hi}} \sum_i X_{hi}.
\end{aligned}
$$

But $(N_h/n_h)\sum_i \delta_{hi}\sigma_{hi}^2$ is the design-unbiased expansion estimator of $\sum_i \sigma_{hi}^2$ and $(N_h/n_h)\sum_i \delta_{hi}X_{hi}$ is the corresponding estimator of $\sum_i X_{hi}$, so the entire expression is the classical ratio estimator of $\sum_i \sigma_{hi}^2$ with $\sum_i X_{hi}$ as the benchmark value of the supplementary variable x.

Since $w_h \sum_i \delta_{hi}\sigma_{hi}^2$ is the classical ratio estimator of $\sum_i \sigma_{hi}^2$, the difference between the two is a sample estimator of zero, and consequently of uncertain sign. Further, both the second and third terms are only of order of magnitude N, as against the leading term's order of magnitude $n^{-1}N^2$.

So when it comes to estimating the prediction variance of $\hat{Y}_{h\bullet R} - Y_{h\bullet}$ under ξ_R in practice, we have a choice. The simpler option is to ignore the second and third terms in (5.1) altogether. The alternative is to construct a model enabling us to estimate the non-sample σ_{hi}^2 (as well as the sample ones, which are needed to construct the leading term itself) and use both sample and non-sample estimates of σ_{hi}^2 to evaluate, in addition, the difference between the second and third terms.

5.3 We will consider the simpler option first. Unbiased estimation of the individual sample σ_{hi}^2 initially looks as though it will be somewhat difficult. The obvious estimator, $\hat{\sigma}_{hi}^2 = (Y_{hi} - \hat{\beta}_h X_{hi})^2$, is always too small by a factor of order $1 - n^{-1}$, on account of $\hat{\beta}_h$ being only an estimator of the true β_h. With our very small sample sizes, we obviously need something more precise than this, but the factor $1 - n^{-1}$ by itself provides only a crude adjustment. To do better, there appears to be an $n_h \times n_h$ matrix to invert, or at least n_h simultaneous equations to be solved. This would not worry us particularly in our immediate setting, because there we have only to deal with the cases $n_B = 2$ and $n_C = 3$, but more generally it could become quite a problem.

Our mentor, however, rises to the occasion. The individual sample σ_{hi}^2 can be estimated unbiasedly under the model ξ_R, even without having to solve a set of n simultaneous equations.

Theorem 5.3.1 A prediction-unbiased estimator of σ_{hi}^2 is $\tilde{\sigma}_{hi}^2 = (\hat{\sigma}_{hi}^2 - g_{hi}^2 H_h)/(1 - 2g_{hi})$, where $g_{hi} = X_{hi}/\sum_k \delta_{hk} X_{hk}$ and $H_h = \sum_i \{\delta_{hi}\hat{\sigma}_{hi}^2/(1 - 2g_{hi})\}/\left[1 + \left\{\sum_i \delta_{hi} g_{hi}^2/(1 - 2g_{hi})\right\}\right]$.

Proof. For each sample unit i in stratum h,

$$
\begin{aligned}
\mathrm{E}_{\xi_R}\hat{\sigma}_{hi}^2 &= \mathrm{E}_{\xi_R}(Y_{hi} - \hat{R}_h X_{hi})^2 \\
&= \mathrm{E}_{\xi_R}\left\{(Y_{hi} - \beta_h X_{hi}) - (\hat{R}_h - \beta_h)X_{hi}\right\}^2 \\
&= \mathrm{E}_{\xi_R}\left\{(Y_{hi} - \beta_h X_{hi})^2 - 2(\hat{R}_h - \beta_h)X_{hi}(Y_{hi} - \beta_h X_{hi}) + (\hat{R}_h - \beta_h)^2 X_{hi}^2\right\} \\
&= \mathrm{V}_{\xi_R}(Y_{hi} - \beta_h X_{hi}) - 2\mathrm{C}_{\xi_R}\{(\hat{R}_h - \beta_h)X_{hi}, (Y_{hi} - \beta_h X_{hi})\} \\
&\quad + X_{hi}^2 \mathrm{V}_{\xi_R}(\hat{R}_h - \beta_h) \\
&= \sigma_{hi}^2 - 2\frac{\sigma_{hi}^2 X_{hi}}{\sum_k \delta_{hk} X_{hk}} + \frac{X_{hi}^2\left(\sum_k \delta_{hk}\sigma_{hk}^2\right)}{\left(\sum_k \delta_{hk} X_{hk}\right)^2}
\end{aligned}
$$

$$= \sigma_{hi}^2 \left\{1 - 2\frac{X_{hi}}{\sum_k \delta_{hk} X_{hk}}\right\} + \frac{X_{hi}^2 \left(\sum_k \delta_{hk}\sigma_{hk}^2\right)}{\left(\sum_k \delta_{hk} X_{hk}\right)^2}$$

$$= \sigma_{hi}^2(1 - 2g_{hi}) + g_{hi}^2 \left(\sum_k \delta_{hk}\sigma_{hk}^2\right). \tag{5.2}$$

So

$$\frac{\mathrm{E}_{\xi_R}\hat{\sigma}_{hi}^2}{1 - 2g_{hi}} = \sigma_{hi}^2 + \frac{g_{hi}^2\left(\sum_k \delta_{hk}\sigma_{hk}^2\right)}{1 - 2g_{hi}}$$

and

$$\mathrm{E}_{\xi_R} \sum_i \left(\frac{\delta_{hi}\hat{\sigma}_{hi}^2}{1 - 2g_{hi}}\right) = \sum_i \delta_{hi}\sigma_{hi}^2 + \frac{\sum_i \delta_{hi} g_{hi}^2}{1 - 2g_{hi}} \sum_k \delta_{hk}\sigma_{hk}^2$$

$$= \sum_i \delta_{hi}\sigma_{hi}^2 \left(1 + \frac{\sum_i \delta_{hi} g_{hi}^2}{1 - 2g_{hi}}\right).$$

It follows that a prediction-unbiased estimator of $\sum_i \delta_{hi}\sigma_{hi}^2$ is

$$H_h = \frac{\sum_i \left\{\delta_{hi}\hat{\sigma}_{hi}^2/(1 - 2g_{hi})\right\}}{1 + \sum_i \delta_{hi} g_{hi}^2/(1 - 2g_{hi})}.$$

Writing this expression (with k replacing i) in place of the $\sum_k \delta_{hk}\sigma_{hk}^2$ in (5.2), we obtain a prediction-unbiased estimator of the individual σ_{hi}^2, namely,

$$\tilde{\sigma}_{hi}^2 = \frac{\hat{\sigma}_{hi}^2 - g_{hi}^2 H_h}{1 - 2g_{hi}}. \tag{5.3}$$

◇

On this occasion we have no plans to go further, but in other situations, where we might want to estimate the difference between the second and third terms in (5.1), we would (as indicated above) need to specify a model for the variance function. Usually we would assume $\sigma_{hi}^2 \propto X_{hi}^{2\gamma}$, where $0.5 \leq \gamma \leq 1$ – a model which our mentor tells us is used quite commonly for such purposes. The parameter γ is called the *coefficient of heteroscedasticity* ('heteroscedasticity' meaning 'inequality in variance'). It takes a large sample (1000+ units) to estimate γ with any useful precision, and for most business populations it is sufficient to work with $\gamma = 0.75$. Trees, however, (and perhaps elephants?) seem to work better with $\gamma = 1$.

5.4 Meanwhile, back to the leading term. As usual, we estimate for the cows' stratum first, as they usually present fewer problems than the bulls do. We know from Section **3.9** that the values of $\hat{\sigma}_{hi}^2$ are 32 for Linda, 10 953 for Pamela and

12 169 for Sara, so common to all three cows we have

$$H_C = \frac{\sum_k \left\{\delta_{Ck}\hat{\sigma}^2_{Ck}/(1-2g_{Ck})\right\}}{1+\sum_k \delta_{Ck}g^2_{Ck}/(1-2g_{Ck})}$$

$$= \frac{[32/\{1-2.2/3.2\}]+[10\,953/\{1-(2.2/3.2)\}]+[12\,169/\{1-(2/3.2)\}]}{1+2[(1.1/3.2)^2/\{1-2.2/3.2\}]+[(1/3.2)^2/\{1-2/3.2\}]}$$

$$\cong \frac{102.4+35\,049.6+32\,450.7}{1+0.756\,25+0.260\,42}$$

$$\cong \frac{67\,602.7}{2.016\,67}$$

$$\cong 33\,522.$$

The corresponding values of $\tilde{\sigma}^2_{Ci}$ are as follows. First, for Linda,

$$\tilde{\sigma}^2_{C12} = \frac{\hat{\sigma}^2_{C12} - g^2_{C12}H_C}{1-2g_{C12}}$$

$$= \frac{32-(121/1024)33\,522}{0.3125}$$

$$\cong \frac{\{32-3961.1\}}{0.3125}$$

$$\cong -12\,573.$$

This is negative, and although a variance cannot be negative, an estimate of variance can be; so since the estimator is unbiased and we have other terms to consider, we leave this one in its negative form.

For Pamela we have

$$\tilde{\sigma}^2_{C16} = \frac{\hat{\sigma}^2_{C16} - g^2_{C16}H_C}{1-2g_{C16}}$$

$$= \frac{10\,953-(1.21/10.24)33\,522}{0.3125}$$

$$\cong \frac{10\,953-3961.1}{0.3125}$$

$$\cong 22\,374.$$

Finally, for Sara,

$$\tilde{\sigma}^2_{C18} = \frac{\hat{\sigma}^2_{C18} - g^2_{C18}H_C}{1-2g_{C18}}$$

$$= \frac{12\,169-(1.00/10.24)33\,522}{0.375}$$

$$= \frac{12\,169 - 3273.6}{0.375}$$
$$= 23\,721.$$

Check: $\sum_i \delta_{Ci}\tilde{\sigma}^2_{Ci} = -12\,573 + 22\,374 + 23\,721 = 33\,522 = H_C$.

Our prediction-unbiased estimator of $V_{\xi_R}(\hat{Y}_{C\bullet R} - Y_{C\bullet})$ is $w_C(w_C - 1) \times \sum_i \delta_{Ci}\sigma^2_{Ci} - (\sum_i w_C\sigma^2_{Ci} - \sum_i \sigma^2_{Ci})$, and we are only considering the leading term, so we write

$$\hat{V}_{\xi_R}(\hat{Y}_{C\bullet R} - Y_{C\bullet}) = w_C(w_C - 1)\sum_i \delta_{Ci}\tilde{\sigma}^2_{Ci}$$
$$= \frac{25.3}{3.2}\left(\frac{25.3}{3.2} - 1\right) 33\,522$$
$$= 7.906\,25 \times 6.906\,25 \times 33\,522$$
$$\cong 1\,830\,000$$
$$\cong 1353^2.$$

This is actually a little smaller than the estimate of design variance from Chapter 3, which was 1 910 000 or 1382^2. The difference is entirely due to the randomization-based raising factor N_h/n_h being replaced by the prediction-based $w_h = \sum_i X_{hi}/\sum_i \delta_{hi}X_{hi}$. The prediction-based estimator of variance is also simpler conceptually, and there is no Taylor series expansion to worry about.

5.5 Once again, however, we hit trouble with the bulls. This time the problem is that, for $n_h = 2$, both the numerator and denominator of H_h are identically zero, so H_B is indeterminate, and consequently so is our expression for $\hat{V}_{\xi_R}(\hat{Y}_{B\bullet R} - Y_{B\bullet})$. Even if we attempt to solve the two simultaneous equations supplied by (5.2), which for the sample consisting of Combo and Flimbo we may write as $\hat{\sigma}^2_{B3} = \tilde{\sigma}^2_{B3}(1 - 2g_{B3}) + g^2_{B3}(\tilde{\sigma}^2_{B3} + \tilde{\sigma}^2_{B6})$ and $\hat{\sigma}^2_{B6} = \tilde{\sigma}^2_{B6}(1 - 2g_{B6}) + g^2_{B6}(\tilde{\sigma}^2_{B6} + \tilde{\sigma}^2_{B3})$, we are still in trouble, for after substituting $g_{B6} = 1 - g_{B3}$ the two equations become identical and the ratio of $\tilde{\sigma}^2_{B3}$ to $\tilde{\sigma}^2_{B6}$ is once again indeterminate.

To obtain a determinate answer it is necessary to *assume* a value for that ratio. We decide that we will make two extreme assumptions and go with the one that yields the larger variance. At one extreme we will assume that $\tilde{\sigma}^2_{B3}$ and $\tilde{\sigma}^2_{B6}$ are equal. At the other we will take $\tilde{\sigma}^2_{Bi} \propto X^2_{Bi}$.

Regardless of which assumption we take, we need first to evaluate $\hat{\sigma}^2_{B3}$ and $\hat{\sigma}^2_{B6}$. For Combo, we have $\hat{\sigma}^2_{B3} = \{4675 - (7707/1.55)0.95\}^2 = 2366$, and for Flimbo we have $\hat{\sigma}^2_{B6} = \{3032 - (7707/1.55)0.60\}^2 = 2366$. (In fact it is true quite generally that, for $n_h = 2$, $\hat{\sigma}^2_{hi} = \hat{\sigma}^2_{hj}$.)

Under the assumption that $\tilde{\sigma}^2_{B3} = \tilde{\sigma}^2_{B6}$ we have $\tilde{\sigma}^2_{Bi} = \hat{\sigma}^2_{Bi}\{(1 - g_{Bi})^2 + g^2_{Bi}\}^{-1}$, $i = 3, 6$, and therefore both $\tilde{\sigma}^2_{B3}$ and $\tilde{\sigma}^2_{B6}$ are equal to $\hat{\sigma}^2_{Bi}(g^2_{B3} + g^2_{B6})^{-1}$, $i = 3, 6$, which comes to $2366 \times 1.55^2(0.95^2 + 0.60^2)^{-1} \cong 4502$. The estimate of $V_{\xi_R}(\hat{Y}_{B\bullet R} - Y_{B\bullet})$

is then

$$\begin{aligned}\hat{\mathrm{V}}_{\xi_R}(\hat{Y}_{B\bullet R} - Y_{B\bullet}) &= \frac{24.35}{1.55}\left(\frac{24.35}{1.55} - 1\right) 2 \times 4502 \\ &\cong 15.71 \times 14.71 \times 9004 \\ &\cong 2\,081\,000 \\ &\cong 1443^2.\end{aligned}$$

(We note in passing that this is slightly smaller than the estimate of 2 149 000 or 1466^2 obtained for the bulls' stratum in Chapter 3.)

Under the alternative assumption that $\tilde{\sigma}_{Bi}^2 \propto X_{Bi}^2$, we have $\tilde{\sigma}_{B6}^2 = \tilde{\sigma}_{B3}^2(X_{B6}^2/X_{B3}^2)$ and therefore that

$$\begin{aligned}\hat{\sigma}_{B3}^2 &= \tilde{\sigma}_{B3}^2(1 - 2g_{B3}) + g_{B3}^2(\tilde{\sigma}_{B3}^2 + \tilde{\sigma}_{B6}^2) \\ &= \tilde{\sigma}_{B3}^2(1 - 2g_{B3}) + g_{B3}^2\left(\tilde{\sigma}_{B3}^2 + \tilde{\sigma}_{B3}^2\frac{X_{B6}^2}{X_{B3}^2}\right) \\ &= \tilde{\sigma}_{B3}^2\left\{(1 - g_{B3})^2 + g_{B3}^2\frac{X_{B6}^2}{X_{B3}^2}\right\};\end{aligned}$$

and, changing the subject of the formula from $\hat{\sigma}_{B3}^2$ to $\tilde{\sigma}_{B3}^2$,

$$\begin{aligned}\tilde{\sigma}_{B3}^2 &= \hat{\sigma}_{B3}^2\left\{(1 - g_{B3})^2 + g_{B3}^2\frac{X_{B6}^2}{X_{B3}^2}\right\}^{-1} \\ &= 2366\left\{\left(\frac{0.60}{1.55}\right)^2 + \left(\frac{0.95}{1.55}\right)^2\left(\frac{0.60^2}{0.95^2}\right)\right\}^{-1} \\ &\cong 2366\{0.3871^2 + 0.6129^2 \times 0.3989\}^{-1} \\ &\cong 2366\{0.1498 + 0.1498\}^{-1} \\ &\cong 7897.\end{aligned}$$

Similarly,

$$\begin{aligned}\tilde{\sigma}_{B6}^2 &= \hat{\sigma}_{B6}^2\left\{(1 - g_{B6})^2 + g_{B6}^2\frac{X_{B3}^2}{X_{B6}^2}\right\}^{-1} \\ &= 2366\left\{\left(\frac{0.95}{1.55}\right)^2 + \left(\frac{0.60}{1.55}\right)^2\left(\frac{0.95^2}{0.60^2}\right)\right\}^{-1} \\ &\cong 2366\{0.3757 + 0.3757\}^{-1} \\ &\cong 3149.\end{aligned}$$

The estimate of $V_{\xi_R}(\hat{Y}_{B\bullet R} - Y_{B\bullet})$ is then

$$\begin{aligned}\hat{V}_{\xi_R}(\hat{Y}_{B\bullet R} - Y_{B\bullet}) &= \frac{24.35}{1.55}\left(\frac{24.35}{1.55} - 1\right)(7897 + 3149) \\ &\cong 15.71 \times 14.71 \times 11\,046 \\ &\cong 2\,553\,000 \\ &\cong 1598^2.\end{aligned}$$

The less favourable assumption is therefore the one in which $\tilde{\sigma}_{Bi}^2 \propto X_{Bi}^2$, and it is this that we adopt. We then have a variance of 2 553 000 for the bulls' stratum and 1 830 000 for the cows' stratum, a total of 4 383 000 or about 2094^2; larger, but only a little larger, than the 2015^2 we obtained for the stratum-by-stratum estimator in Chapter 3.

5.6 The estimated standard deviations of the estimated totals in Chapter 3 (design-based) and this chapter (model-based) are very similar. For the bulls, Chapter 3 gave 1466 kg and this chapter gave 1598 kg. For the cows, the comparable figures are 1382 kg and 1353 kg. This numerical similarity may be considered surprising when we consider how radically different they are in concept, the former being defined in terms of the variability over all possible samples and the latter over all possible realizations of the model ξ_R. All is intelligible, however, when we consider that, as mentioned at the end of **5.4**, the only difference between the estimators is the replacement of N_h/n_h by $w_h = \sum_i X_{hi} / \sum_i \delta_{hi} X_{hi}$. So although the two variances are conceptually very different, numerically they are likely to be quite similar. In fact, it was shown by Isaki and Fuller (1982) that when the estimator of total is unbiased under both approaches, the design expectation of the prediction variance is equal to the prediction expectation of the design variance.

5.7 Finally we have to produce the confidence interval that we promised the circus owner, and here we hit yet another a snag, one that we should have recognized earlier but did not bargain for.

It is this. When we made our calculations back in **1.2** we were counting on being able to use four degrees of freedom. Unfortunately, once we stratified into bulls and cows, we only had two degrees of freedom for the cows and one for the bulls. This does not just mean a loss of one degree of freedom; it means that we need to use two degrees of freedom when forming a confidence interval for the cows and only one when dealing with the bulls. That factor of 4.60 that we used when we thought we had four degrees of freedom becomes 5.84 for three degrees of freedom, 9.92 for two and 63.66 for one! At that rate, there is just no way we will be able to fulfil our commitment to the circus owner. Whatever can we do?

My colleague once again comes to the rescue. What we can still do, she explains, is pool the population variance estimates for cows and bulls, weighting them by the number of degrees of freedom supplied by each stratum. We can then also add the two degrees of freedom for the cows to the one for the bulls, to arrive at a total of three degrees of freedom.

Since the prediction-based estimates of population variance are, on balance, slightly larger than the randomization-based, it is those that we should use. (They are not, of course, the 'raw' population variances that measure the variabilities of the elephants' weights, but the population variances of the residuals $Y_{hi} - \hat{R}_h X_{hi}$, or equivalently $Y_{hi} - \hat{\beta}_h X_{hi}$, obtained in the course of ratio estimation.)

Because of the form of the variance estimator we used for prediction-based inference, which we may now write as $w_h(w_h - 1)\sum_i \delta_{hi}\tilde{\sigma}_{hi}^2$, we have as yet no explicit estimator of the population variances. But $\sum_i \delta_{hi}\tilde{\sigma}_{hi}^2$ is obviously a mixed randomization/prediction-unbiased estimator of n_h times what Isaki and Fuller (1982) called the *anticipated* population variance (the design expectation of the prediction-based population variance). So we just divide the 33 522 by 3 to get 11 174 as our estimator of the population variance for the cows' stratum. For the bulls, we similarly divide their 11 046 by 2 to arrive at 5523. (All these population variances are, of course, in square kilograms.)

It is tempting to say that the 11 174 is an estimate with two degrees of freedom and 5523 an estimate with one degree of freedom, and therefore that the pooled estimate should be $(2 \times 11\,174 + 5523)/3 \cong 9920$, but there is a further complication. There is some evidence that the population variances are proportional to the square of the elephants' weights; and as our estimate of the weight of 25 cows is 76 414 kg and of 25 bulls 121 704 kg, we should really multiply the bulls' 5523 by $(76\,414/121\,074)^2$ or 0.3983 to obtain a comparable estimate of 2200 to apply to the cows. And, similarly, we should multiply the cows' 11 174 by $(121\,074/76\,414)^2$ or 2.5105 to obtain a comparable estimate of 28 052 to apply to the bulls. So our pooled estimate of the cows' population variance should in fact be $(2 \times 11\,174 + 2200)/3 \cong 8183\ \text{kg}^2$ with three degrees of freedom, and the comparable estimate for the bulls should be $(2 \times 28\,052 + 5523)/3 \cong 20\,542\ \text{kg}^2$, also with three degrees of freedom. The estimated variances for the estimates of total are then $7.906\,25 \times 6.906\,25 \times 3 \times 8183$ or 1 340 400 for the cows and $15.71 \times 14.71 \times 2 \times 20\,542$ or 9 899 600 for the bulls, making 11 240 000, or 3353^2, for the two strata combined.

The shortest 99% confidence interval for the t distribution with three degrees of freedom is, as previously indicated, 5.84 estimated standard deviations on either side of the sample mean. This means a half-width for the confidence interval of 5.84×3353 kg or 19.6 tonnes. Our final estimate is therefore 197.5 ± 19.6 or between 177.9 and 217.1 tonnes with 99% confidence. We are not exactly comfortably within the bounds set by our target, but we have just squeaked inside them. A salutary reminder as to just how unstable estimates of precision can be when based on very few degrees of freedom!

It seems we now *are* finally home and dry! We have determined the total weight of the herd within 10% either way, we have achieved our required 99% confidence interval and there is no worry about bias. *Just so long as we can defend our use of prediction-based inference for the variance!*

I wonder about that as I prepare for bed. I remember reading once, 'I know what I think when I read what I write.' That seems very pertinent here. Tomorrow, I promise myself, we will write a long report for our immediate supervisor, with whom it pays to be strictly honest, warts and all, and a draft of a short one for the circus owner, where we will probably need to put our best foot forward.

Exercises

5.1 When using Poisson sampling, the sample size, $n = \sum_{i=1}^{N} \delta_i$, is a random variable. The Horvitz–Thompson estimator of total (HTE) is $\hat{Y}_{\bullet HT} = \sum_{i=1}^{N} \delta_i Y_i \pi_i^{-1}$, so the size of the Horvitz–Thompson *estimate* of total is strongly influenced by the number of units that happen to be selected in the sample, and the variance of the HTE is typically dominated by a component that depends solely on the variability of the achieved sample size.

It is therefore better to use the Horvitz–Thompson ratio estimator of total (HTRE), $\hat{Y}_{\bullet HTR}$, instead, where

$$\begin{aligned}\hat{Y}_{\bullet HTR} &= \left(\sum_{i=1}^{N} \delta_i \pi_i \pi_i^{-1}\right)^{-1} \left(\sum_{i=1}^{N} \delta_i Y_i \pi_i^{-1}\right)\left(\sum_{i=1}^{N} \pi_i\right) \\ &= \left(\sum_{i=1}^{N} \delta_i\right)^{-1} \left(\sum_{i=1}^{N} \delta_i Y_i \pi_i^{-1}\right) \mathrm{E}n \\ &= \hat{Y}_{\bullet HT}\left(\frac{\mathrm{E}n}{n}\right).\end{aligned}$$

Because this has the form of the classical ratio estimator (CRE), with the inclusion probabilities π_i as the supplementary variable and their population total $\mathrm{E}n = \sum_{i=1}^{N} \pi_i$ as benchmark, it is possible to use the ratio estimation theory of Chapter 3 to estimate its variance

There are still problems, however. If the achieved sample size is zero, the HTRE is indeterminate. Moreover, when the achieved sample size is either zero or one, the CRE-based estimator of variance for the HTRE also yields an indeterminate estimate.

Because of these difficulties, it has been suggested that the HTRE be treated instead as the HTE *conditioned on the achieved sample size*. That is, the HTRE should be thought of as though it were an HTE of the form $\sum_{i=1}^{N} \delta_i Y_i \pi_i'^{-1}$ where $\pi_i' = (n/\mathrm{E}n)\pi_i$, and these 'adjusted inclusion probabilities', π_i', should be treated as though they were the real inclusion probabilities.

(a) Modify the prediction model ξ_R of Section **5.2** in such a way as to arrive at one that could provide the inferential support for the use of the HTRE given above as $\hat{Y}_{\bullet HTR} = \hat{Y}_{\bullet HT}(\mathrm{E}n/n)$.

(b) If your model has Y_i dependent on the value of π_i, consider the implications. It means that if π_i is changed in an arbitrary fashion, Y_i changes with it. (This is not just a quibble. Remember that the circus statistician lost his job as a result of taking such an assumption to its logical but totally unrealistic conclusion.) So modify your model to make it reflect the likely reality more closely.

(c) Show that under your model, $\hat{Y}_{\bullet HTR}$ is unbiased for $Y_{\bullet}$. (If it is not, there is something wrong with your model.)

(d) Following the pattern of Theorem 5.2.2, derive an expression for the model variance of $\hat{Y}_{\bullet HTR} - Y_{\bullet}$.

5.2 If we drop the subscript h, $V_{\xi R}(\hat{Y}_{\bullet \xi R} - Y_{\bullet})$ is the variance of $\hat{Y}_{\bullet \xi R} = \sum_i \delta_i Y_i + \hat{\beta} \sum_i (1 - \delta_i) X_i$, regarded as an estimator of the population total $Y_{\bullet}$. We have shown that $V_{\xi R}(\hat{Y}_{\bullet R} - Y_{\bullet}) \cong w(w - 1) \sum_i \delta_i \sigma_i^2$, where $w = X_{\bullet} / \sum_k \delta_k X_k$ and σ_i^2 is the prediction model variance of Y_i. It is also shown that a prediction-unbiased estimator of σ_i^2 is $\tilde{\sigma}_i^2 = (\hat{\sigma}_i^2 - g_i^2 H)/(1 - 2g_i)$, where $\hat{\sigma}_i^2 = (Y_i - \hat{R} X_i)^2, \hat{R} = \hat{Y}_{\bullet}/\hat{X}_{\bullet}, g_i = X_i / \sum_k \delta_k X_k$ and $H = \sum_i \{\delta_i \hat{\sigma}_i^2 / (1 - 2g_i)\} / [1 + \{\sum_i \delta_i g_i^2 / (1 - 2g_i)\}]$.

(a) Show that in the special case where $X_i = 1$ for $i = 1, 2, \ldots, N$ and the σ_i^2 are all equal at σ^2, a prediction-unbiased estimator of the $V_{\xi R}(\hat{Y}_{\bullet \xi R} - Y_{\bullet})$ is approximately $w(w - 1) \sum_i \delta_i \hat{\hat{\sigma}}_i^2$ where $\hat{\hat{\sigma}}^2 = n^{-1} \sum_i \delta_i \hat{\sigma}_i^2 = n^{-1} \times \sum_i \delta_i (Y_i - \hat{R} X_i)^2$.

(b) Use the result in (a) to estimate the variance of the poststratification estimate arrived at in Exercise 2.1.

(c) Suggest reasons why the variance estimates arrived at in this exercise and in Exercise 2.1 might differ, and comment on the extent of that difference.

5.3 Take the formulae given in the preamble to Exercise 5.2, and consider the case where there are only two units in the sample.

(a) Show that the expressions for H and $\tilde{\sigma}_i^2$ given by these formulae are indeterminate, and that in consequence they cannot be used to estimate the approximate expression for $V_{\xi R}(\hat{Y}_{\bullet \xi R} - Y_{\bullet})$.

(b) Use the model assumption $\tilde{\sigma}_i^2 \propto X_i^{2\gamma}$ in this case to arrive at a usable estimator for the two sample values of σ_i^2.

6

The Reporting

Report to Supervisor 95
Draft of a Report for the Circus Owner 98
Comments from Supervisor 98
Action Consequential on Supervisor's Comments 99
Randomization-Based and Prediction-Based Sampling Inferences are Complementary 101
More about the Background to Our Assignment 104

Report to Supervisor

6.1 This has been a most instructive learning experience for us. Everything has come out well in the end, but we made a number of mistakes in the process and even now we are going to have some difficulty with the presentation. We are attaching a draft report for the client, which we hope you will find satisfactory. Our presentation problems are not so much with him as with our colleagues, including perhaps even yourself.

The idea of sending us out together without either of us actually being in charge, but with access to you if we were completely at loggerheads, has worked well in this case. We spark each other off quite usefully.

We started out by making several elementary mistakes. Instead of taking time to get to know our clients and become familiar with the subject matter, we dashed straight in to treat the technical sampling problem. Had we appreciated earlier how much professional expertise the elephant trainer had, how useful it was going to be for us, and how sensitive he was about 'experts' in other areas ignoring his own expertise, we would also have realized much sooner how unrepresentative the elephant Flimbo was, or perhaps we should say 'appeared to be', and would have saved ourselves a great deal of trouble. We were in fact very lucky that, despite having already alienated the elephant trainer, we were still able to tap into that expertise of his through the good offices of the circus owner. Without it we would have found ourselves in very deep trouble.

Again, because we did not initially consider the possibility that the difference between cows and bulls would be of such significance, we went ahead selecting five elephants without regard to this distinction, and were lucky that we did not end up with all bulls or all cows. We were actually unlucky in the short run, in that we selected the atypical elephant Flimbo; but in the longer run it was to our advantage, as we were thereby alerted to the need to be familiar with the herd's composition.

Yet again, had we appreciated from the beginning the extreme cumbersomeness of the weighing procedure, we would have thought twice before insisting that five elephants was the smallest pilot sample worth contemplating, particularly since 5 is not divisible by 2. Yet , perversely, we were lucky, because we really needed that many elephants in our pilot sample, and they did the job for us in the end.

6.2 Turning to the more technical sampling aspects of our assignment, we experienced considerable difficulties along the way. Before we had any auxiliary variable information to draw on, the fact that Flimbo was a highly atypical bull reduced our effective sample size for the bulls' stratum to a single elephant, and we had to impute the relevant population variance. As indicated above, we were subsequently able to tap into the elephant trainer's expertise and were supplied with an extremely valuable set of estimated relative weights, which made all the difference. After conditioning on this auxiliary variable, Flimbo's weight became a completely well-behaved variable and we were able to deal with the bulls' stratum on the basis of a sample size of two, rather than just one. Even with a sample size of two, however, we experienced certain unexpected difficulties.

Chief among these was that when we attempted to use the classical ratio estimator, the available expressions for bias and variance were asymptotic and therefore unreliable for our sample sizes (three elephants for the cows' stratum and only two for the bulls'). Attempts which we made to circumvent this problem by using unequal inclusion probabilities (retaining the elephants originally selected as far as possible using the Keyfitz technique) led us up one blind alley after another, chiefly as a result of our being unable to retain Flimbo in sample once the random number drawn for him had failed to fall in the retention range.

These difficulties eventually caused us to reconsider the appropriateness of design-based inference in circumstances where the small sample size (whether of the target sample or the achieved sample or both) brought into question the implicit assumption on which design-based inference depends, namely that for any unit in sample for which the inclusion probability is π, or one in $\varpi = \pi^{-1}$, that portion of the population not included in sample should be regarded (at least to a first approximation) as containing $\varpi - 1$ units whose properties were similar to those of the sample unit. This way of thinking about the population could be what some people mean when they refer to a 'randomization model'.

Then there were the problems that we struck when we were trying to change our elephants' probabilities of inclusion in sample, so as to be able to use different estimators. We got very confused as to whether we should be using unconditional probabilities of inclusion or probabilities conditioned on achieved sample sizes. We should have been consistent about using one or the other, and we have little doubt now that we should have used the conditional ones. They may not accord with the pure randomization theory so well, but they give more realistic estimates.

A related problem was the way in which the composition of our sample then depended on quite deliberately random outcomes that seemed to have only the most tenuous connections to the values we were trying to estimate. At one point we were even trying to arrive at the joint probabilities of inclusion of pairs of units, before we realized what a pointless exercise that had become. At that stage our confidence in the whole notion of randomization-based inference was being really severely shaken, and it was only restored when we began to think how useful it could be with large samples.

6.3 The above considerations eventually led us to the decision to use prediction-based, or so-called model-based, inference instead. (We prefer to use the description 'prediction-based' ourselves. As we noted above, there is a way in which even design-based inference is built on a model.) We are now convinced that design-based (or randomization-based) inference and prediction-based inference should not be regarded as competing but as complementary. It is perhaps worth pointing out that model-assisted survey sampling already uses prediction models to optimize its design-based estimators; and that our sample sizes were so small that the standard ratio model we used could not possibly be falsified by sample evidence.

Conversely, however, when the sample size is large, there is an appreciable risk that the deficiencies of the standard ratio model will be detectable – or, worse still, not detectable in terms of standard hypothesis tests but still sufficiently large to disturb the estimates appreciably (Hansen *et al.*, 1983). The randomization model described above is unusual in that it is not falsifiable by sample information but, on the contrary, relies for the completeness of its definition on sample information and becomes more reliable rather than less as the sample size increases.

It was probably such considerations that led Godambe to suggest, in the course of a discussion at the International Statistical Institute Congress in New Delhi in 1977, that what was needed was a way of finding estimators that made sense using either approach. (We believe that this was the first time such a suggestion had been made publicly.) Later they certainly led authors such as Särndal and Wright (1984) and Brewer (1999a) to address the implementation of Godambe's suggestion.

Fortunately, in our situation we were able to employ an estimator of total, namely the classical ratio estimator, that is indeed supported by both these inference frameworks. We were less fortunate with regard to the estimation of variances or mean squared errors, where the design-based estimates are not regarded as reliable for such small samples. We did nevertheless begin by estimating the design-based variances, but later we also estimated the corresponding prediction variances.

In the event, the two variance estimation formulae and the numerical values of the two sets of estimates both turned out to be surprisingly close. Additionally, each set met criteria that the other failed to meet. The estimates of randomization variance were not vulnerable to prediction-model breakdown and the prediction-based estimates did not depend on asymptotic theory. Perhaps we may be allowed a courtroom analogy. When two entirely independent witnesses are in broad agreement, then even if each of them separately has to be treated with suspicion (for quite different reasons) their combined testimony must command a certain measure of respect.

The most important of our numerical estimates have been included in the attached draft report for the client. In summary, we finally just managed to achieve all that was asked of us. The attachment contains a full account of the procedures we used to obtain our classical ratio estimates, their estimated variances and the confidence interval we found for the herd as a whole. [Since these calculations have already been presented in Chapters 3 and 5, this attachment has been omitted here. KB]

Draft of a Report for the Circus Owner

6.4 We have pleasure in submitting our report regarding the weight of your herd of 50 Indian elephants. We are particularly pleased that we have been able to achieve the objective you specified without the need to weigh any more elephants beyond the five that were included in the initial weighing.

The successful completion of this project was greatly facilitated by your own ready co-operation and by the quite indispensable input supplied by your elephant trainer in the provision of eye estimated weights for all 50 elephants. But for this list, or one containing equally useful information, we would have needed to weigh many additional elephants in order to be able to complete our assignment.

The weights in kilograms of the five sample elephants were found to be as follows: Combo, 4675; Flimbo, 3032; Linda, 3328; Pamela, 3427; Sara, 2910. The total weight of your herd, as estimated using the standard or classical ratio estimator (with the elephant trainer's eye estimates as the auxiliary variable), is 197.5 tonnes. This is made up of 121.1 tonnes for the 25 bulls and 76.4 tonnes for the 25 cows.

The standard errors of these estimates are themselves estimated as 3.1 tonnes for the bulls, 1.2 tonnes for the cows and 3.4 tonnes for the entire herd. The 99% confidence interval for the true weight of the herd (assuming the weights of bulls and cows are each normally distributed, and taking into account the small sample sizes on which the estimates were based) is between 177.9 and 217.1 tonnes. Since the best point estimate of 197.5 tonnes is less than 19.75 tonnes distant from both these limits, your requirement that the herd's total weight be ascertained within 10% with 99% confidence has been achieved without the need to weigh any further elephants.

We appreciate your giving us your custom. As you are aware, the task you set us proved to be more of a challenge than we had anticipated. We were obliged to try out a number of different approaches before finding the one that was most appropriate, but that was a valuable exercise for us in skill development, and we have quite a sense of achievement in having completed it successfully. Please accept our assurance that we would be prepared to tackle with equal dedication any further statistical work you should ask us to do.

Comments from Supervisor

6.5 I appreciate the honesty displayed in the first part of your report. Don't feel too bad about the mistakes. I am sure you will learn from them.

The more technical part of your report made fascinating reading. I have to agree that the use of design-based information is problematical for small samples. Your persistence in trying to resolve the problems is commendable, and I would like to discuss your experiences with you first thing Monday morning. In the meantime, although I am half convinced that your resort to prediction-based inference was justifiable in the circumstances, I am relieved that it merely confirmed the results you had already obtained using design-based inference. One further point: could you not have obtained the necessary assurance of negligible bias within the design-based framework, simply by assuming that the regression of Y_i on X_i went almost through the origin?

Another thing that I would like to discuss with you next Monday is your argument that the prediction model and what you refer to as the 'randomization model' are complementary. I have always regarded design-based inference as model-free, but I can understand now why you choose to regard it as a model. I think Kyburg (1987) might describe it as an inverse inference model, since it is based essentially on sample (that is, empirical) information and changes as the sample changes. But Kyburg sees this as a weakness and you are arguing that it is a strength. There is much to think about here. Would you please prepare a longer note about the merits of these two forms of inference that I would be able to think about over the weekend?

Action Consequential on Supervisor's Comments

6.6 We are generally heartened by our supervisor's comments. We had not expected him to be an immediate convert to prediction-based inference, or even to its being treated on an equal footing with design-based, but he is clearly open to reasonable argument. Monday will indeed be interesting, and writing the longer note will be a challenge.

The matter of the classical ratio estimator's design bias when the regression of Y_i on X_i is linear through the origin is best analysed first in terms of randomization inference, and then in terms of prediction inference.

So let us remind ourselves of what we found in **3.8**. The asymptotic formula for the design bias of the classical ratio estimator, $\hat{Y}_{\bullet R}$, is found there, to be proportional to $\sum_i\{X_i(\bar{R}X_i - Y_i)\}$. Now if we take the entire finite population and regress Y_i with ordinary least squares (OLS) on X_i, the regression coefficient we obtain may be written as $B = \left(\sum_i Y_iX_i - N\bar{Y}\bar{X}\right)/\left(\sum_i X_i^2 - N\bar{X}^2\right)$, and the intercept as $A = \bar{Y} - B\bar{X}$. The condition that the regression goes through the origin is then simply $A = 0$, which implies that $B = \bar{Y}/\bar{X} = \bar{R}$. Substituting this into the original expression for B yields $B = \left(\sum_i Y_iX_i - NB\bar{X}^2\right)/\left(\sum_i X_i^2 - N\bar{X}^2\right)$. Cross-multiplying, $B\sum_i X_i^2 - NB\bar{X}^2 = \sum_i Y_iX_i - NB\bar{X}^2$; so $B = \sum_i Y_iX_i/\sum_i X_i^2$. It follows that the bias must contain a factor

$$\sum_i\{X_i(\bar{R}X_i - Y_i)\} = \sum_i\{X_i(BX_i - Y_i)\} = B\sum_i X_i^2 - \sum_i Y_iX_i = 0.$$

So our supervisor is right so far; when the OLS regression of Y_i on X_i is linear through the origin, the asymptotic formula for the design bias of the classical ratio estimator does indeed collapse to zero.

However, the assumption that the regression goes through the origin can hardly be applied to bias without being applied to the mean squared error as well, where it is less helpful. The asymptotic formula for the *relative* bias is given in (3.4) as $\mathrm{V}\hat{\bar{X}}/\bar{X}^2 - \mathrm{C}(\hat{\bar{Y}},\hat{\bar{X}})/\bar{Y}\bar{X}$, where $\mathrm{V}\hat{\bar{X}}/\bar{X}^2$ is the relative variance of $\hat{\bar{X}}$ and $\mathrm{C}(\hat{\bar{Y}},\hat{\bar{X}})/\bar{Y}\bar{X}$ is the relative covariance of $\hat{\bar{Y}}$ and $\hat{\bar{X}}$. If the absolute bias is asymptotically zero, so is the relative bias, and the equation expressing this condition is $\mathrm{V}\hat{\bar{X}}/\bar{X}^2 = \mathrm{C}(\hat{\bar{Y}},\hat{\bar{X}})/\bar{Y}\bar{X}$. Substituting this expression in (3.5) we have that $\mathrm{V}\hat{R}/R^2 \cong \mathrm{V}\hat{\bar{Y}}/\bar{Y}^2 - \mathrm{V}\hat{\bar{X}}/\bar{X}^2$. In words, zero randomization bias for the classical ratio estimator implies that the relative variance of the estimated ratio $\hat{R}$, and of the ratio estimator, is approximately equal to the difference between the relative variance of the sample mean of the survey variable and the relative variance of the sample mean of the auxiliary variable.

Now in our assignment, Y_i is the true weight of an elephant and X_i is an eye estimate of that weight, so we would expect the relative variance of the Y_i to be *less* than that of the X_i, implying therefore that we are unlikely to find, even from a large sample, that $\mathrm{V}\hat{\bar{X}}/\bar{X}^2 = \mathrm{C}(\hat{\bar{Y}},\hat{\bar{X}})/\bar{Y}\bar{X}$ or, equivalently, that the OLS regression of the Y_i on the X_i would pass through the origin or, again equivalently, that the randomization bias is (even asymptotically) zero. If we want to assert that the regression of Y_i on X_i should go through the origin, it is much better that we make the assumption explicitly, by way of a model like ξ_R, than try to demonstrate it using asymptotic randomization theory.

Next, it will help to take a detour through normal distribution theory. Consider two jointly normally distributed random variables, x and y, that have positive means, $\bar{x}$ and $\bar{y}$ respectively, and are positively correlated. The major axes of the elliptical contours of their joint density distribution all lie along the same straight line. We will call the equation of that straight line, which is of the form $y - \bar{y} = \lambda(x - \bar{x})$, the *natural relationship* between x and y. If $\lambda = \bar{y}/\bar{x}$, so that the natural relationship is the straight line that passes through the origin and the point ($\bar{x}$, $\bar{y}$), we will say that their natural relationship is a *ratio relationship*.

It is well known that if y is regressed on x in that situation, using OLS, the line of best fit has a slope less than $\bar{y}/\bar{x}$ and a positive intercept on the y-axis. (Conversely, if x is OLS regressed on y, the line of best fit has a slope greater than $\bar{y}/\bar{x}$ and a positive intercept on the x-axis.)

A similar result obviously holds for at least some well-behaved distributions other than the normal. We extend the concept here to finite populations. Suppose a straight line L is drawn through the scattergram of the N points (X_i, Y_i), in such a way as to minimize the sum of squares of the lengths of all lines that pass through a point (X_i, Y_i) and are orthogonal to L. Then L will be referred to as the *natural relationship* between the X_i and the Y_i. If, in such circumstances, Y_i is regressed OLS on X_i, there would usually be a positive intercept on the y-axis. So if the result of Y_i being regressed OLS on X_i is a line of best fit through the origin – which in **3.8** we found was the condition for the ratio estimator to have zero bias – it is reasonable to guess that the natural relationship between the X_i and the Y_i has a *negative* intercept on the y-axis.

How does this relate to our assignment? At no stage did we regress using OLS. Our prediction model specified a regression without any intercept term on the y-axis. This is tantamount to specifying that the natural relationship is a ratio relationship, and that it would be inappropriate to use OLS. Our choice of the ratio $\bar{Y}/\bar{X}$ to estimate the slope, which is specified under the randomization approach by the use of the classical ratio estimator, and is also permissible (though not mandatory) under the prediction approach, ensured that our line of best fit would pass through the origin. It also ensured simultaneously that our estimator of total would be free from prediction bias. It seems then, from the analysis above, that the classical ratio estimator is unlikely to be free from randomization bias. In any case, it could not be free from both kinds of bias simultaneously.

The straightforwardness of the prediction-based inference on the one hand, together with the contorted paradoxes of the randomization-based inference on the other hand, lead us to conclude that the prediction bias in this case is zero, and that randomization bias is no more than a red herring – negligible when the sample is large, and an issue which is best ignored when the sample is small.

Our supervisor's request for a 'longer note about the merits of these two forms of inference' required rather more thought. The following is what we eventually came up with.

Randomization-Based and Prediction-Based Sampling Inferences are Complementary

6.7 Neyman's (1934) design-based or randomization approach to survey sampling has been the dominant one since the end of World War II. During the early 1970s, however, Richard Royall, with the help from time to time of several co-authors, challenged it with great determination. He claimed that although it made no assumptions regarding unknown probability distributions, and therefore appeared to be non-parametric and robust, it was subject to serious shortcomings. Two 'notorious examples' of such shortcomings, cited in Royall (1971, p. 260), are:

1. the surprising complications encountered in the study and execution of probability-proportional-to-size sampling plans and
2. the awkwardness of almost all probabilistic calculations concerning the estimates of ratios.

(In the last few days we have ourselves had abundant evidence as to the existence of these two shortcomings!)

In the same paper, Royall also pointed to several other authors who had, from Godambe (1955) onwards, either pointed out the inadequacies of the conventional theory or else attempted to remedy them by 'erecting atop the conventional model' various probabilistic superstructures or superpopulation models. The latter of these two approaches has since led to a new orthodoxy known as model-assisted survey sampling (Särndal *et al.*, 1992), which still depends exclusively on randomization-based inference and estimators, but optimizes them under the explicit assumption that the finite population under study is itself a sample drawn from a superpopulation generated by a specific stochastic model.

Royall's own suggestion was more radical than this. He proposed to abandon randomization-based inference entirely in favour of estimators whose useful properties (unbiasedness, consistency, optimality etc.) were defined in terms of whatever ratio or regression model appeared appropriate. This meant that concepts such as bias and variance were no longer defined as expectations over all possible samples that could be drawn under the specified sample design, but rather as averages over all possible realizations of the population units (whether included in sample or not) under the assumed superpopulation model. Randomized sampling then became irrelevant, and Royall's earliest papers proposed choosing purposively whatever sample led to the most accurate estimates of the finite population total, which in practice meant selecting all the largest units!

Not surprisingly, this suggestion of Royall's appeared to promise very substantial improvements in precision as compared with conventional sampling strategies. Still less surprisingly though, inadequacies in the superpopulation models adopted resulted in unacceptable biases. Royall met this difficulty by suggesting instead the selection of *balanced samples*, defined as subsets of the finite population for which the sample moments of the auxiliary variables were equal to those of the finite population itself (Royall and Herson, 1973a, 1973b).

This was an attractive idea, since every orthodox sampling statistician is delighted when his random sample is nearly balanced, and understandably disturbed when it is clearly a long way from being balanced. The spectacular reductions in model variance obtained by choosing all the largest units were, however, no longer to be had, and Brewer (1999a) showed that the difference between the design expectation of prediction variance obtained using a random sample and the actual prediction variance obtained using a balanced sample of the same size was a small quantity of the second order.

Brewer also pointed out in the same paper that although balanced sampling designs held some advantage over comparable random samples in terms of robustness against prediction model breakdown, the random sampling designs could make up most of the difference by regressing on whatever variables the balanced sample schemes were balanced on. The choice was therefore essentially between a complicated sampling procedure (balanced sampling) with a simple estimator ($\hat{Y}_{\bullet R}$) and a simple sampling procedure (random sampling) with a more complicated estimator.

Additional points made by Brewer included the more ready public understanding of the fairness of random sampling and (perhaps even more importantly) the relative advantage of prediction-based inference for small samples and of randomization-based inference for large samples. It is this last point which is most relevant in our present situation, and therefore deserves special consideration.

6.8 It is immediately obvious that, being based on the assumption that a particular model is true, prediction inference will come under increasing stress as the sample size increases. As observed by Box (1979, p. 202), 'All models are wrong but some are useful', and while prediction models can be very useful for small samples, the fact that they are wrong becomes more and more demonstrable as the sample size increases. The choice then comes between elaborating the model to the extent that it becomes once again useful for the new sample size, and abandoning it altogether.

It is less obvious that design- or randomization-based inference itself involves the use of a model, although it is interesting to note that Royall (1971) referred explicitly to 'the conventional model' when attacking it. The nature of this model is somewhat unusual and needs to be spelt out. We may start with a quote from Brewer (1999a):

> In its pure form, design-based inference rests on what may be termed the *Representative Principle*, namely that *every unit in sample is to be treated as representing itself plus a group of non-sample units, whose properties are close to those of the sample unit, and whose number can be estimated from that unit's inclusion probability*. For stratified random sampling, that estimated number is the reciprocal of the relevant stratum's sampling fraction, minus one. For example, a sample unit in a one-in-ten stratum represents itself plus an estimated nine non-sample units.
>
> More generally, ... the Representative Principle requires that the weight given to each unit included in sample should be the reciprocal of its probability of inclusion. The estimator of total based exclusively on these weights is the Horvitz–Thompson (HT) estimator.

Taking Brewer's argument a little further, we may say that his Representative Principle, which leads directly to the HT estimator, is essentially using a model of the population as one consisting of precisely $\sum_i \delta_i \pi_i^{-1}$ units (where $i = 1, 2, \ldots, n$) and that the π_i^{-1} population units corresponding to the ith sample unit have precisely the same characteristics as the ith sample unit itself (again where $i = 1, 2, \ldots, n$). There are of course certain logical problems where π_i^{-1} is not an integer and/or where $\sum_i \delta_i \pi_i^{-1} \neq N$, but these are peripheral issues which we need not go into here. The important point is that it is indeed a model, and we have just made it an explicit model. The next most important point is that it differs radically from the prediction model, and perhaps from every other statistical model, in being based exclusively on sample observations instead of on *a priori* assumptions. Such assumptions may be – and, if the sample is large enough, almost certainly will be – overturned by sample evidence.

You referred to Kyburg's (1987) paper, and you are right; he does say 'Inverse inference proceeds from the particular to the general, direct inference from the general to the particular'. On that distinction, randomization inference is inverse inference and prediction inference is direct inference. We might add that Kyburg's paper is basically a vindication of direct inference and an attack on inverse inference (both in general and on Bayesian inference as a special case of inverse inference in particular). If you are taking your cues from Kyburg, you should not be questioning but welcoming our use of prediction inference!

It is unusual, however, to find Bayesian and randomization inference ranged together on one side of an argument, or of a definition, with frequentist and prediction inference together on the other. At one stage Royall's population modelling approach was described as looking 'exactly like a Bayesian formulation of the surveyor's background knowledge or information' (Basu, 1971, p. 242), and there is at least one sampling textbook (Bolfarine and Zacks, 1992) that is both prediction-oriented and Bayesian in its approach.

Fortunately, it is not in general necessary to make a choice of one kind of inference and reject the other. There are certainly occasions, and our recently completed assignment is one of them, where a recourse to prediction inference seems to be inescapable. Characteristically, they are occasions when the sample sizes involved are very small. But there are also situations where randomization inference works so well that there appears to be no need for any other. These will usually occur when the sample is large. Brewer (1999a) points out, however, that the tendency these days is to use randomization-based inference for large domains and synthetic sampling (which is prediction-based) for small domains *within the same population and the same study*. He advocates the use of 'cosmetically calibrated estimators' that are randomization-based and prediction-based simultaneously. [The description of such estimators as 'cosmetic' originated with Särndal and Wright (1984). They chose this word, they explained, because the fact that these estimators could be viewed or interpreted as predictors from a regression made them look attractive.]

The classical ratio estimator, which we are using here, is a very simple case of a cosmetically calibrated estimator. It is asymptotically true that the design expectation of its prediction variance and the prediction expectation of its design variance are equal. Since the approximation we are using for the design variance is an asymptotic expression, we are not surprised to find that the two variance estimates are close, despite the fact that they estimate radically different kinds of variance. We believe our recent assignment has demonstrated convincingly that the two forms of inference can indeed be used together, and that they are complementary rather than competitive in nature.

More about the Background to Our Assignment

6.9 On Monday morning we duly present ourselves in our supervisor's office. He is now happy with our text and it will duly be sent to the client. He is also receptive to the points we raised regarding regression through the origin, though we get the impression that he might want to come back to it later. The main thing he wants to talk about, however, is that 'longer note' that we gave him last Friday concerning the complementary nature of randomization-based and prediction-based inference. What he particularly wants to do is find out what light it sheds on the former circus statistician's misfortunes.

He has been in touch with the circus owner on the phone and (without giving too much away) has given him the gist of our two reports. He (our supervisor) tells us that the owner was very surprised. He had only looked cursorily at the elephant trainer's eye estimates, confirmed that Sambo's sat on the 'average' of 1.0 and given it no further thought. (Indeed, however hard the owner might have looked at the eye estimates and nothing else, he would not have picked up any clue that bulls weighed substantially more than cows. For that, he would have needed to look at the elephants themselves instead, or, better still, as well).

Apparently what had happened in the circus before we were called in was this. The owner had asked the elephant trainer which one was 'the average elephant in the herd'. The trainer had said that he always regarded Sambo as 'very typical'.

'Average in regard to weight?' pressed the owner.

'Oh yes, very typical in his weight,' replied the trainer, 'I always think of him as right on average.'

The operative words so far as the owner was concerned were 'average' and 'weight'. For the trainer, they were 'typical' and 'his'. (Yes, he was unconsciously being sexist, but no more than most of his generation.) For the trainer, an elephant coming in at the arithmetic mean of the weights of the 50 elephants would either be a very small bull like Timbo (only Flimbo being smaller) or a cow larger than any cow in the herd. Either way it would not be typical of the herd as a whole. So the owner and the trainer had quite different concepts in their minds for the word 'average', and particularly for the phrase 'average in regard to weight'. Had they eventually done what the owner had been planning to do, the estimate of the total herd weight would have been of the order of 240 tonnes, about 20% too high; but this scheme was put on hold as a result of the circus statistician's intervention. The question 'Was he perhaps sacked unfairly?' comes to mind.

But our supervisor continues with his account of the events leading to our being called in. 'So the owner plans to weigh Sambo', he tells us, 'and take $50\,Y_{35}$ (where Y_{35} is the present weight of Sambo) as an estimate of the total weight, $Y_{\bullet} = Y_1 + \cdots + Y_{50}$, of the 50 elephants. But the circus statistician is horrified when he learns of the owner's purposive sampling plan. With the help of a table of random numbers they devise a plan that allots a selection probability of 99/100 to Sambo and equal selection probabilities of 1/4900 to each of the other 49 elephants. Naturally, Sambo is selected and the owner is happy. "How are you going to estimate $Y_{\bullet}$?", asks the statistician. "Why? The estimate ought to be $50\,Y_{35}$ of course", says the owner. "Oh! No! That cannot possibly be right," says the statistician. "I recently read an article in the *Annals of Mathematical Statistics* where it is proved that the Horvitz–Thompson estimator is the unique hyperadmissible estimator in the class of all generalized polynomial unbiased estimators." "What is the Horvitz–Thompson estimator in this case?" asks the owner, duly impressed. "Since the selection probability for Sambo in our plan was 99/100," says the statistician, "the proper estimate of $Y_{\bullet}$ is $100\,Y_{35}/99$ and not $50\,Y_{35}$." "And, how would you have estimated $Y_{\bullet}$", inquires the incredulous owner, "if our sampling plan made us select, say, the big elephant Jumbo?" "According to what I understand of the Horvitz–Thompson estimation method," says the unhappy statistician, "the proper estimate of $Y_{\bullet}$ would then have been $4900\,Y_{20}$, where Y_{20} is Jumbo's weight." That is how the statistician lost his circus job (and perhaps became a teacher of statistics!)' (Basu, 1971, p. 213).

While we are still sitting there trying to take all this in, we are rudely jerked back to the present by our supervisor asking us to prepare yet another report as a follow-on from a point we had made in our 'longer note'. This new report is to be a think-piece on the advisability or otherwise of introducing an intercept term into the population model when using this combined inference. No peace for the wicked . . .

7

The Simple Regression Estimator and Synthetic Estimation

Report for Supervisor: Introduction 107
Circumstances Favourable for Simple Regression Estimation 108
Questionable Reasons for Using Simple Regression Estimation 109
Properties of the Simple Regression Estimator 112
Some Empirical Evidence 119
Summary 121
Conclusions 121
Response from Supervisor 121
Exercises 121

Report for Supervisor: Introduction

7.1 You have asked us to consider the question as to whether and in what circumstances it would be appropriate to introduce an intercept term into the ratio-type population model that we used to arrive at a suitable estimate of the weight of the circus elephants. The model we used was the one introduced at the start of **5.2**, namely,

$$\xi_R: \quad Y_i = \beta X_i + U_i; \quad \mathrm{E}_{\xi_R} U_i = 0; \quad \mathrm{E}_{\xi_R} U_i^2 = \sigma_i^2; \quad \mathrm{E}_{\xi_R}(U_i U_j) = 0, \quad j \neq i; \quad i = 1, 2, \ldots, N. \tag{7.1}$$

(The subscript h has been dropped for this report, as we will not be considering more than a single stratum at a time).

It is customary to introduce the intercept term into this model by using a very simple form of ordinary least squares known as simple regression estimation. This model is specified as

$$\xi_O: \quad Y_i = \alpha_O + \beta_O X_i + U_i; \quad \mathrm{E}_{\xi_O} U_i = 0; \quad \mathrm{E}_{\xi_O} U_i^2 = \sigma^2; \quad \mathrm{E}_{\xi_O}(U_i U_j) = 0, \quad j \neq i; \quad i, j = 1, 2, \ldots, N. \tag{7.2}$$

This differs from ξ_R in two ways. The first is the additional parameter, α_O, which is the coefficient on the intercept term. Its corresponding regressor variable is a column vector of ones. The second is that the residual or error term, U_i, is now specified to be *homoscedastic* (Greek for 'uniformly spread'), which is to say that all the U_i now have the same variance, σ^2. When using ξ_R, we estimated each of the

σ_i^2 individually (although we only used the sum of the estimates when estimating the variance of the ratio estimator $\hat{Y}_{\bullet R}$ of the population total, $Y_{\bullet}$). With ξ_O we estimate only a single variance parameter, σ^2, but we may still choose to estimate the squared error terms individually and pool them, as we did in Chapter 1.

The best linear unbiased estimators of the parameters for model ξ_O are

$$\hat{\beta}_O = \frac{n\sum_i \delta_i Y_i X_i - \left(\sum_i \delta_i Y_i\right)\left(\sum_i \delta_i X_i\right)}{n\sum_i \delta_i X_i^2 - \left(\sum_i \delta_i X_i\right)^2} \tag{7.3}$$

and

$$\hat{\alpha}_O = \hat{\bar{Y}} - \hat{\beta}_O \hat{\bar{X}} = \frac{\left(\sum_i \delta_i Y_i\right)\left(\sum_i \delta_i X_i^2\right) - \left(\sum_i \delta_i Y_i X_i\right)\left(\sum_i \delta_i X_i\right)}{n\sum_i \delta_i X_i^2 - \left(\sum_i \delta_i X_i\right)^2}. \tag{7.4}$$

Using these estimators, the regression estimator of the same population total, $Y_{\bullet}$, is

$$\hat{Y}_{\bullet O} = \frac{N}{n}\sum_i \delta_i Y_i + \left(N - \frac{N}{n}\sum_i \delta_i\right)\hat{\alpha}_O + \left(X_{\bullet} - \frac{N}{n}\sum_i \delta_i X_i\right)\hat{\beta}_O,$$

or equivalently (since $\sum_i \delta_i = n$),

$$\hat{Y}_{\bullet O} = \frac{N}{n}\sum_i \delta_i Y_i + \left(X_{\bullet} - \frac{N}{n}\sum_i \delta_i X_i\right)\hat{\beta}_O. \tag{7.5}$$

Note that when the entire population is in sample, $\hat{Y}_{\bullet O} = Y_{\bullet}$, so the simple regression estimator is Cochran consistent. It is our considered opinion, however, that the circumstances in which simple regression estimation is preferable to classical ratio estimation do not occur very often.

Circumstances Favourable for Simple Regression Estimation

7.2 In other fields of interest, notably econometrics, simple regression and the generalized form of it known as ordinary least squares are used fairly commonly. They are likely to be useful if the following three conditions hold simultaneously:

1. The range of the data is limited to a region far removed from the origin.
2. Linear dependency holds to a fair degree of approximation within the data range.
3. There is no reason to believe that the dependency of the Y_i on the X_i is simply proportional (a ratio relationship) whether it passes through the origin or not.

These three conditions do sometimes hold also in the context of survey sampling. Australian farm surveys provide a good example of this, in the relationship between value of production and farm size. Where there is no land, there is no

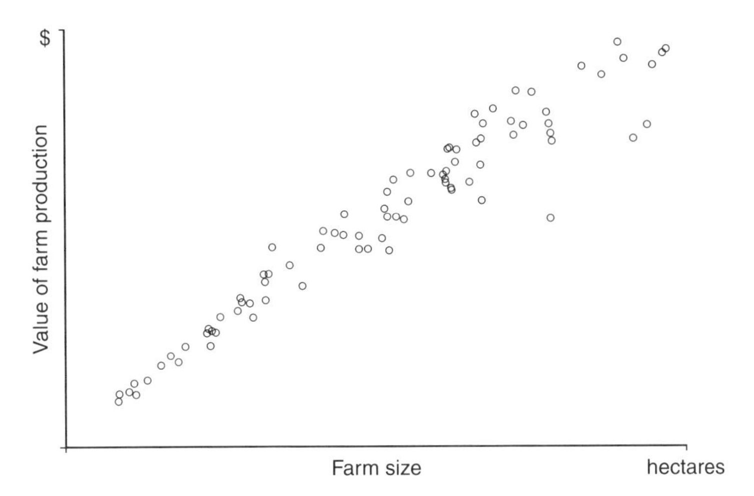

Figure 7.1 A heuristic representation of Australian broadacre farm data exhibiting heteroscedasticity and a non-linear relationship passing through the origin.

production; so the relationship necessarily passes through the origin. But there is also an inverse relationship between farm area and land quality, so the slope of the relationship is a decreasing function of farm size, and it is not appropriate to omit the intercept term, when carrying out regressions of production on farm size over limited ranges of that size variable, except where a stratum contains only very small farms (Figure 7.1).

Another example of where these three conditions can hold is the estimation of total household consumption using a consumption function (relationship between consumption expenditure and income) estimated from a household survey. Consumption expenditure is a survey variable, measured only for the sample households. Income is a census variable and known for nearly all households, so a useful supplementary variable as well as a necessary input into the consumption function. It is well known that consumption is nearly a linear function of income with a considerable positive intercept on the consumption axis when the households are similar in size and composition. The intercept can be interpreted as the amount a household would need to dis-save if it were suddenly left without any source of income (Figure 7.2).

Questionable Reasons for Using Simple Regression Estimation

7.3 We will next examine whether there are any other reasons for using model ξ_O that might hold water.

1. A belief that the introduction of a second parameter makes the model more flexible and therefore potentially more realistic.

While this belief seems to persist in some quarters, there is no good case for it. It is well known that regressor variables, when introduced for reasons other than

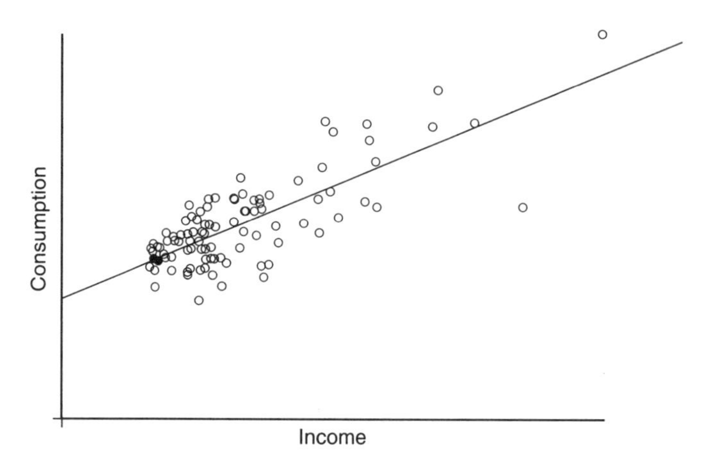

Figure 7.2 A heuristic representation of a household consumption function.

that they may have appreciable explanatory power, tend to increase rather than decrease the estimates of variance. Under OLS, they take up a degree of freedom, but explain very little.

It is more often the case than not, in survey sampling, that the most appropriate supplementary variable is close to being proportional to its corresponding survey variable, and that their natural relationship or line of best fit is a straight line through the origin. If the range of the supplementary variable is limited (and it often is limited by the process of stratification on size) then the inclusion of an intercept term permits the estimated relationship to stray well away from the origin, with a consequent loss of efficiency.

2. The wish to be able to calibrate the estimates on the known total number of population units, N, as well as on the known total, $X_{\bullet}$, of the principal supplementary variable.

There are two cases to be considered here. The first is the kind of survey in which each survey variable can be associated with a particular most suitable supplementary variable. An example would be a retail establishment survey where current sales of groceries are paired with known census sales of groceries, and the same pairing is used for other items (survey variables) such as clothing, footwear and hardware. In this case, the weight accorded to a sample unit can vary from item to item, and no harm is done, because the only outcome is the publication of estimated totals for these items. In this case, there is no reason to introduce any intercept term.

The other case is where the survey data are to be made available (usually stripped of any identification) to a wider public. That wider public includes, most importantly, secondary analysts who wish to explore relationships between items, and for whom a multitude of different survey weights for different items within the same sample record is a serious inconvenience. It is then important to produce a single *case weight* for all items, one for each sample unit. This is achieved by regressing on a considerable set of explanatory variables simultaneously, and that set may or may not include an intercept term. But here we are a long way away from the concept of simple regression.

3. The wish to have estimated residuals that sum exactly to zero, either so as to be able to use certain statistics for hypothesis testing, notably the F statistic, or to ensure that the model being fitted is not manifestly unsuitable.

Although hypothesis testing is seldom carried out in the context of finite-population sampling, situations do occasionally arise that call for it. However, a zero mean for the estimated residuals can only be achieved by way of including an intercept term if the model used reflects an assumption that the residuals themselves are homoscedastic. The model ξ_O certainly incorporates that assumption, but making the assumption of homoscedasticity does not make the actual residuals homoscedastic.

In fact, homoscedasticity is the exception rather than the rule for sample survey populations. Typically, the model variances of the units that constitute most finite populations increase with size. At the end of **5.2** we noted that $\sigma_i^2 \propto X_i^{2\gamma}$, with $0.5 \leq \gamma \leq 1$, was a commonly used and not unreasonable way to model heteroscedasticity, and now is a good time to explain why.

Consider a population, say of retail stores, containing both large and small units. In this particular population, the large units consist of loose aggregations of what were originally small units, and effectively each original component of any such aggregation acts independently of each other such component. Variances are additive under independence, so $\sigma_i^2 \propto X_i$ and $\gamma = 0.5$. A smaller value than 0.5 would imply that components within such aggregations differed among themselves more than they differed from components of other units. A mechanism for such behaviour is difficult to imagine, so a reasonable lower limit for γ is 0.5.

At the other extreme, consider another population containing both large and small units in which the actions of each unit are tightly controlled by its own central management. There will then be a tendency for the σ_i^2 to increase more rapidly with size than they did in the population previously considered. Again, however, it is difficult to imagine a situation in which the *proportionate* variability (as measured by σ_i^2/X_i^2 or σ_i/X_i) increases with size, because random shocks usually tend to affect small units proportionally more than they do large units. This indicates an upper limit of 1.0 for γ. Putting these two considerations together, we arrive at $0.5 \leq \gamma \leq 1$.

When $\gamma = 0.5$ (i.e. $\sigma_i^2 \propto X_i$), the BLUE of the regression coefficient β is $\hat{\beta}_R = \sum_i \delta_i Y_i / \sum_i \delta_i X_i$, so that the classical ratio estimator, $\hat{Y}_{\bullet R} = \hat{\beta}_R X_{\bullet}$, is also the best linear predictor of the population total $Y_{\bullet}$ (see Exercise **7.1**). For this estimator, the mean of the residuals is not generally equal to zero. But as just explained, the mean of the residuals does not automatically become zero when this extra term is introduced. For that to happen, we need to specify, in addition, that $\sigma_i^2 = \sigma^2$ for all $i = 1, \ldots, N$ (again see Exercise **7.1**). But, of course, the true residuals are not homoscedastic, so the value of such a specification must be questionable.

Why, in fact, should we ever need to insist that the mean of the estimated residuals be zero? If the intercept term is not included, the mean of the estimated residuals may be a long way from zero, and this is usually a symptom of the assumed model being incorrect. If that mean is in fact both appreciably and significantly different from zero, something should be done about finding a better model, but it may not be clear what that something is.

An easy way out is to stipulate that the population model is a homoscedastic one with an intercept term, since this guarantees that the mean of the estimated residuals will be zero. But this amounts to no more than getting rid of an embarrassing symptom without doing what really needs to be done – namely, find a genuinely realistic model for the population. When we do that, we might, for instance, find that the realistic model is a heteroscedastic ratio one with $\gamma = 0.5$. In that case, the classical ratio estimator with $\hat{R} = \sum_i \delta_i Y_i / \sum_i \delta_i X_i$ is actually optimal; in other words, it is the BLUE for the β in the model

$$\xi_{0.5}\colon\quad Y_i = \beta X_i + U_i; \quad \mathrm{E}_{\xi_{0.5}} U_i = 0; \quad \mathrm{E}_{\xi_{0.5}} U_i^2 = \sigma^2 X_i; \quad \mathrm{E}_{\xi_{0.5}} (U_i U_j) = 0, \quad j \neq i; \quad i = 1, 2, \ldots, N$$

(see Exercise 7.2). In such circumstances the adoption of the OLS model ξ_O is clearly inappropriate. The correct way to ensure that the residuals have zero mean is to introduce instead a regressor variable for which the values are proportional to the σ_i, but there is no obvious meaning that could be attached to the coefficient on it. It hardly seems an objective worth pursuing.

7.4 Although we are quite convinced that the simple regression estimator is inappropriate in most sample survey contexts, it may reasonably be asked how this estimator has managed to survive in survey sampling textbooks and (we imagine) also occasionally in practice. If it is as bad as we are painting it, why is it not notoriously the case that it does not work and should not be used?

The answer may well be that, to the extent that it has been used at all, it has been used almost exclusively in contexts where it could not do much harm. It has probably been used primarily in large samples with estimators that have a design- or randomization-based validity. It is only when such a sample is divided among small domains, and hence effectively loses the support provided by design-based inference, that the weakness of the simple regression estimator becomes particularly apparent, but even in contexts where it does relatively little harm, it seldom does any appreciable good. In the remainder of this report we provide mathematical and empirical evidence for these assertions.

Properties of the Simple Regression Estimator

7.5 As noted in **7.2**, finite populations are only rarely homoscedastic, and in consequence the equation $\mathrm{E}_{\xi_O} U_i^2 = \sigma^2$ in (7.2) is unrealistic. Also, more often than not, the relationship between Y_i and X_i clearly has to go through the origin. A better choice of model in such circumstances is the ξ_R of (7.1).

The optimal estimator for the β of (7.1) is one that uses *weighted* least squares (WLS):

$$\hat{\beta} = \frac{\sum_i \delta_i Y_i X_i \sigma_i^{-2}}{\sum_i \delta_i X_i^2 \sigma_i^{-2}} \tag{7.6}$$

(Exercise 7.2). If we substitute $Y_i = \beta X_i + U_i$ from (7.1) into (7.6) we obtain

$$\hat{\beta} = \beta + \frac{\sum_i \delta_i U_i X_i \sigma_i^{-2}}{\sum_i \delta_i X_i^2 \sigma_i^{-2}}. \tag{7.7}$$

Since $\mathrm{E}_\xi U_i = 0$, the $\hat{\beta}$ of (7.6) and (7.7) is a prediction-unbiased estimator of β; also the random error term has the minimum possible variance under ξ, and the line of best fit goes through the origin. If, however, we substitute that same $Y_i = \beta X_i + U_i$ from (7.1) into the OLS formulae (7.3) and (7.4), we obtain

$$\hat{\beta}_O = \beta + \frac{n \sum_i \delta_i U_i X_i - \left(\sum_i \delta_i U_i\right)\left(\sum_i \delta_i X_i\right)}{n \sum_i \delta_i X_i^2 - \left(\sum_i \delta_i X_i\right)^2} \tag{7.8}$$

and

$$\hat{\alpha}_O = \hat{\bar{Y}} - \hat{\beta}_O \hat{\bar{X}} = \frac{\left(\sum_i \delta_i U_i\right)\left(\sum_i \delta_i X_i^2\right) - \left(\sum_i \delta_i U_i X_i\right)\left(\sum_i \delta_i X_i\right)}{n \sum_i \delta_i X_i^2 - \left(\sum_i \delta_i X_i\right)^2}. \tag{7.9}$$

If $\hat{\beta}_O$ is regarded as an estimator of β, it is still ξ_R-unbiased, but the random error term in (7.8) is larger than the one in (7.7). In addition, even though the prediction expectation of $\hat{\alpha}_O$ in (7.9) is zero, $\hat{\alpha}_O$ itself is not generally equal to zero, so the line of best fit through the sample data almost never goes through the origin. The OLS model is therefore suboptimal, but the fact that β is still estimated without model bias may indicate that all is reasonably well under control.

A third reason for concern appears when we examine more closely the suitability of model ξ_R itself. The primary equation in that model, $Y_i = \beta X_i + U_i$, may also be written $X_i = \beta^{-1} Y_i - \beta^{-1} U_i = \beta^{-1} Y_i + U_{2i}$. In the context of our sampling of elephants, this is actually a better way of looking at the situation, because the eye estimate X_i is a random function of the true weight Y_i, rather than the other way around. But if we substitute

$$\xi_{R2}\colon\quad X_i = \beta^{-1} Y_i + U_{2i};\quad \mathrm{E}_{\xi_{R2}} U_{2i} = 0;\quad \mathrm{E}_{\xi_{R2}} U_{2i}^2 = \sigma_{2i}^2;\quad \mathrm{E}_{\xi_{R2}} U_{2i} U_{2j} = 0,$$
$$j \neq i;\quad i, j = 1, 2, \ldots, N \tag{7.10}$$

into (7.3), we obtain

$$
\begin{aligned}
\mathrm{E}_{\xi R2}\hat{\beta}_O &= \mathrm{E}_{\xi R2}\left[\frac{n\sum_i \delta_i Y_i X_i - \left(\sum_i \delta_i Y_i\right)\left(\sum_i \delta_i X_i\right)}{n\sum_i \delta_i X_i^2 - \left(\sum_i \delta_i X_i\right)^2}\right] \\
&= \mathrm{E}_{\xi R2}\left[\frac{\beta^{-1}\left\{n\sum_i \delta_i Y_i^2 - \left(\sum_i \delta_i Y_i\right)^2\right\} + n\sum_i \delta_i Y_i U_{2i} - \left(\sum_i \delta_i Y_i\right)\left(\sum_i \delta_i U_{2i}\right)}{n\sum_i\{\beta^{-1}Y_i + U_{2i}\}^2 - \left\{\sum_i(\beta^{-1}Y_i + U_{2i})\right\}^2}\right] \\
&< \mathrm{E}_{\xi R2}\left[\frac{\beta^{-1}\left\{n\sum_i \delta_i Y_i^2 - \left(\sum_i \delta_i Y_i\right)^2\right\} + n\sum_i \delta_i Y_i U_{2i} - \left(\sum_i \delta_i Y_i\right)\left(\sum_i \delta_i U_{2i}\right)}{\beta^{-2}\left\{n\sum_i \delta_i Y_i^2 - \left(\sum_i \delta_i Y_i\right)^2\right\}}\right] \\
&= \beta + \beta^2 \mathrm{E}_{\xi R2}\left[\frac{n\sum_i \delta_i Y_i U_{2i} - \left(\sum_i \delta_i Y_i\right)\left(\sum_i \delta_i U_{2i}\right)}{n\sum_i \delta_i Y_i^2 - \left(\sum_i \delta_i Y_i\right)^2}\right]. \qquad (7.11)
\end{aligned}
$$

But the expectation of U_{2i} is zero, so $\mathrm{E}_{\xi R2}\hat{\beta}_O < \beta$.

It may fairly be objected that this bias is a consequence of the rather unusual situation where X_i is stochastically dependent on Y_i rather than the other way round. What is more common, however, is for neither to be strictly dependent on the other, but for the two to be co-dependent. We have already mentioned in **6.6** that if two continuously distributed variables, x and y, both having positive means, are positively correlated, and if the natural relationship between them passes through the origin, then the regression of y on x has a positive intercept on the x-axis and the regression of x on y has a positive intercept on the y-axis (Figure 7.3). Many

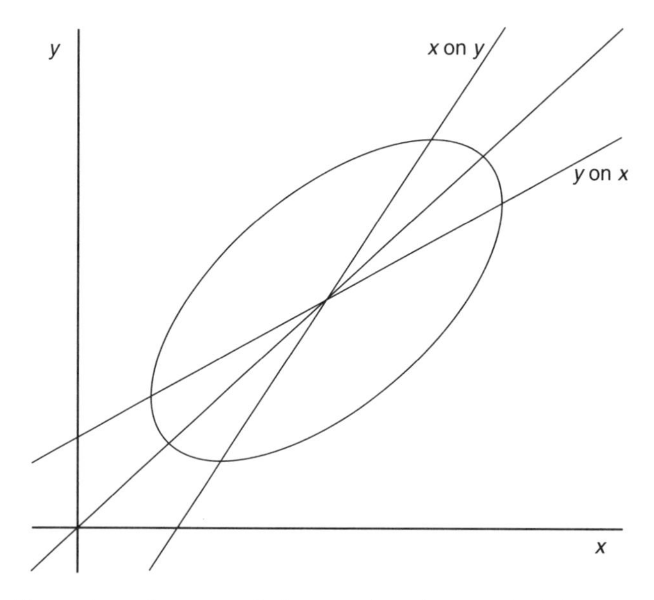

Figure 7.3 Regressions of y on x and of x on y when the natural relationship between them passes through the origin.

survey sampling situations resemble this, and the result $E_{\xi_{R2}}\hat{\beta}_O < \beta$ will still hold in such cases.

Note that this bias does not tend to diminish as the sample size increases, so (wherever such a bias exists) it is necessary to rely on something more than a large sample size to ensure that inferences based on the OLS model are acceptable. It is true that $\hat{Y}_{\bullet O}$ is Cochran consistent, that its design bias is only of order n^{-1} (Cochran, 1977, pp. 198–199) and that for large samples it usually estimates $Y_{\bullet}$ reasonably well. As we shall see, however, 'reasonably well' is not the same as 'efficiently', and if not supported by design-based inference, even estimators that look very similar to $\hat{Y}_{\bullet O}$ can be highly unreliable.

7.6 The existence of this negative bias in $\hat{\beta}_O$ when used to estimate β is a matter for some concern, but for small samples it is less serious than the extent of the variance of $\hat{\beta}_O$. Consider what would have happened had we fitted the ξ_O of (7.2) to the sample consisting of Linda, Pamela and Sara. We would then have estimated the slope by

$$\begin{aligned}\hat{\beta}_O &= \frac{3328 \times 1.1 + 3427 \times 1.1 + 2910 - 9665 \times 3.2/3}{1.1^2 + 1.1^2 + 1^2 - 3.2^2/3} \\ &= \frac{10\,340.5 - 30\,928/3}{3.42 - 10.24/3} \\ &= 4675,\end{aligned}$$

and the intercept by

$$\hat{\alpha}_O = \hat{\bar{Y}} - \hat{\beta}_O\hat{\bar{X}} = \frac{9665}{3} - \frac{4675 \times 3.2}{3} = -1765.$$

(Note that 4675 is the sample estimate (in kilograms per 'Sara') of the regression slope for the cows' stratum. It depends completely and exclusively on the weights of Linda, Pamela and Sara. It so happens that Combo's weight is also 4675 kg, a number you are probably quite familiar with by now. But all the occurrences of the number 4675 in the remainder of this chapter relate only to the cows' stratum and have nothing to go with Combo, so please do not get confused!) Substituting these values of $\hat{\beta}_O$ and $\hat{\alpha}_O$ into the expression $\hat{\alpha}_O + \hat{\beta}_O X_i$, we can obtain prediction-estimated weights for every elephant in the cows' stratum. When we do that, however, we find that the estimated weight of Amanda, the largest cow, is $1.2 \times 4675 - 1765$ or 3845 kg while that of, say, Edna, one of the smallest, is $0.85 \times 4675 - 1765$ or 2209 kg. That makes the largest cow 1.74 times as heavy as the smallest. The elephant trainer's estimate of the ratio is $1.2/0.85$ or 1.41. We may not be elephant trainers ourselves, but just by casual observation, we are reasonably sure that 1.74 is an overestimate.

Attacking the estimation problem from that direction, it may come as something of a surprise that the estimated total weight of the 25 cows would, using that equation, be $25.3 \times 4675 - 25 \times 1765$ or 74 153 kg. This is only about 2250 kg below the general drift of estimates we were getting for the cows' stratum, and within tolerable limits. How can the estimate of total come out so acceptably when the predicted weights for the individual cows are so suspect?

7.7 This question can be answered from either the design-based or the prediction-based standpoint. We will use the design-based approach first. From that point of view, the relevant individual (metric) weights are those of the three sample cows, and these are known without any appreciable error. Each cow is also given a sample weight or case weight (not measured in kilograms!) indicating how many of the 25 cows in the stratum it represents, and these case weights are required to sum to 25. How could the estimate of total possibly be badly out?

To discover what these case weights are, we write (7.5) in the form

$$\begin{aligned}
\hat{Y}_{\bullet O} &= \frac{N}{n}\sum_i \delta_i Y_i + \left(X_{\bullet} - \frac{N}{n}\sum_i \delta_i X_i\right)\hat{\beta}_O \\
&= \frac{N}{n}\sum_i \delta_i Y_i + \frac{\{X_{\bullet} - (N/n)\sum_i \delta_i X_i\}\left\{\sum_i \delta_i Y_i X_i - n^{-1}(\sum_i \delta_i Y_i)(\sum_i \delta_i X_i)\right\}}{\sum_i \delta_i X_i^2 - n^{-1}(\sum_i \delta_i X_i)^2} \\
&= \frac{N}{n}\sum_i \delta_i Y_i + K_s\left\{\sum_i \delta_i Y_i X_i - n^{-1}\left(\sum_i \delta_i Y_i\right)\left(\sum_i \delta_i X_i\right)\right\},
\end{aligned}$$

where $K_s = \left\{X_{\bullet} - (N/n)\sum_i \delta_i X_i\right\} / \left\{\sum_i \delta_i X_i^2 - n^{-1}\left(\sum_i \delta_i X_i\right)^2\right\}$. Then

$$\hat{Y}_{\bullet O} = \sum_i \delta_i Y_i \left\{\frac{N}{n} + K_s X_i - n^{-1} K_s \left(\sum_k \delta_k X_k\right)\right\}. \tag{7.12}$$

The case weights W_{si} (for the unit i included in the sample s) are defined by

$$\hat{Y}_{\bullet O} = \sum_i \delta_i Y_i W_{si}. \tag{7.13}$$

Comparing coefficients of (7.12) and (7.13)

$$W_{si} = \frac{N}{n} + K_s\left(X_i - n^{-1}\sum_k \delta_k X_k\right) \tag{7.14}$$

For the cows' stratum, $N = 25$, $n = 3$, $X_{\bullet} = 25.3$, $\delta_i X_i = (1.1, 1.1, 1.0)$, $\sum_k \delta_k X_k = 3.2$ and $\sum_k \delta_k X_k^2 = 3.42$. Substituting these values into $K_s = \{X_{\bullet} - (N/n)\sum_i \delta_i X_i\} / \left\{\sum_i \delta_i X_i^2 - n^{-1}\left(\sum_i \delta_i X_i\right)^2\right\}$, we obtain

$$K_s = \frac{25.3 - 3.2 \times 25/3}{3.42 - 10.24/3} = -205.$$

Substituting into (7.14), we obtain

$$W_{C12} = W_{C16} = \frac{25}{3} - 205\left(1.1 - \frac{1}{3} \times 3.2\right) = 1.5$$

and

$$W_{C18} = \frac{25}{3} - 205\left(1.0 - \frac{1}{3} \times 3.2\right) = 22.$$

The sum of the case weights is indeed 25, which is reasonable, but the discrepancy between the 1.5 for Linda and Pamela and the 22 for Sara constitutes a warning that the estimate is likely to be inefficient. By contrast, the case weights for the classical ratio estimate are each 25.3/3.2 or 7.906 25. With equal weights, the estimator is close to being fully efficient, and if we limit ourselves to the context of sampling *srswr*, it is fully efficient.

This may be seen as follows. A convenient approximation to the efficiency of a weighted sample mean with unequal weights W_i based on a sample of n units drawn using *srswr* can be constructed as follows. When the relevant random variable (Y_i, say) has the same variance, σ^2, for each sample unit, the best estimator of the population mean is the unweighted sample mean, $\sum_i \nu_i Y_i n^{-1}$. Since there is no finite-population correction, the variance of that sample mean is $\sigma^2 n^{-1}$. With unequal weights W_i, however, the weighted sample mean is $\sum_i \nu_i W_i Y_i / \sum_i \nu_i W_i$, and again with no finite-population correction its variance is $\sum_i \nu_i^2 W_i^2 \sigma^2 / \left(\sum_i \nu_i W_i\right)^2$. In this circumstance the approximate efficiency of the weighted estimate is the ratio of $\sigma^2 n^{-1}$ to $\sum_i \nu_i^2 W_i^2 \sigma^2 / \left(\sum_i \nu_i W_i\right)^2$ or $\left(\sum_i \nu_i W_i\right)^2 / n \sum_i \nu_i^2 W_i^2$. Substituting the weights 1.5, 1.5 and 22, we find that $\sum_i \nu_i W_i = 25$ and $\sum_i \nu_i^2 W_i^2 = 488.5$, so the approximate efficiency of the regression estimate (as compared with the ratio estimate) is $625/1465.5 = 0.4265$. The support provided by design-based inference in the context of this model breakdown may be saving us from complete disaster, but not from a fairly serious inefficiency.

Here we have been dealing with a sample of only three cows, and it is not surprising to see that α and β have been poorly estimated, given that the sample is so small. If the sample size is progressively increased, the efficiency with which these two parameters are estimated will improve, up to the point where the potential biases demonstrated at the end of **7.5** will start to show up (if they exist at all). With large sample sizes, the variances of $\hat{\alpha}$ and $\hat{\beta}$ are no problem, but it must be emphasized that we are talking here about the sample size we are using to estimate the α and β within a particular stratum, and that can be something much smaller than the sample size for the entire survey.

So far we have been considering the situation from the point of view of model-assisted design-based inference (equal inclusion probabilities implying equal weights). From the point of view of prediction-based inference, it is the strong negative correlation between the estimates of slope and intercept that has saved the day, even though the sample size is small, but the notion that we can obtain additional accuracy by estimating two parameters instead of one cannot be sustained in a situation like this. From a prediction-based viewpoint, estimates should never be based on a model that is clearly less realistic than another model of equal or greater simplicity. Model ξ_O is less simple and in most instances less realistic than the ξ_R of (7.2). In the next section we will consider what would happen if such unrealistic individual predictions were used to estimate domains within a population or stratum.

7.8 We have already noted that the validity of design-based or randomization-based inference is based on the Representative Principle, according to which the ith population unit, if it is included in sample, is regarded as representing itself and about $\pi_i^{-1} - 1$ other reasonably similar population units that have not been included in sample (π_i being the inclusion probability of that ith population unit). In any given situation there is a minimum size of sample below which it is unsafe to rely on the Representative Principle. That minimum depends on what is required to be estimated, the precision required for the estimate, the estimator being used, and the intrinsic variability of the population in terms of that estimator.

In the case of the elephants that we were weighing recently, we had a sample size of 5 only. By any standards, that is a very small sample, and the Representative Principle cannot be guaranteed to work effectively. And once we found that we had to use prediction-based inference, there was no escape from the need to find the best available model.

7.9 Consider now the case where we might have wanted to estimate the combined weight of the seven heaviest cows, that of the middle-sized ten, and that of the lightest eight, as indicated by the elephant trainer's eye estimates. We will first use synthetic estimates based on the simple regression estimator for this purpose, and then compare them with synthetic estimates that have been based on the classical ratio estimator instead.

To use the simple regression estimator, we develop (7.5) in prediction form as follows:

$$\begin{aligned}\hat{Y}_{\bullet O} &= \frac{N}{n}\sum_i \delta_i Y_i + \left(X_\bullet - \frac{N}{n}\sum_i \delta_i X_i\right)\hat{\beta}_O, &(7.5)\\ &= N\hat{\alpha}_O + \left(\frac{N}{n}\sum_i \delta_i X_i\right)\hat{\beta}_O + \left(X_\bullet - \frac{N}{n}\sum_i \delta_i X_i\right)\hat{\beta}_O\\ &= N\hat{\alpha}_O + X_\bullet\hat{\beta}_O\\ &= \sum_i (\hat{\alpha}_O + X_i\hat{\beta}_O). &(7.15)\end{aligned}$$

Since the ξ_O of (7.2) is being used as the prediction model, the BLUPs for the individual population units are given by $\hat{Y}_i = \hat{\alpha}_O + X_i\hat{\beta}_O$ and the simple regression estimator is the sum of those BLUPs over the population (or stratum).

If we now sum these BLUPs for the cow elephants over the three size groups just mentioned, we find that the seven heaviest cows have an estimated total weight of

$$\begin{aligned}&7\hat{\alpha}_O + (1.20 + 1.10 + 1.15 + 1.10 + 1.10 + 1.10 + 1.10)\hat{\beta}_O\\ &\quad = 7 \times (-1765) + 7.85 \times 4675 \cong 24\,344\ \text{kg},\end{aligned}$$

an average of 3478 kg per cow.

The ten cows of medium size have an estimated total weight of

$$10\,\hat{\alpha}_O + (1.00 + 1.00 + 1.05 + 1.00 + 1.05 + 1.00 + 1.00 + 1.00 + 1.00 + 1.05)\hat{\beta}_O = 10 \times (-1765) + 10.15 \times 4675) \cong 29\,801\ \text{kg},$$

an average of 2980 kg per cow.

Finally, the eight lightest cows have an estimated total weight of

$$8\,\hat{\alpha}_O + (0.85 + 0.95 + 0.90 + 0.95 + 0.95 + 0.90 + 0.90 + 0.90)\hat{\beta}_O = 8 \times (-1765) + 7.3 \times 4675 \cong 20\,008\ \text{kg},$$

an average of 2501 kg per cow.

The total for the stratum is, as before, a fraction over 74 150 kg, but the estimates for the largest and the smallest size group indicate a greater dispersion in size than that indicated by the elephant trainer's eye estimates.

Carrying out the same exercise for the classical ratio estimator, we obtain an appreciably different set of synthetic estimates: 23 709 kg for the seven heaviest cows, 30 656 kg for the ten of medium size and 22 048 kg for the eight lightest. The simple regression estimates are not startlingly different from these, but we know now that they are less efficient. And precisely because they are not obviously wrong, they can be subtly misleading. We are all the more convinced from this exercise of the importance of putting the regression line through the origin.

7.10 It should be noted that such synthetic estimates can still be unreliable, even if based on large sample sizes. At the end of **7.5** we mentioned a bias in the estimation of β that was due to co-dependence between Y_i and X_i or, in the more extreme case, counter-dependence of X_i on Y_i. We noted also that the bias did not diminish with sample size. Suppose, then, that a large sample is selected from such a population, that the simple regression estimator is used to estimate the total, and finally that synthetic estimation is used to estimate domains or subpopulations within that population. In those circumstances, the 'co-dependence bias' might possibly be large enough to make those domain estimates unreliable, in the same way as the small-sample estimates of α_O and β_O made the synthetic estimates unreliable in **7.9**.

Some Empirical Evidence

7.11 There is not a great deal of empirical evidence available to us on this topic, which is perhaps not surprising considering that it is somewhat heretical to suggest that an intercept term does more harm than good, but a recent conference paper (Brewer and Gregoire, 2001) does present some relevant results.

Brewer and Gregoire were carrying out a Monte Carlo study of 14 443 loblolly pine trees in Alabama. The aim of their exercise was to estimate as accurately as possible the total volume of timber obtainable from these trees given samples of 145, 48 and 16 drawn using different selection procedures and different estimators.

For estimation purposes, they first constructed a number of regression models of the entire population (excluding for that purpose nine trees that were clearly atypical). Some of these models were better than others. The performance of the poorer models was usually improved by the introduction of an intercept term, acting here as a substitute or proxy in the absence of any more relevant regressor, but the better the model, the less it was improved by the intercept term.

Their best-fitting model was one in which the two regressor variables were $A_i^{4/3}$ and H_i^4, where A_i was bole area 4 feet above ground level for the ith tree and H_i was its eye-determined height. This rather unlikely choice of regressor variables calls for some explanation. These particular trees become progressively thicker as they grow, and A_i was empirically found to be proportional to the cube of H_i (rather than its square). Hence volume, being proportional to A_iH_i, had to be proportional to H_i^4 as well as to $A_i^{4/3}$.

The heteroscedasticity of the residuals in their best-fitting regression equations was of a strictly multiplicative kind ($\gamma = 1$). This being so, Brewer and Gregoire might have chosen to log-transform all the variables in the regression, in which case the logarithm of the proportionality constant would have become an intercept term itself. They did not do this, however, because small trees with large negative logarithms for $A_i^{4/3}$ and H_i^4 would then have become highly influential, which would not be appropriate for a study where the emphasis was on estimating total volume. Instead, using untransformed data obtained from random systematic samples (Goodman and Kish, 1950), they came up with the following percentage root mean squared errors (RMSEs) and percentage biases for the best-fitting regression models:

	Sample size 145		Sample size 48		Sample size 16	
Model regressors	%RMSE	%Bias	%RMSE	%Bias	%RMSE	%Bias
$A_i^{4/3}$	2.17	0.03	4.15	0.01	7.48	0.11
$A_i^{4/3}$, 1	2.19	0.10	4.22	0.26	7.93	1.06
$A_i^{4/3}$, H_i^4	1.65	0.12	3.03	0.39	5.06	0.94
$A_i^{4/3}$, H_i^4, 1	1.69	0.15	2.96	0.33	5.19	1.15

Comparing these rows in pairs, the introduction of an intercept term into the equation with the single regressor $A_i^{4/3}$ increased all three RMSEs and all three biases, while its introduction into the model with the regressors $A_i^{4/3}$ and H_i^4, increased two of the three RMSEs and two of the three observed biases. For these well-fitting models, the additional degree of freedom used up produced virtually no improvement in the estimate for any sample size. Similar results were also obtained using ordered systematic sampling, Poisson sampling and collocated sampling. (For a description of collocated sampling, see Brewer *et al.*, 1972; 1984.)

Summary

7.12 In normal circumstances, survey variables are better catered for by the classical ratio estimator than by the simple regression estimator. This happens because those variables are better described by a mildly heteroscedastic model *without* an intercept term than by a homoscedastic model *with* an intercept term. The introduction of an intercept term can help if the model chosen is relatively poor, but can actually increase the bias and variance of the estimator if the model is well chosen in other respects. If the sample size is large enough, and/or if design-based inference is being used, these problems become much less pressing. In consequence, the most serious problems arise when the inference relates to a small domain and the estimator is synthetic (i.e. not supported by design-based inference).

Conclusions

7.13 We may draw four practical conclusions. First, and fairly firmly, where the true relationship between the survey variable and the supplementary variable is naturally a straight line through the origin, it is better not to introduce an intercept term. Second, and tentatively, when that relationship is through the origin, but not a straight line, it may be advisable to estimate the relationship in an explicitly non-linear fashion across all sizes. Third, and firmly, it is particularly important to avoid introducing an intercept term unnecessarily when the sample size is very small (as with our elephant-weighing problem) as it not only wastes but actually misuses a whole degree of freedom. Fourth, firmly and most importantly, any estimator used in survey sampling should be based on the best model that can conveniently be constructed and, wherever possible, on prediction-based inference and randomization-based inference at the same time.

Response from Supervisor

7.14 You have made a good case for three of the conclusions set out in **7.13**, and even your second conclusion is intuitively plausible. I for one will think twice or three times in future before I decide to introduce an intercept term into any sample survey regression analysis.

I think also that the time has now come when we must examine the consequences of attempting to combine design-based and prediction-based inference in the more general contexts of unequal probability sampling and multivariate regression. I realize that this will probably require you to use matrix notation, but do your best to make it easy for me to follow.

Exercises

7.1 Show that when the model fitted is ξ: $Y_i = \alpha + \beta X_i + U_i$ with $E_\xi U_i = 0$; $E_\xi U_i^2 = \sigma_i^2$ (known) and $E_\xi(U_i U_j) = 0$, $j \neq i$; $i, j = 1, 2, \ldots, N$, the mean of the residuals is not generally equal to zero unless the σ_i^2 are all equal to the same constant σ^2.

7.2 Show that when the model fitted is $\xi_{0.5}$ of Section **7.3**, the BLUE of β is identical to $\hat{R} = \sum_i \delta_i Y_i / \sum_i \delta_i X_i$, so that the classical ratio estimator in this situation is also the BLUP of $Y_{\bullet}$.

8

Regression Estimation with More Than One Supplementary Variable

Report for Supervisor: Introduction 123
Combining the Inferences When Using Simple Random Sampling without Replacement 123
Combining the Inferences When Sampling with Unequal Probabilities 127
Generalization to p Regressor Variables 128
The Problem of Unacceptably Small Case Weights 133
Design Variance and Anticipated Variance of any Generalized Regression Estimator 135
Prediction Variance of any Prediction-Unbiased Linear Estimator Based on a Probability Sample 138
Estimation of the Prediction Variances of Individual Sample Units 139
Response from Supervisor 143
Exercises 143

Report for Supervisor: Introduction

8.1 You have asked us to examine the consequences of attempting to combine design-based and prediction-based inference in the contexts of unequal probability sampling and more than one supplementary variable. In this we shall be drawing largely on Brewer (1999b). Matrix notation cannot be avoided, but we will lead into it gently.

We will proceed by treating first the special case where there is only a single regressor variable, x, to assist in the estimation of the total of the survey variable, y. We have already used the notation $Y_{\bullet} = \sum_{i=1}^{N} Y_i$ for this total. In the early chapters of this book we described x simply as 'a supplementary variable', but by the time we were introduced to the prediction form of the classical ratio estimator in Chapter 5, it was clear that the essential nature of the role played by x was that of a regressor variable.

Combining the Inferences When Using Simple Random Sampling without Replacement

8.2 Consider first the case where sampling is *srswor*. It is then possible to form regression estimators that are supported both by design-based (randomization-based) inference and by model-based (prediction-based) inference. For the former, we may write

$$\hat{Y}_{\bullet REG} = n^{-1}N\sum_i \delta_i Y_i + \left(X_{\bullet} - n^{-1}N\sum_i \delta_i X_i\right)\hat{\beta}_{REG}. \tag{8.1}$$

The first term in this expression is immediately recognizable as the (design-unbiased) expansion estimator of $Y_{\bullet}$, but it is also the particular form that the Horvitz–Thompson estimator (HTE) takes when the inclusion probabilities are all equal at $\pi_i = nN^{-1}$.

The second term is one that decreases in relative importance as n increases. In fact, when $n = N$ (in other words, when every population unit is included in the sample) the first term is exactly equal to $Y_{\bullet}$ and the second term is zero; so $\hat{Y}_{\bullet REG}$ is Cochran consistent. Usually, $n^{-1}N\sum_i \delta_i Y_i$ is the predominant or leading term, and $(X_{\bullet} - n^{-1}N\sum_i \delta_i X_i)\hat{\beta}_{REG}$ is a small adjustment term that ensures that if the Y_i are exactly proportional to the X_i, $\hat{Y}_{\bullet REG} = Y_{\bullet}$, even for samples as small as $n = 1$. For that reason, we describe $\hat{Y}_{\bullet REG}$ as being *calibrated* on x, and $(X_{\bullet} - n^{-1}N\sum_i \delta_i X_i)\hat{\beta}_{REG}$ as the *calibration term*.

The calibration term is the product of the known expression $X_{\bullet} - n^{-1}N\sum_i \delta_i X_i$ and an as yet unspecified estimator of β, namely $\hat{\beta}_{REG}$. This estimator is necessarily a measure of the average ratio between the y and x variables, and the only available source for such a measure is the set of sample values (Y_i, X_i) for all i such that $\delta_i = 1$. There are n individual estimates, Y_i/X_i, available from this source. Any linear combination of these estimates is of the form $\left(\sum_{i=1}^N \delta_i b_i X_i\right)^{-1}\sum_{i=1}^N \delta_i b_i Y_i$, where the b_i may be functions of the X_i, but not of the Y_i.

It is not immediately obvious what choice of b_i would be optimal, the estimator $\hat{Y}_{\bullet REG}$ being Cochran consistent for all such choices. If, however, the Y_i are capable of being modelled as dependent on the X_i through the model

$$\begin{aligned} \xi_R: \qquad & Y_i = \beta X_i + U_i; \quad \mathrm{E}_{\xi_R} U_i = 0; \quad \mathrm{E}_{\xi_R} U_i^2 = \sigma_i^2; \\ & \mathrm{E}_{\xi_R}(U_i U_j) = 0, \quad j \neq i, \end{aligned} \tag{8.2}$$

where the σ_i^2 are known within a constant multiplier, then there is a particularly attractive choice for the b_i. This is $b_i = X_i\sigma_i^{-2}$, for then $\hat{\beta}_{REG} = \left\{\sum_i \delta_i X_i^2 \sigma_i^{-2}\right\}^{-1}\sum_i \delta_i Y_i X_i \sigma_i^{-2}$, which is the best linear unbiased estimator (BLUE), $\hat{\beta}_{BLUE}$, of the parameter β in ξ_R. The formula for $\hat{Y}_{\bullet REG}$ is then:

$$\begin{aligned} \hat{Y}_{\bullet REG} &= n^{-1}N\sum_i \delta_i Y_i + \left(X_{\bullet} - n^{-1}N\sum_i \delta_i X_i\right)\hat{\beta}_{BLUE} \\ &= n^{-1}N\sum_i \delta_i Y_i + \left(X_{\bullet} - n^{-1}N\sum_i \delta_i X_i\right) \\ &\quad \times \left(\sum_i \delta_i X_i^2 \sigma_i^{-2}\right)^{-1}\sum_i \delta_i Y_i X_i \sigma_i^{-2}. \end{aligned} \tag{8.3}$$

8.3 Using prediction-based inference, however, we treat the sample sum of the Y_i as known 'without error', and add predictions of each of the non-sample Y_i to write, instead:

$$\hat{Y}_{\bullet PRED} = \sum_i \delta_i Y_i + \left(X_{\bullet} - \sum_i \delta_i X_i \right) \hat{\beta}_{PRED}. \tag{8.4}$$

In this instance, there can be no hesitation in choosing $\hat{\beta}_{REG} = \hat{\beta}_{BLUE}$, because this is (by definition) the best linear unbiased estimator of β, and in consequence

$$\hat{Y}_{\bullet BLUP} = \sum_i \delta_i Y_i + \left(X_{\bullet} - \sum_i \delta_i X_i \right) \hat{\beta}_{BLUE} \tag{8.5}$$

is the *best linear unbiased predictor* of $Y_{\bullet}$.

The term 'predictor' deserves a little explanation. When y is regressed on x (outside the context of survey sampling) the question is often asked, 'What is the most likely value of y for a given value of x that is not the x-value for any of the original sample observations?' In the context of model ξ_R, the answer is $\hat{\beta}_{BLUE}$ times the given value of x. So we would predict the value of Y_i for a given non-sample value of X_i to be $X_i\hat{\beta}_{BLUE}$, and describe $X_i\hat{\beta}_{BLUE}$ as the best linear unbiased predictor of Y_i. The BLUP of $Y_{\bullet}$ itself is then the sum of the known sample values of the Y_i, plus the non-sample sum of the $X_i\hat{\beta}_{BLUE}$. This is clearly the same as the $\hat{Y}_{\bullet BLUP}$ of (8.5).

8.4 How can we combine these two methods of inference in a single estimator? Neither the $\hat{Y}_{\bullet REG}$ of (8.3) nor the $\hat{Y}_{\bullet BLUP}$ of (8.5) is suitable by itself, for the former cannot easily be written as the sample sum of the Y_i plus a simple estimator of β times the non-sample sum of the X_i, and the latter cannot be expressed as the HTE of the Y_i plus a simple estimator of β times the difference between $X_{\bullet}$ and its HTE. Some compromise between the two is necessary. A simple way to achieve such a compromise is to require that

$$\begin{aligned} \hat{Y}_{\bullet REG} &= n^{-1}N \sum_i \delta_i Y_i + \left(X_{\bullet} - n^{-1}N \sum_i \delta_i X_i \right) \hat{\beta} = \hat{Y}_{\bullet PRED} \\ &= \sum_i \delta_i Y_i + \left(X_{\bullet} - \sum_i \delta_i X_i \right) \hat{\beta}, \end{aligned} \tag{8.6}$$

and find what condition (8.6) imposes on the estimator $\hat{\beta}$. In fact this condition is $\hat{\beta} = \left[\sum_{i=1}^{N} \delta_i\{(N/n) - 1\}X_i\right]^{-1} \sum_{i=1}^{N} \delta_i\{(N/n) - 1\}Y_i$, or, more simply,

$$\hat{\beta} = \left(\sum_{i=1}^{N} \delta_i X_i \right)^{-1} \sum_{i=1}^{N} \delta_i Y_i. \tag{8.7}$$

In this case the compromise estimator that is supported by both forms of inference is the classical ratio estimator (CRE),

$$\hat{Y}_{\bullet R} = \left(\sum_i \delta_i X_i\right)^{-1} \left(\sum_i \delta_i Y_i\right) X_{\bullet}. \tag{8.8}$$

8.5 What does the design-oriented statistician lose in embracing (8.8) rather than (8.3)? Almost nothing. Not only is (8.8) the very familiar CRE; it is also simpler and almost indistinguishable in efficiency from (8.3). This is because the calibration term is small compared with the leading term and hence the difference between using $\hat{\beta}_{BLUE}$ and using the $\hat{\beta}$ of (8.7) to multiply the relatively small difference between $X_{\bullet}$ and its HTE is itself relatively small. (This is asymptotic reasoning, of course. If the sample is too small for the asymptotics to take over, the loss in efficiency may be appreciable. But estimates from very small samples are mostly very imprecise in any case, and usually the best remedy for that is to increase the sample size.)

Our model-oriented mentor, however, might justifiably feel that, in using (8.8) rather than (8.5), she was losing rather more in efficiency than her design-oriented counterpart. This is because the difference between $\hat{\beta}_{BLUE}$ and the $\hat{\beta}$ of (8.7) would in her case be applied to the leading term in (8.5), and the CRE of (8.8) is not in general a BLUP.

The CRE is, nevertheless, a simpler estimator and one with a well-established reputation. Indeed, the thrust for prediction-based estimation in the early 1970s started with a plea that the CRE be interpreted from a model-oriented standpoint (Royall, 1970; Royall and Herson, 1973a, 1973b). It was also, as these authors pointed out, an unbiased estimator of $Y_{\bullet}$ under the ξ_R of (8.2), regardless of the values of the σ_i^2. More than that, it was the BLUP itself when $\sigma_i^2 \propto X_i$. Since (for reasons set out at the end of **5.3**) the variance function can legitimately be modelled as $\sigma_i^2 \propto X_i^{2\gamma}$, where $0.5 \leq \gamma \leq 1$, the CRE would seldom be very different from the BLUP.

To these considerations we might add (though our model-oriented mentor might not agree with us) that, for large n, even the most general form of ξ_R is likely to show signs of ceasing to be an adequate model of the population, and hence the value of being a BLUP under ξ_R could be somewhat compromised. Still more likely is the possibility that she might argue, with Royall and Herson (1973a, 1973b), that the most likely manner in which ξ_R might show signs of breaking down would still leave (8.5) as an unbiased predictor of $Y_{\bullet}$. To this we could counter that (8.8) would also produce an unbiased predictor in those circumstances, and would in fact be even more robust than (8.5), because for large enough samples the Representative Principle (which underlies all design-based inference) needs no other model than the randomization model itself to produce a valid estimator.

In summary, a design-oriented statistician could have no quarrel at all with the use of (8.8), and even a model-oriented statistician would find it difficult to establish the proposition that (8.5) was appreciably better.

Combining the Inferences When Sampling with Unequal Probabilities

8.6 How much of the analysis of **8.2–8.5** can be taken over into the more general case where the units are selected with unequal probabilities ($\pi pswor$)? For a start, we may generalize (8.1) as

$$\hat{Y}_{\bullet REG} = \sum_i \delta_i Y_i \pi_i^{-1} + \left(X_{\bullet} - \sum_i \delta_i X_i \pi_i^{-1} \right) \hat{\beta}_{REG}, \tag{8.9}$$

where, as usual, π_i is the probability of the ith population unit being included in sample. Once again, the first term is the HTE of $Y_{\bullet}$ and the second is a (typically small) calibration term that ensures that $\hat{X}_{\bullet REG} \equiv X_{\bullet}$.

From the prediction-oriented standpoint, we can actually retain (8.5) without change as the BLUP of $Y_{\bullet}$ under model ξ_R. Hence, replacing both the $\hat{\beta}_{REG}$ of (8.9) and the $\hat{\beta}_{BLUE}$ of (8.5) by a common $\hat{\beta}$ and equating those two modified equations, we can obtain $\sum_i \delta_i Y_i \pi_i^{-1} + (X_{\bullet} - \sum_i \delta_i X_i \pi_i^{-1})\hat{\beta} = \sum_i \delta_i Y_i + (X_{\bullet} - \sum_i \delta_i X_i)\hat{\beta}$, implying that

$$\hat{\beta} = \left\{ \sum_i \delta_i X_i (\pi_i^{-1} - 1) \right\}^{-1} \sum_i \delta_i Y_i (\pi_i^{-1} - 1), \tag{8.10}$$

and that an estimator of $Y_{\bullet}$ supported by both randomization-based and prediction-based inference is

$$\hat{Y}_{\bullet C} = \sum_i \delta_i Y_i \pi_i^{-1} + \left(X_{\bullet} - \sum_i \delta_i X_i \pi_i^{-1} \right) \times \left\{ \sum_i \delta_i X_i (\pi_i^{-1} - 1) \right\}^{-1} \sum_i \delta_i Y_i (\pi_i^{-1} - 1) \tag{8.11}$$

$$\equiv \sum_i \delta_i Y_i + \left(X_{\bullet} - \sum_i \delta_i X_i \right) \times \left\{ \sum_i \delta_i X_i (\pi_i^{-1} - 1) \right\}^{-1} \sum_i \delta_i Y_i (\pi_i^{-1} - 1). \tag{8.12}$$

The subscript C here refers to *cosmetic* calibration. $\hat{Y}_{\bullet C}$ is the cosmetically calibrated estimator (CCE) of $Y_{\bullet}$, (8.11) being its regression form and (8.12) being its prediction form.

'Cosmetic' was the word chosen by Särndal and Wright (1984) to describe estimators that were supported by both randomization- and design-based inference. We are beginning to see that they not only look nice but really do have pleasant properties. If, for instance, we use (8.11) and (8.12) to write down the weights w_i that attach to the sample Y_i in these two equations, we obtain, respectively,

$$w_i = \pi_i^{-1} + \left(X_{\bullet} - \sum_i \delta_i X_i \pi_i^{-1}\right)\left\{\sum_i \delta_i X_i (\pi_i^{-1} - 1)\right\}^{-1} (\pi_i^{-1} - 1) \quad (8.13)$$

and

$$w_i = 1 + \left(X_{\bullet} - \sum_i \delta_i X_i\right)\left\{\sum_i \delta_i X_i (\pi_i^{-1} - 1)\right\}^{-1} (\pi_i^{-1} - 1). \quad (8.14)$$

You will see that if the ith population unit is certain of being included in sample (that is, if $\pi_i = 1$), then the second terms of both (8.13) and (8.14) are zero, and $w_i = \pi_i^{-1} = 1$. This weight is obviously suitable for a unit that is included in sample with certainty. More than that, the second term in (8.13) indicates that the contribution of the ith population unit to the calibration term is also zero. Neither of these pleasant properties is possessed by the BLUP of (8.5) or by any other ordinary predictor. And, as we shall see in the remainder of this chapter, this property has particularly important consequences for the w_i when we regress on more than a single explanatory variable.

Generalization to *p* Regressor Variables

8.7 A more general regression model, of which (8.2) is a special case, may be written in matrix notation as

$$\xi_{REG}\colon\quad Y_i = \mathbf{X}_i'\beta + U_i; \quad \mathrm{E}_{\xi_{REG}} U_i = 0; \quad \mathrm{E}_{\xi_{REG}} U_i^2 = \sigma_i^2; \quad \mathrm{E}_{\xi_{REG}}(U_i U_j) = 0,$$
$$j \neq i; \quad i,j = 1, 2, \ldots, N, \quad (8.15)$$

where $\mathbf{X}_i$ is the column p-vector with the entry X_{ik} in the kth position, $k = 1, \ldots, p$, and β is the corresponding column p-vector containing the entries β_k.

Once again we require an estimator, $\hat{Y}_{\bullet C}$, that is interpretable in both the design-based and the prediction-based approaches to inference. For design-based inference we require it to be a generalized regression estimator (GREG) (Särndal *et al.*, 1992, Chapter 6) of the form

$$\hat{Y}_{\bullet GREG} = \mathbf{1}_N' \boldsymbol{\pi}^{-1} \boldsymbol{\delta} \mathbf{y} + \mathbf{1}_N'(\mathbf{I}_N - \boldsymbol{\pi}^{-1}\boldsymbol{\delta})\mathbf{X}\hat{\boldsymbol{\beta}}_{GREG}, \quad (8.16)$$

where $\mathbf{1}_N'$ is a row N-vector of ones, $\boldsymbol{\pi}$ is the diagonal $N \times N$ matrix of the inclusion probabilities π_i, $\boldsymbol{\delta}$ is the diagonal $N \times N$ matrix of the sample inclusion indicators δ_i, $\mathbf{y}$ is the column N-vector of the Y_i, $\mathbf{X}$ is the $N \times p$ matrix of the X_{ik} and $\hat{\boldsymbol{\beta}}_{REG}$ is an as yet unspecified estimator of $\boldsymbol{\beta}$.

It will be more convenient for matrix manipulation if, for the sample terms only, we replace the $N \times N$ matrices (which are only of rank n) by $n \times n$ matrices of full rank. For conformity, the sample N-dimensional vectors and $N \times p$ matrices will also be replaced by n-vectors and $n \times p$ matrices. Specifically, we will replace the $N \times N$ diagonal matrix $\boldsymbol{\pi}^{-1}\boldsymbol{\delta}$ of sample values π_i^{-1}, $i = 1, 2, \ldots, n$, by the $n \times n$ full rank matrix $\boldsymbol{\pi}_s^{-1}$, the $N \times p$ matrix of sample values $\boldsymbol{\delta}\mathbf{X}$ by the $n \times p$ full rank matrix $\mathbf{X}_s$, and the N-vector $\boldsymbol{\delta}\mathbf{y}$ of sample values, y_i, by the n-vector $\mathbf{y}_s$. We may then rewrite (8.16) as

$$\hat{Y}_{\bullet GREG} = \mathbf{1}'_n \boldsymbol{\pi}_s^{-1} \mathbf{y}_s + (\mathbf{1}'_N \mathbf{X} - \mathbf{1}'_n \boldsymbol{\pi}_s^{-1} \mathbf{X}_s) \hat{\boldsymbol{\beta}}_{GREG}. \tag{8.17}$$

Once again we can recognize the first term as the HTE of $Y_\bullet$, and the second term as the difference between $\mathbf{1}'_N\mathbf{X}$ and its HTE, multiplied by $\hat{\boldsymbol{\beta}}_{GREG}$. The leading term is the HTE of $Y_\bullet$, and the remaining term ensures calibration on the p supplementary variables in the $\mathbf{X}$ matrix. In this context, calibration means that if the Y_i are exactly equal to any linear combination of these supplementary variables, $\hat{Y}_{\bullet C}$ will estimate their total, $Y_\bullet$, without error. As the sample size increases, the GREG estimator approaches the HTE, and the proportionate difference between them (that is, the ratio of the difference between them to the HTE itself), is $O(n^{-1})$.

For prediction-based inference we require that $\hat{Y}_{\bullet C}$ be a predictor of the form

$$\hat{Y}_{\bullet PRED} = \mathbf{1}'_n \mathbf{y}_s + (\mathbf{1}'_N \mathbf{X} - \mathbf{1}'_n \mathbf{X}_s) \hat{\boldsymbol{\beta}}_{PRED}. \tag{8.18}$$

This formula has some resemblance to (8.17) but its rationale is entirely different. The first term is the sample sum or 'sample take' of the Y_i, and appears because the sample values are known exactly and hence there is no need to estimate them. The second term is essentially an estimator of the sum of the non-sample Y_i, obtained by using the relationship between the sample Y_i and the sample $\mathbf{x}'_i$. In most situations, the estimate of the non-sample sum is much greater than the sample take; so the ratio of the second term to the first is typically large in (8.18), although it was small in (8.17).

Setting $\hat{Y}_{\bullet REG} = \hat{Y}_{\bullet PRED} = \hat{Y}_{\bullet C}$ and $\hat{\boldsymbol{\beta}}_{REG} = \hat{\boldsymbol{\beta}}_{PRED} = \hat{\boldsymbol{\beta}}_C$ in (8.17) and (8.18), and then subtracting the one from the other, we obtain the following condition on $\hat{\boldsymbol{\beta}}_C$:

$$0 = \mathbf{1}'_n (\boldsymbol{\pi}_s^{-1} - \mathbf{I}_n)(\mathbf{y}_s - \mathbf{X}_s \hat{\boldsymbol{\beta}}_C). \tag{8.19}$$

In (8.19), the non-zero (diagonal) entries in $\boldsymbol{\pi}_s^{-1}$ typically exceed those in $\mathbf{I}_n$ by a factor of order N/n, but the entries in $\mathbf{y}_s$ and $\mathbf{X}_s\hat{\boldsymbol{\beta}}_C$ are similar in size and tend to cancel.

Any $\hat{\boldsymbol{\beta}}_C$ that meets requirement (8.19) is a Cosmetically Calibrated Estimator (CCE) of $\boldsymbol{\beta}$. One formula for such an estimator is supplied by the following theorem.

Theorem 8.7.1 Let $\mathbf{Z}_s$ be a diagonal $n \times n$ matrix such that $\mathbf{Z}_s \mathbf{1}_n = \mathbf{X}_s \boldsymbol{\alpha}$ is a linear combination of the columns of $\mathbf{X}_s$ and $\boldsymbol{\alpha}$ is a p-vector of weights. Then the estimator $\hat{\boldsymbol{\beta}}_C = (\mathbf{Q}'_s \mathbf{X}_s)^{-1} \mathbf{Q}'_s \mathbf{y}_s$, where $\mathbf{Q}'_s = \mathbf{X}'_s \mathbf{Z}_s^{-1} (\boldsymbol{\pi}_s^{-1} - \mathbf{I}_n)$, satisfies (8.19).

Proof.

$$
\begin{aligned}
\mathbf{1}_n'(\boldsymbol{\pi}_s^{-1} - \mathbf{I}_n)(\mathbf{y}_s - \mathbf{X}_s\hat{\boldsymbol{\beta}}_C) &= \boldsymbol{\alpha}'\mathbf{X}_s'\mathbf{Z}_s^{-1}(\boldsymbol{\pi}_s^{-1} - \mathbf{I}_n)(\mathbf{y}_s - \mathbf{X}_s\hat{\boldsymbol{\beta}}_C) \\
&= \boldsymbol{\alpha}'\mathbf{Q}_s'(\mathbf{y}_s - \mathbf{X}_s\hat{\boldsymbol{\beta}}_C) \\
&= \boldsymbol{\alpha}'\mathbf{Q}_s'\{\mathbf{y}_s - \mathbf{X}_s(\mathbf{Q}_s'\mathbf{X}_s)^{-1}\mathbf{Q}_s'\mathbf{y}_s\} \\
&= \boldsymbol{\alpha}'\{\mathbf{Q}_s' - \mathbf{Q}_s'\mathbf{X}_s(\mathbf{Q}_s'\mathbf{X}_s)^{-1}\mathbf{Q}_s'\}\mathbf{y}_s \\
&= 0.
\end{aligned}
$$

◇

Remark 8.7.1 This formula for $\hat{\boldsymbol{\beta}}_C$ is not the only one that would satisfy (8.19), but it is probably the simplest and almost certainly the most convenient. An alternative formula, using instrumental variables, may be found in Brewer (1995), but it has been found too unstable to be useful in the (admittedly demanding) context of Australian farm surveys, where there are many explanatory variables and relatively few farms in the sample.

8.8 What does this theorem imply? We already know that the p components of the vector $\boldsymbol{\alpha}$ are the weights attached to the p regressor variables to form the single n-vector $\mathbf{Z}_s\mathbf{1}_n = \mathbf{X}_s\boldsymbol{\alpha}$. In other words, the p entries in $\boldsymbol{\alpha}$ indicate which linear combination of the columns of the $\mathbf{X}_s$ matrix make up the diagonal matrix $\mathbf{Z}_s$. That last matrix, together with $\boldsymbol{\pi}_s^{-1}$ and $\mathbf{X}_s$, determines the form of the projection matrix $\mathbf{Q}_s$.

Alternatively, we might say that there are infinitely many ways of satisfying condition (8.19), and that by choosing the vector $\boldsymbol{\alpha}$ we effectively choose one of those ways. We shall see shortly that a good choice of $\boldsymbol{\alpha}$ is one which fashions the n diagonal entries z_i within $\mathbf{Z}_s$ into approximate measures of size for the selected sample units.

Ideally, we would have liked to choose $\hat{\boldsymbol{\beta}}_C$ to be the best linear unbiased estimator, $\hat{\boldsymbol{\beta}}_{BLUE} = (\mathbf{X}_s'\boldsymbol{\Sigma}_s^{-1}\mathbf{X}_s)^{-1}\mathbf{X}_s'\boldsymbol{\Sigma}_s^{-1}\mathbf{y}_s$, where $\boldsymbol{\Sigma}_s$ is the (diagonal) variance matrix of $\mathbf{y}_s - \mathbf{X}_s\hat{\boldsymbol{\beta}}_{BLUE}$; but unfortunately this does not generally satisfy (8.19). An interesting question is how close $\hat{\boldsymbol{\beta}}_C$ can get to mimicking $\hat{\boldsymbol{\beta}}_{BLUE}$. To answer that, we first write the formula for $\hat{\boldsymbol{\beta}}_C$ in the familiar projection form as

$$
\hat{\boldsymbol{\beta}}_C = (\mathbf{Q}_s'\mathbf{X}_s)^{-1}\mathbf{Q}_s'\mathbf{y}_s = \left[\mathbf{X}_s'\mathbf{Z}_s^{-1}(\boldsymbol{\pi}_s^{-1} - \mathbf{I}_n)\mathbf{X}_s\right]^{-1}\mathbf{X}_s'\mathbf{Z}_s^{-1}(\boldsymbol{\pi}_s^{-1} - \mathbf{I}_n)\mathbf{y}_s, \quad (8.20)
$$

and the corresponding formulae for $\hat{Y}_{\bullet C}$ as

$$
\begin{aligned}
\hat{Y}_{\bullet C} &= \mathbf{1}_n'\boldsymbol{\pi}_s^{-1}\mathbf{y}_s + (\mathbf{1}_N'\mathbf{X} - \mathbf{1}_n'\boldsymbol{\pi}_s^{-1}\mathbf{X}_s) \\
&\quad \times \left[\mathbf{X}_s'\mathbf{Z}_s^{-1}(\boldsymbol{\pi}_s^{-1} - \mathbf{I}_n)\mathbf{X}_s\right]^{-1}\mathbf{X}_s'\mathbf{Z}_s^{-1}(\boldsymbol{\pi}_s^{-1} - \mathbf{I}_n)\mathbf{y}_s \qquad (8.21) \\
&= \mathbf{1}_n'\mathbf{y}_s + (\mathbf{1}_N'\mathbf{X} - \mathbf{1}_n'\mathbf{X}_s)\left[\mathbf{X}_s'\mathbf{Z}_s^{-1}(\boldsymbol{\pi}_s^{-1} - \mathbf{I}_n)\mathbf{X}_s\right]^{-1}\mathbf{X}_s'\mathbf{Z}_s^{-1} \\
&\quad \times (\boldsymbol{\pi}_s^{-1} - \mathbf{I}_n)\mathbf{y}_s, \qquad (8.22)
\end{aligned}
$$

expression (8.21) being the GREG form and (8.22) the prediction (PRED) form of $\hat{Y}_{\bullet C}$.

Writing $\hat{Y}_{\bullet C} = \mathbf{w}_s'\mathbf{y}_s$, it may be seen from (8.21) that the row vector of the weights w_i may be written as

$$\begin{aligned}\mathbf{w}_s' &= \mathbf{1}_n'\boldsymbol{\pi}_s^{-1} + (\mathbf{1}_N'\mathbf{X} - \mathbf{1}_n'\boldsymbol{\pi}_s^{-1}\mathbf{X}_s)(\mathbf{Q}_s'\mathbf{X}_s)^{-1}\mathbf{Q}_s' \\ &= \mathbf{1}_n'\boldsymbol{\pi}_s^{-1} + (\mathbf{1}_N'\mathbf{X} - \mathbf{1}_n'\boldsymbol{\pi}_s^{-1}\mathbf{X}_s)[\mathbf{X}_s'\mathbf{Z}_s^{-1}(\boldsymbol{\pi}_s^{-1} - \mathbf{I}_n)\mathbf{X}_s]^{-1}\mathbf{X}_s'\mathbf{Z}_s^{-1} \\ &\quad \times \left(\boldsymbol{\pi}_s^{-1} - \mathbf{I}_n\right). \qquad (8.23)\end{aligned}$$

Similarly, from (8.22), the same weights may be written as

$$\begin{aligned}\mathbf{w}_s' &= \mathbf{1}_n' + (\mathbf{1}_N'\mathbf{X} - \mathbf{1}_n'\mathbf{X}_s)(\mathbf{Q}_s'\mathbf{X}_s)^{-1}\mathbf{Q}_s' \\ &= \mathbf{1}_n' + (\mathbf{1}_N'\mathbf{X} - \mathbf{1}_n'\mathbf{X}_s)[\mathbf{X}_s'\mathbf{Z}_s^{-1}(\boldsymbol{\pi}_s^{-1} - \mathbf{I}_n)\mathbf{X}_s]^{-1}\mathbf{X}_s'\mathbf{Z}_s^{-1} \\ &\quad \times \left(\boldsymbol{\pi}_s^{-1} - \mathbf{I}_n\right). \qquad (8.24)\end{aligned}$$

As we have seen, the choice of $\mathbf{Z}_s$ is to some extent arbitrary, but one case is of particular interest here. Suppose that all three of the following conditions are fulfilled:

(i) The σ_i are proportional to the non-zero elements z_i of the diagonal matrix $\mathbf{Z}_s$; in other words, $\sigma_i^2 \propto z_i^{2\gamma}$ and $\gamma = 1$. (To fulfil this condition we suggest that the z_i be fashioned into approximate measures of size.)
(ii) The π_i are chosen to be proportional to the σ_i (aiming to minimize the design variance of the GREG).
(iii) All the π_i are small compared with unity, so that $\pi_i^{-1} - 1 \approx \pi_i^{-1}$.

In those circumstances, $z_i^{-1}(\pi_i^{-1} - 1) \approx z_i^{-1}\pi_i^{-1} \propto \sigma_i^{-\gamma^{-1}}\sigma_i^{-1} = \sigma_i^{-(1+\gamma^{-1})} = \sigma_i^{-2}$ and $\hat{\boldsymbol{\beta}}_C$ is close to $\hat{\boldsymbol{\beta}}_{BLUE}$.

In practice, it often happens that all three of these conditions hold up reasonably well. Condition (i) holds up particularly well for most populations of businesses, except that γ is usually somewhat less than unity. (A reasonable guess for most business populations would be $\gamma = 0.75$.) Condition (ii) is aimed at by all competent randomization-oriented sample designers. Condition (iii) looks at first glance as though it would be quite unlikely to hold, but in fact it usually does so for all but a small set of large units and, more often than not, those units are completely enumerated. (We shall show in **8.9** that completely enumerated units have no influence on the value of $\hat{\boldsymbol{\beta}}_C$.) So $\hat{\boldsymbol{\beta}}_C$ is a reasonable approximation to $\hat{\boldsymbol{\beta}}_{BLUE}$ in many practical circumstances. Moreover, even where it is not, the efficiency of $\hat{Y}_{\bullet C}$ is not particularly sensitive to the choice of the estimate used for $\boldsymbol{\beta}$, because $\hat{Y}_{\bullet C}$ is a GREG.

In summary, the estimator $\hat{Y}_{\bullet C}$ is almost as precise as the most efficient $\hat{Y}_{\bullet REG}$ that can be described by (8.18), namely the one where $\hat{\boldsymbol{\beta}}_{REG} = \hat{\boldsymbol{\beta}}_{BLUE}$, and it is not all that much lower in efficiency than the BLUP itself. (The BLUP is the particular $\hat{Y}_{\bullet PRED}$ of (8.19) for which $\hat{\boldsymbol{\beta}}_{PRED} = \hat{\boldsymbol{\beta}}_{BLUE}$.) That modest sacrifice of efficiency is the price paid for the additional robustness supplied by randomization-based inference – a robustness that can be and often is important for large samples.

Remark 8.8.1 When there is only a single supplementary variable, it is necessarily true that $z_i \propto x_i$.

Remark 8.8.2 If n is fixed, the HTE itself is a special case of the CCE. In its GREG form the same scalar X_i is both the auxiliary variable in the model that supplies the prediction inference, and the one to which the inclusion probabilities are chosen to be proportional.

8.9 Equation (8.23) looks a bit daunting, but well repays close attention. There are row n-vectors on both sides of the equation. On the left-hand side we have the row n-vector of cosmetically calibrated weights. The term $\mathbf{1}'_n \boldsymbol{\pi}_s^{-1}$ on the right-hand side is the vector of HTE weights. The second term on the right contains the additional weights required to calibrate the estimator to the *benchmark*, $\mathbf{1}'_N \mathbf{X}$. This last is a row p-vector, as is also the factor $\mathbf{1}'_N \mathbf{X} - \mathbf{1}'_n \boldsymbol{\pi}_s^{-1} \mathbf{X}_s$, which is the difference between the benchmark vector and its HTE.

The remaining factors in the second term constitute the row n-vector of the coefficients of the sample y_i in the formula for $\hat{\boldsymbol{\beta}}_C$. Note in particular that the last of these factors, $\boldsymbol{\pi}_s^{-1} - \mathbf{I}_n$, is a diagonal $n \times n$ matrix with the important property that if any of the π_i, say π_1, is equal to unity, then the corresponding diagonal entry in $\boldsymbol{\pi}_s^{-1} - \mathbf{I}_n$, namely $\pi_1^{-1} - 1$, must be equal to zero. So, as we saw in the single regressor variable case with (8.13) and (8.14), a sample unit included with certainty makes no contribution to the value of $\hat{\beta}_C$ and no contribution to the calibration term. That is, any sample unit that has weight unity in the HTE also has weight unity in the CCE.

Intuitively, this result may be seen to be a consequence of the prediction form estimating only for the non-sample units. If $\pi_i = 1$, the ith unit makes no contribution to the total of the non-sample units and therefore has no influence on the formula for $\hat{\boldsymbol{\beta}}_C$. However, this is a property only of the CCE, and not of other GREG or PRED estimators. In fact, wherever the estimation process for $\boldsymbol{\beta}$ involves the entire population, as is the case with the original formulation of the GREG (Cassel *et al.*, 1976; see also Chapter 6 of Särndal *et al.*, 1992) there is no corresponding requirement for $\pi_i = 1$ to imply $w_i = 1$.

It is similarly the case that the calibration term for a particular sample unit in (8.23) will be small if the corresponding non-zero diagonal entry in $\boldsymbol{\pi}_s^{-1} - \mathbf{I}_n$ is small. That result, which is also peculiar to cosmetic calibration, makes excellent sense from the randomization-based viewpoint. The Representative Principle suggests that when the ith population unit is included in sample, it is appropriate to assume that there are approximately $\pi_i^{-1} - 1$ units in the non-sample portion of the population more or less resembling it. (This is most likely to be the case, of course, when the sample and the population are both large.) In (8.20), the factor $\boldsymbol{\pi}_s^{-1} - \mathbf{I}_n$ ensures that the ith unit contributes to the estimation of $\hat{\boldsymbol{\beta}}_C$ only to the extent that it represents, at least in principle, $\pi_i^{-1} - 1$ units in the non-sample portion of the population. In particular, if π_i^{-1} barely exceeds unity, the contribution of the ith population unit to the estimation of $\hat{\boldsymbol{\beta}}_C$ is, and should be, trivial.

It seldom happens in practice, though, that any population unit is assigned an inclusion probability close to but not exactly unity. If the inclusion probabilities are originally chosen to be more or less proportional to size, it is usual for a cut-off size to be set, above which it is not considered worthwhile bothering to sample. An inclusion probability of 0.5 might be as large as most sampling statisticians would be prepared to use as an upper limit.

The Problem of Unacceptably Small Case Weights

8.10 An important feature of the sample weights in equations (8.23) and (8.24) is that they are specific to an individual sample unit, but constant over all survey variables. Such sample weights are known as *case weights*. This is in contrast to the situation where every survey variable has its own CRE with its own supplementary variable. Each supplementary variable then implies its own sample weight, and these differ from one survey variable to another for the same sample unit.

With cosmetic calibration, the leading term in the GREG form of the CCE is the HTE, so the case weights for units in large samples are usually close to the reciprocals of their inclusion probabilities. For small and medium-sized samples, however, the case weights can depart substantially from the π_i^{-1}, especially where there are more than two or three supplementary variables to calibrate on.

The departures can then become problematical. Small inclusion probabilities for units actually selected in sample imply large case weights and therefore high sample variances, but it is common knowledge that a sensible minimum needs to be set for the π_i. As a result, small and negative case weights are more often the greater nuisance. Sample units with large case weights can be considered as typical in that they 'represent' large numbers of population units. Sample units with smaller weights can also be regarded as typical; they just 'represent' fewer population units. But a sample unit with weight unity is only on the borderline of being typical. It represents itself alone, and no other population unit. A sample unit with a weight less than one is definitely atypical. It does not even represent itself, and it makes a negative contribution to the second term in the prediction form of $\hat{Y}_{\bullet C}$ in (8.22). A sample unit with a negative weight is even more perversely atypical and, in effect, counter-representative. For a small enough domain, negative sample weights can actually produce negative estimates of total for variables that are intrinsically non-negative (such as the combined weight, measured in tonnes, of a specific group of elephants).

Clearly something needs to be done to minimize the problems caused by weights that are negative or less than one, but exactly what to do has been a vexed question. Brewer (1999b) suggested the following:

> A sample unit taking a weight less than unity is a 'rare event'. Yet it must be part of the population, or it would not be in the sample. The obvious procedure to adopt for such a unit is to delete it both from the sample and the sample frame, to recalculate the [case weights] so that the remaining sample units are calibrated on the totals of the remaining population units, and then

> add the deleted unit on as an atypical extra. This, of course, is precisely what many design-oriented survey statisticians have been doing with 'outlying observations' for decades. It is also the natural thing to do with sample units that are allocated weights in the unacceptable range.
>
> If, however, we start with an ordinary GREG that has not been cosmetically calibrated and attempt to remove the unacceptable weights by setting them at unity and recalculating the remainder, we typically find that many of the newly recalculated weights are themselves unacceptable. If the procedure is taken through further iterations, the number of units whose weights have been set to unity increases steadily, and the larger positive weights that are needed for those that remain lead to a substantial increase in prediction-variance.

Brewer then showed that the problem could be substantially reduced by using cosmetic calibration. Wherever a sample contains one or more units with such unacceptable weights, each of the corresponding π_i values can (by a convenient fiction) be set equal to unity, and the calculation then repeated. The factor $(\boldsymbol{\pi}_s^{-1} - \mathbf{I}_n)^{-1}$ in both (8.23) and (8.24) then ensures that wherever π_i is set equal to unity, the corresponding case weight, w_i, is also unity.

Removing negative and unacceptably small positive weights in this fashion provides no absolute guarantee that the remaining weights do not include some large ones. There is then the danger of introducing a substantial design bias, but the results of an empirical study of Australian farm data presented in Brewer (1999b) indicate that this danger is less than might be feared. Where the inclusion probabilities increased only modestly with size, cosmetic calibration greatly reduced and in favourable circumstances eliminated the incidence of unacceptable weights for a GREG estimator, without materially increasing its design variance or introducing any appreciable squared bias term into its design MSE.

The only serious problems encountered during the process of eliminating negative weights occurred when the inclusion probabilities increased rapidly with size. Selection with probability proportional to the 0.75 and 0.6 powers of size, which are optimal when $\gamma = 0.75$ and $\gamma = 0.6$ respectively, provided few and no problems respectively in the form of negative or unacceptably small positive sample weights, but when selection was with probability proportional to the 0.9 power of size, these problems became insuperable.

The few problems encountered with the 0.75 power of size were traced to a small subpopulation of dairy farms. In Australia, dairy farms are relatively small compared with other types of farm, so they had correspondingly small inclusion probabilities for these samples. Situations arose several times where only three dairy farms were included in a sample of 100 farms, and all three were above average in size.

The eleven supplementary variables on which the estimator was being calibrated included both number of dairy cattle and number of dairy farms. Since all three sample dairy farms were above average size, it was logically impossible to calibrate exactly on both those variables without giving at least one of the farms a negative sample weight. Similar events were almost certainly happening in other situations where the inclusion probabilities rose rapidly with size.

Remark 8.10.1 In the example just cited, the zero–one variable, number of dairy farms, was effectively an intercept term. This can therefore be taken as a further instance of the danger of including an intercept term when the item of principal interest (in this case income from dairy cattle) is related to its natural supplementary variable (number of dairy cattle) by a function passing through the origin. There is no point in including an intercept term unless there are other survey variables that clearly need one in their own explanatory models.

Design Variance and Anticipated Variance of any Generalized Regression Estimator

8.11 The CCE, $\hat{Y}_{\bullet C}$, is a special case of the GREG estimator, and any GREG estimator that is prediction-unbiased under the model ξ_{REG} of (8.15), as $\hat{Y}_{\bullet C}$ is, can be written as $\hat{Y}_{\bullet GREG} = \mathbf{1}'_n\boldsymbol{\pi}_s^{-1}\mathbf{y}_s + (\mathbf{1}'_N\mathbf{X} - \mathbf{1}'_n\boldsymbol{\pi}_s^{-1}\mathbf{X}_s)\hat{\boldsymbol{\beta}}_{GREG}$, where $\hat{\boldsymbol{\beta}}_{GREG}$ is any prediction-unbiased and prediction-consistent estimator of $\boldsymbol{\beta}$. If the sample size is fixed at n, the design variance of $\hat{Y}_{\bullet HT}$ is (Sen, 1953; Yates and Grundy, 1953)

$$\mathrm{V}\hat{Y}_{\bullet HT} = \sum_{i=1}^{N-1}\sum_{j=i+1}^{N}(\pi_i\pi_j - \pi_{ij})\left(Y_i\pi_i^{-1} - Y_j\pi_j^{-1}\right)^2, \tag{8.25}$$

where π_{ij} is the joint probability of the inclusion of units i and j in sample. If the model ξ_{REG} of (8.15) holds, $\hat{Y}_{\bullet GREG} = \mathbf{1}'_n\boldsymbol{\pi}_s^{-1}\mathbf{y}_s + (\mathbf{1}'_N\mathbf{X} - \mathbf{1}'_n\boldsymbol{\pi}_s^{-1}\mathbf{X}_s)\hat{\boldsymbol{\beta}}_{GREG} = \mathbf{1}'_N\mathbf{X}\hat{\boldsymbol{\beta}}_{GREG} + \hat{U}_{\bullet HT}$, where $U_{\bullet}$ is the population sum of the U_i. Also $\hat{\boldsymbol{\beta}}_{GREG}$ approaches $\boldsymbol{\beta}$ as n^{-1}, whereas $\hat{U}_{\bullet HT}$ approaches $U_{\bullet}$ only as $n^{-0.5}$; so, asymptotically, $\hat{Y}_{\bullet GREG} \cong \mathbf{X}_{\bullet}\boldsymbol{\beta} + \hat{U}_{HT}$. It then follows from (8.25) that

$$\mathrm{V}\hat{Y}_{\bullet GREG} \cong \mathrm{V}\hat{U}_{\bullet HT} = \sum_{i=1}^{N-1}\sum_{j=i+1}^{N}(\pi_i\pi_j - \pi_{ij})\left(U_i\pi_i^{-1} - U_j\pi_j^{-1}\right)^2. \tag{8.26}$$

The design variances of the HTE and GREG estimators are therefore both functions of the π_{ij}. Important problems that this fact raises were discussed in some detail by Särndal (1996). Basically they are that the π_{ij} tend to be difficult to evaluate and that their use involves a cumbersome double summation. To this we may add that if any of them are zero, (8.25) is downwardly biased.

Särndal's proposals were to circumvent these problems, either by relaxing the requirement that the first-order inclusion probabilities be exactly as initially prescribed, or else by relaxing the demand that the number of population units included in sample be fixed at n.

Neither of these suggestions is ideal. Changing the inclusion probabilities away from their most desirable values (proportional to the square root of the variance function) means that they will no longer be optimal in terms of variance minimization, a point which will better be appreciated later in this section, when we come to equation (8.27).

Allowing the number of units included in sample to be variable is even more serious. The HT estimate (meaning the realized value of the HT estimator for a particular achieved sample) is made up of n contributions, one from each sample unit, and typically these contributions are of nearly equal size. So the value of any HT estimate tends to be proportional to the achieved sample size, and in consequence the design variance of the HT estimat*or* is substantially smaller when the sample size is fixed than when it is not fixed.

Because of these considerations, Brewer (1999b) suggested another way to circumvent these problems, namely to use the *anticipated variance*, defined by Isaki and Fuller (1982), as a substitute for the design variance itself. The anticipated variance is the prediction expectation of the design variance and therefore a hybrid of the two inferential approaches; but it does not depend on the π_{ij}.

It must be borne in mind, however, that if the sample is selected systematically from a deliberately ordered population, with a view to exploiting some feature of that population that makes such a systematically selected sample resemble a stratified sample more nearly than a purely random sample, there is no reason to suppose that population model (8.15) will hold even approximately (a relevant regressor variable being missing), and hence none to suppose that the anticipated variance will be meaningful either.

But in circumstances where the anticipated variance *is* meaningful, it is equal to the model expectation of the design variance, that is, it is equal to

$$\begin{aligned}\mathrm{E}_{\xi_{REG}}\mathrm{V}\hat{Y}_{\bullet GREG} &= \sum_{i=1}^{N-1}\sum_{j=i+1}^{N}(\pi_i\pi_j - \pi_{ij})\left(\pi_i^{-2}\sigma_i^2 + \pi_j^{-2}\sigma_j^2\right)\\ &= \frac{1}{2}\sum_{i=1}^{N}\sum_{\substack{j=1\\ j\neq i}}^{N}\left(\pi_j\pi_i^{-1}\sigma_i^2 + \pi_i\pi_j^{-1}\sigma_j^2 - \pi_{ij}\pi_i^{-2}\sigma_i^2 - \pi_{ij}\pi_j^{-2}\sigma_j^2\right).\end{aligned}$$

Now when the number of units included in sample is fixed at n, $\sum_j \pi_j = n$ and

$$\sum_{j\neq i}\pi_j = n - \pi_i.$$

Also (because there are $n-1$ opportunities for the jth unit to accompany an already selected ith unit in sample)

$$\sum_{j\neq i}\pi_{ij} = (n-1)\pi_i. \tag{4.7a}$$

Hence,

$$\begin{aligned}\mathrm{E}_{\xi_{REG}}\mathrm{V}\hat{Y}_{\bullet GREG} &= \sum_{i=1}^{N}\left[(n-\pi_i)\pi_i^{-1} - (n-1)\pi_i^{-1}\right]\sigma_i^2\\ &= \sum_{i=1}^{N}\left(\pi_i^{-1} - 1\right)\sigma_i^2. \end{aligned} \tag{8.27}$$

This is the same expression as was shown (Godambe, 1955; Godambe and Joshi, 1965) to be the minimum possible value of the model-expected design variance (given the values of π_i) for any design-unbiased estimator of $Y_{\bullet}$. It also provides the justification for the choice of $\pi_i \propto \sigma_i$ when seeking to minimize the design variance, for if we differentiate (8.27) with respect to π_i under the constraint that the population sum of π_i is n, and set that derivative equal to zero, we obtain the requirement that $\pi_i^{-2}\sigma_i^2$ be the same for all i, and hence that $\pi_i \propto \sigma_i$.

Given the simplicity of (8.27), and also its plausibility if (8.15) is indeed a useful working model, it often makes sense to estimate $\mathrm{E}_{\xi_{REG}} \mathrm{V}\hat{Y}_{\bullet GREG}$ rather than the design variance of $\hat{Y}_{\bullet GREG}$. From (8.27), a prediction-consistent estimator of $\mathrm{E}_{\xi_{REG}} \mathrm{V}\hat{Y}_{\bullet GREG}$ is $\sum_{i=1}^{N} (\pi_i^{-1} - 1)\hat{\sigma}_i^2$, where the $\hat{\sigma}_i^2$ are prediction-consistent estimators of the σ_i^2. These can be obtained either in the same way as we found estimates of the individual σ_i^2 for Linda, Pamela and Sara in Chapters 3 and 5 (see, in particular, Theorem 5.3.1), or by using a model of the variance function such as $\sigma_i^2 = \sigma^2 Z_i^{2\gamma}$, where the Z_i are known measures of size and γ is assumed to be known. Moreover, the individual estimates in Chapter 5 are prediction-unbiased, and they are also easy to calculate if there is only one regressor variable. If there is more than one such variable, however, even though the individual estimates can still be estimated using simultaneous equations or matrix inversion (see **8.14**), the modelling process may be preferred.

Let us follow the modelling route. If, for each assumed value of γ, the sample $Z_i^{2\gamma}$ are normalized to sum to n, the values of $\hat{\sigma}^2$ will be comparable, but the best choice of γ is unlikely to be the one that minimizes that $\hat{\sigma}^2$, because the corresponding σ^2 varies very sensitively with γ. It is true that a reasonably robust estimator of γ can be obtained by finding the value of $\hat{\gamma}$ for which the correlation (over the units included in sample) between $(y_i - \mathbf{x}_i\hat{\boldsymbol{\beta}})^2/z_i^{2\hat{\gamma}}$ and the size rank of z_i is equal to zero, but such estimates of γ, except where they come from samples of 1000 or more, are typically subject to high variance, and should be treated with caution, especially if they lie outside the range $0.5 \leq \gamma \leq 1$. (This is one instance where a Bayesian estimation procedure would be particularly appropriate, if the survey statistician has any inclination in that direction.)

The value $\gamma = 0.5$ is the case where variance increases linearly with size and, since variances are additive under independence, $\gamma = 0.5$ also corresponds to the situation where large units behave like random aggregations of small units. Situations where $\gamma < 0.5$ are rare, and estimates of γ less than 0.5 are more commonly an indication of a poorly estimated parameter than of a genuinely low value. Correspondingly, estimates of γ greater than unity are more commonly an indication of a poorly estimated parameter than of a genuinely high value, for the latter would imply that the (model) standard deviations of individual Y_i-values increased faster than the Z_i themselves.

As a default option, almost all economic populations have values of γ in the range $0.5 \leq \gamma \leq 1$, and usually within striking distance of $\gamma = 0.75$. Certain tree populations, for which Y_i denotes available timber and Z_i an eye estimate of size, seem to obey the rule $\gamma = 1$ reasonably closely. Demographic populations may behave differently, however. One example of interest and importance is that where Y_i is the proportion of female adults to total adults and Z_i is the total number of adults in the ith household. In this case, because of the prevalence of bonded pairs, the Y_i for households of a given size tend to vary less among themselves than they would among random aggregations of similarly small numbers of individuals. This causes the value of γ relevant for comparing individuals and households to be somewhat less than 0.5.

Prediction Variance of any Prediction-Unbiased Linear Estimator Based on a Probability Sample

8.12 (Note that we will not need matrix algebra here and in **8.13**, so we will temporarily resume our use of the symbol δ_i to denote the sample inclusion indicator for the ith population unit.) It is appropriate to estimate $\mathrm{E}_{\xi_{REG}} \mathrm{V}\hat{Y}_{\bullet}$ for sample design purposes but, for the analysis of any particular sample, the prediction variance $\mathrm{V}_{\xi_{REG}}(\hat{Y}_{\bullet} - Y_{\bullet})$ is a more logical choice. More generally, the prediction variance of $\hat{Y}_{\bullet PRED} - Y_{\bullet}$ where $\hat{Y}_{\bullet PRED}$ is *any* prediction-unbiased estimator of the form $\hat{Y}_{\bullet PRED} = \sum_{i=1}^{N} \delta_i w_i Y_i$ is, by definition,

$$
\begin{aligned}
\mathrm{V}_{\xi_{REG}}(\hat{Y}_{\bullet PRED} - Y_{\bullet}) &\equiv \mathrm{E}_{\xi_{REG}} \left(\sum_{i=1}^{N} \delta_i w_i Y_i - Y_{\bullet} \right)^2 \\
&= \mathrm{E}_{\xi_{REG}} \left\{ \sum_{i=1}^{N} \delta_i (w_i - 1) Y_i - \sum_{i=1}^{N} (1 - \delta_i) Y_i \right\}^2 \\
&= \mathrm{E}_{\xi_{REG}} \left\{ \sum_{i=1}^{N} \delta_i (w_i - 1)(\beta X_i + U_i) \right. \\
&\qquad \left. - \sum_{i=1}^{N} (1 - \delta_i)(\beta X_i + U_i) \right\}^2 \\
&= \mathrm{E}_{\xi_{REG}} \left\{ \sum_{i=1}^{N} \delta_i (w_i - 1) U_i - \sum_{i=1}^{N} (1 - \delta_i) U_i \right\}^2 \\
&= \sum_{i=1}^{N} \delta_i (w_i - 1)^2 \sigma_i^2 + \sum_{i=1}^{N} (1 - \delta_i) \sigma_i^2 \\
&= \sum_{i=1}^{N} \delta_i (w_i^2 - 2w_i + 1) \sigma_i^2 + \sum_{i=1}^{N} (1 - \delta_i) \sigma_i^2 \\
&= \sum_{i=1}^{N} \delta_i w_i (w_i - 2) \sigma_i^2 + \sum_{i=1}^{N} \delta_i \sigma_i^2 + \sum_{i=1}^{N} (1 - \delta_i) \sigma_i^2
\end{aligned}
$$

$$= \sum_{i=1}^{N} \delta_i w_i (w_i - 1)\sigma_i^2 + \sum_{i=1}^{N} \sigma_i^2 - \sum_{i=1}^{N} \delta_i w_i \sigma_i^2 \tag{8.28}$$

$$= \sum_{i=1}^{N} \delta_i w_i (w_i - 1)\sigma_i^2 + \left(\sum_{i=1}^{N} \sigma_i^2 - \sum_{i=1}^{N} \delta_i \pi_i^{-1} \sigma_i^2 \right)$$
$$- \left(\sum_{i=1}^{N} \delta_i w_i \sigma_i^2 - \sum_{i=1}^{N} \delta_i \pi_i^{-1} \sigma_i^2 \right). \tag{8.29}$$

Some simplification is possible here. The expression $\sum_{i=1}^{N} \sigma_i^2 - \sum_{i=1}^{N} \delta_i \pi_i^{-1} \sigma_i^2$ in (8.29) is the difference between the population sum of the σ_i^2 and its HTE, and has design expectation zero. Further, since w_i tends asymptotically to π_i^{-1}, the expression $\sum_{i=1}^{N} \delta_i w_i \sigma_i^2 - \sum_{i=1}^{N} \delta_i \pi_i^{-1} \sigma_i^2$ in (8.29) is asymptotically zero and negligible for large samples. Hence a simpler but still prediction-cum-design-consistent estimator of the prediction variance, $V_{\xi_{REG}}(\hat{Y}_{\bullet PRED} - Y_{\bullet})$, is $\sum_{i=1}^{N} \delta_i w_i (w_i - 1)\hat{\sigma}_i^2$. This is just the leading term in (8.28) and (8.29) with σ_i^2 replaced by $\hat{\sigma}_i^2$. Both this leading term and the sums of the remaining terms in (8.28) and (8.29) conveniently take the value zero when every unit in the population is also in sample, with $w_i = 1$ for all i.

Estimation of the Prediction Variances of Individual Sample Units

8.13 It remains to estimate the sample σ_i^2, and where possible their non-sample counterparts, to a sufficient degree of accuracy. For large samples it might be considered sufficient to use the simple prediction-consistent estimator, $\hat{\sigma}_i^2 = (Y_i - X_i \hat{\beta}_{PRED})^2$, but provided the estimator uses only a single regressor variable it is almost as simple to use a prediction-unbiased estimator of the kind that we ended up using when we were estimating the accuracy of $\hat{Y}_{\bullet R}$ for the circus owner (again see Theorem 5.3.1).

The way it would work in the unequal probability situation is as follows. Where there is only a single regressor variable, the simple but downwards-biased estimator of σ_i^2 becomes $\hat{\sigma}_i^2 = (Y_i - X_i \hat{\beta}_{PRED})^2$, and if we write $\hat{\beta}_{PRED} = \sum_j \delta_j c_j Y_j$ where $\sum_j \delta_j c_j X_j = 1$, the expectation of $\hat{\sigma}_i^2$ over the univariate population model ξ_R of (8.2) is

$$E_{\xi_R} \hat{\sigma}_i^2 = E_{\xi_R} \left(\beta X_i + U_i - \beta X_i - \sum_j \delta_j c_j U_j X_i \right)^2$$
$$= E_{\xi_R} \left\{ U_i (1 - c_i X_i) - \sum_{j \neq i} \delta_j c_j U_j X_i \right\}^2$$

$$= \sigma_i^2(1 - c_i X_i)^2 + \sum_{j \neq i} \delta_j c_j^2 \sigma_j^2 X_i^2$$

$$= \sigma_i^2\left(1 - 2c_i X_i + c_i^2 X_i^2\right) + \sum_{j \neq i} \delta_j c_j^2 \sigma_j^2 X_i^2$$

$$= \sigma_i^2(1 - 2c_i X_i) + X_i^2 \sum_j \delta_j c_j^2 \sigma_j^2 .$$

Hence

$$\mathrm{E}_{\xi_R}(1 - 2c_i X_i)^{-1}\hat{\sigma}_i^2 = \sigma_i^2 + X_i^2(1 - 2c_i X_i)^{-1} \sum_j \delta_j c_j^2 \sigma_j^2 . \tag{8.30}$$

It follows that

$$\begin{aligned} \mathrm{E}_{\xi_R} \sum_i \delta_i c_i^2 (1 - 2c_i X_i)^{-1}\hat{\sigma}_i^2 &= \sum_i \delta_i c_i^2 \sigma_i^2 \\ &\quad + \sum_i \delta_i c_i^2 X_i^2 (1 - 2c_i X_i)^{-1} \sum_j \delta_j c_j^2 \sigma_j^2, \\ &= \sum_i \delta_i c_i^2 \sigma_i^2 \left\{ 1 + \sum_i \delta_i c_i^2 X_i^2 (1 - 2c_i X_i)^{-1} \right\}, \end{aligned}$$

and hence that

$$\sum_i \delta_i c_i^2 \sigma_i^2 = \left\{ 1 + \sum_i \delta_i c_i^2 X_i^2 (1 - 2c_i X_i)^{-1} \right\}^{-1} \mathrm{E}_{\xi_R} \sum_i \delta_i c_i^2 (1 - 2c_i X_i)^{-1} \hat{\sigma}_i^2,$$

so that a prediction-unbiased estimator of $\sum_i \delta_i c_i^2 \sigma_i^2$ is

$$S = \left\{ 1 + \sum_i \delta_i c_i^2 X_i^2 (1 - 2c_i X_i)^{-1} \right\}^{-1} \sum_i \delta_i c_i^2 (1 - 2c_i X_i)^{-1} \hat{\sigma}_i^2 . \tag{8.31}$$

Substituting (8.31) into (8.30), we have

$$\mathrm{E}_{\xi_R}(1 - 2c_i X_i)^{-1}\hat{\sigma}_i^2 = \sigma_i^2 + X_i^2 (1 - 2c_i X_i)^{-1} \mathrm{E}_{\xi_R} S,$$

and therefore that a prediction-unbiased estimator of σ_i^2 under the univariate population model ξ_R of (8.2) is

$$\tilde{\sigma}_i^2 = (1 - 2c_i X_i)^{-1}\left(\hat{\sigma}_i^2 - X_i^2 S\right). \tag{8.32}$$

8.14 In the multivariate case, however, we will effectively need to solve $F = p(p+1)/2$ simultaneous linear equations, where p is the length of the vector $\boldsymbol{\beta}$. The following derivation comes from Dr P.S. Kott (private communication). It is somewhat more difficult to follow than the matrix algebra used so far, and you may wish to omit it at your first reading. (When you do come to read it, however, please note that because of the matrix notation we will be making our summations over the sample rather than over the entire population, thereby dispensing once more with the need for the symbol δ to denote a sample inclusion indicator.)

Let $\hat{\sigma}_i = \hat{u}_i = y_i - \mathbf{x}_i'\hat{\boldsymbol{\beta}}_{PRED} = u_i - \mathbf{x}_i'\mathbf{C}_s\mathbf{u}_s = u_i - \mathbf{g}_i'\mathbf{u}_s$ where $\mathbf{u}_s$ is the n-vector of the sample u_i, $\mathbf{C}_s$ is the $p \times n$ matrix of coefficients defined by $\hat{\boldsymbol{\beta}}_{PRED} = \mathbf{C}_s\mathbf{y}_s$ and $\mathbf{g}_i' = \mathbf{x}_i'\mathbf{C}_s$. Then

$$\begin{aligned}\mathrm{E}_{\xi_{REG}}\hat{\sigma}_i^2 &= \mathrm{E}_{\xi_{REG}}(y_i - \mathbf{x}_i'\hat{\boldsymbol{\beta}}_{PRED})^2 = \mathrm{E}_{\xi_{REG}}(u_i - \mathbf{g}_i'\mathbf{u}_s)^2 \\ &= (1 - 2g_{ii})\sigma_i^2 + \sum_{k=1}^{n} g_{ik}^2\sigma_k^2.\end{aligned}$$

It follows that

$$\begin{aligned}&\mathrm{E}_{\xi_{REG}}\left\{\hat{\sigma}_i^2(1 - 2g_{ii})^{-1}\right\} \\ &= \sigma_i^2 + (1 - 2g_{ii})^{-1}\sum_{k=1}^{n} g_{ik}^2\sigma_k^2 \\ &= \sigma_i^2 + (1 - 2g_{ii})^{-1}\sum_{k=1}^{n}\left(\sum_{t} x_{it}c_{tk}\right)^2\sigma_k^2 \\ &= \sigma_i^2 + (1 - 2g_{ii})^{-1}\sum_{k=1}^{n}\sigma_k^2\left\{\sum_{t=1}^{p} x_{it}^2c_{tk}^2 + 2\sum_{t=1}^{p-1} x_{it}c_{tk}\sum_{t'=t+1}^{p} x_{it'}c_{t'k}\right\}.\end{aligned}$$

This may be written

$$\mathrm{E}_{\xi_{REG}}\check{\boldsymbol{\sigma}}^2 = \boldsymbol{\sigma}^2 + \mathbf{EH}\boldsymbol{\sigma}^2 = (\mathbf{I}_n + \mathbf{EH})\boldsymbol{\sigma}^2,$$

where $\boldsymbol{\sigma}^2$ and $\check{\boldsymbol{\sigma}}^2$ are the n-vectors of the σ_i^2 and the $\hat{\sigma}_i^2(1 - 2g_{ii})^{-1}$, respectively; $\mathbf{E}$ is an $n \times F$ matrix with $F = p(p + 1)/2$; the element in the ith row and fth column of $\mathbf{E}$ (see below for the definition of f) is $(1 - 2g_{ii})^{-1}(2 - \Delta_d)x_{it}x_{it'}$, where $d = t' - t$, and $\Delta_d = 1$ when $d = 0$ but $\Delta_d = 0$ otherwise; and $\mathbf{H}$ is an $F \times n$ matrix whose element in the fth row and kth column is $c_{tk}c_{t'k}$.

It is necessary for the subscript f to be uniquely defined by (t, t'). One way in which this unique definition may be specified is $f = t + pd - \{d(d - 1)/2\}$. This corresponds to f numbering first down the main diagonal, then down the first superdiagonal, and so on, finishing in the top right-hand corner, where $t' = p = d + 1$ and f takes its maximum value, namely F.

An unbiased estimator of $\boldsymbol{\sigma}^2$ is then

$$\begin{aligned}\tilde{\boldsymbol{\sigma}}^2 &= (\mathbf{I}_n + \mathbf{EH})^{-1}\check{\boldsymbol{\sigma}}^2 \\ &= [\mathbf{I}_n - \mathbf{EH} + (\mathbf{EH})^2 - (\mathbf{EH})^3 + \cdots]\check{\boldsymbol{\sigma}}^2 \\ &= [\mathbf{I}_n - \mathbf{E}\{\mathbf{I}_F - \mathbf{HE} + (\mathbf{HE})^2 + \cdots\}\mathbf{H}]\check{\boldsymbol{\sigma}}^2 \\ &= [\mathbf{I}_n - \mathbf{E}\{\mathbf{I}_F + \mathbf{HE}\}^{-1}\mathbf{H}]\check{\boldsymbol{\sigma}}^2. \end{aligned} \tag{8.33}$$

The matrix to invert here, $\mathbf{I}_F + \mathbf{HE}$, is of order $F \times F$ where $F = p(p+1)/2$ is usually much smaller than n, so that $\mathbf{I}_F + \mathbf{HE}$ itself is typically much smaller than the $n \times n$ matrix requiring inversion in the direct solution of $\hat{\sigma}_i = \hat{u}_i = u_i - \mathbf{g}_i'\mathbf{u}$.

8.15 (No more matrix notation now, so back come the δ_i.) As a result of the theory just presented, we are now in a position to estimate the prediction variance of $\hat{Y}_{\bullet PRED}$, and therefore also that of $\hat{Y}_{\bullet C}$, using the estimator $\sum_{i=1}^{N} \delta_i w_i(w_i - 1)\tilde{\sigma}_i^2$. To use $\sum_{i=1}^{N} \delta_i w_i(w_i - 1)\tilde{\sigma}_i^2 + \sum_{i=1}^{N} \tilde{\sigma}_i^2 - \sum_{i=1}^{N} \delta_i w_i \tilde{\sigma}_i^2$, however, (where the non-sample $\tilde{\sigma}_i^2$ are defined in such a fashion as to be comparable with the sample ones), it will be necessary to assume that the σ_i^2 are related to the supplementary variables in some functional fashion. We will again assume that $\sigma_i^2 = \sigma^2 Z_i^{2\gamma}$, where the Z_i are measures of size defined as some linear combination of the supplementary variables and γ is a coefficient of heteroscedasticity in the range $0.5 \leq \gamma \leq 1$.

If the value of γ is accurately chosen, the expected values of $\tilde{\sigma}_i^2/Z_i^{2\gamma}$ will not change with Z_i, so the correlation of $\tilde{\sigma}_i^2/Z_i^{2\gamma}$ with any function of the Z_i should be zero. For estimation purposes, the chosen function should obviously be monotonic, and the problem of highly influential observations can be avoided by choosing that function of Z_i to be its rank order.

As indicated earlier, however, at least 1000 observations are typically required to estimate γ with any degree of accuracy, so it is not uncommon to choose a value of γ on the basis of past experience. As mentioned in **8.5** and **8.11**, it is usual for $0.5 \leq \gamma \leq 1$. The middle-of-the-range value 0.75 is a reasonable choice for many if not most economic variables. For tree populations $\gamma = 1$ is more likely to be suitable.

Given the value of γ, the appropriate proportionality factor, σ^2, may be estimated as $\hat{\sigma}^2 = n^{-1} \sum_i \delta_i \tilde{\sigma}_i^2 / Z_i^{2\gamma}$. If the value of γ is well chosen, each sample value will make the same expected contribution. If, however, it were found that the larger (smaller) units were dominating the estimation process, there would be good reason to suppose that γ had been underestimated (overestimated) and therefore to choose a higher (lower) value for that parameter.

The value of σ^2 is highly sensitive to the choice of γ, but if we wished to establish some degree of comparability between the proportionality factors for different values of γ, we could define variance function values $\sigma_\gamma^2 a_{\gamma i}^2$ with σ_γ^2 chosen such that the values of the sample estimates $\hat{a}_{\gamma i}^2$ of $a_{\gamma i}^2$ for any given value of γ summed to n. The best choice of γ would then result in a small (though not necessarily the smallest) value of σ_γ^2. With the resulting estimates, $\tilde{\sigma}_{\gamma i}^2 = \sigma_\gamma^2 \hat{a}_{\gamma i}^2$, of the non-sample $\sigma_{\gamma i}^2$, it is straightforward to estimate the prediction variance of $\hat{Y}_{\bullet C}$ using $\sum_{i=1}^N \delta_i w_i(w_i - 1)\tilde{\sigma}_{\gamma i}^2 + \sum_{i=1}^N \tilde{\sigma}_{\gamma i}^2 - \sum_{i=1}^N \delta_i w_i \tilde{\sigma}_{\gamma i}^2$.

Response from Supervisor

8.16 You have done what I asked in examining the consequences of combining randomization-based and prediction-based inference in the context of unequal probability sampling, but there is one consequence that I had not foreseen and it disturbs me.

You mention that the variance of the HTE is a function of the joint probabilities, π_{ij}, of the inclusion of units *i* and *j* in sample; also that these π_{ij} 'tend to be difficult to evaluate', that they are 'not conducive to the efficient estimation of variance' and that their use 'involves a cumbersome double summation'.

In consequence of these difficulties, you appear to abandon entirely any idea of estimating the randomization variance of the HT estimator or any estimator based on it, such as the GREG. You fall back instead on the anticipated variance to do the job that is normally done by the randomization variance in the planning of future sample surveys.

I am not convinced that this is either wise or necessary. It could be unwise in two regards. First, there are still many survey users and operators that regard randomization as the only acceptable basis for survey inference. Secondly, it depends on the appropriateness of the prediction model to a greater extent than is required for, say, classical ratio estimation.

It is also strange that the π_{ij} should be seen as a necessary input into the variance estimation process. We know that certain unequal probability sample designs yield very similar HT variances even though they have quite different π_{ij} (Hartley and Rao, 1962; Asok and Sukhatme, 1976). Is it not possible to estimate the variance of the HTE in such circumstances without recourse to the π_{ij}?

Exercises

8.1 In what circumstances and why might it be particularly important to use:

(a) prediction inference rather than randomization inference?
(b) randomization inference rather than prediction inference?
(c) both simultaneously?

8.2 In Section **8.4**, the cosmetically calibrated estimator was defined by

$$\hat{Y}_{\bullet REG} = n^{-1}N\sum_i \delta_i Y_i + \left(X_{\bullet} - n^{-1}N\sum_i \delta_i X_i\right)\hat{\beta} = \hat{Y}_{\bullet PRED}$$

$$= \sum_i \delta_i Y_i + \left(X_{\bullet} - \sum_i \delta_i X_i\right)\hat{\beta}.$$

Suppose an alternative estimator had been defined from the simpler set of equations

$$\hat{Y}_{\bullet REG} = n^{-1}N\sum_i \delta_i Y_i + \left(X_{\bullet} - n^{-1}N\sum_i \delta_i X_i\right)\hat{\beta} = \hat{Y}_{\bullet RAT} = X_{\bullet}\hat{\beta}$$

instead.

(a) Follow through the derivation of this alternative estimator using Sections **8.4**, **8.5** and **8.6** as a pattern.
(b) Continue the alternative derivation through Sections **8.7**, **8.8** and **8.9**, now using $\hat{Y}_{\bullet RAT} = \mathbf{1}'_N\mathbf{X}\hat{\boldsymbol{\beta}}_{PRED}$ in place of $\hat{Y}_{\bullet PRED} = \mathbf{1}'_n\mathbf{y}_s + (\mathbf{1}'_N\mathbf{X} - \mathbf{1}'_n\mathbf{X}_s)\hat{\boldsymbol{\beta}}_{PRED}$.
(c) Indicate what you would regard as the advantages and disadvantages of using this alternative approach (instead of the cosmetically calibrated estimator) throughout Chapter 8.

8.3 Starting with the prediction model ξ_R of (8.2), show how to obtain prediction-consistent estimators $\hat{\sigma}_i^2$ of both the sample and non-sample σ_i^2, under the additional model assumption that $\sigma_i^2 = \sigma^2 a_i^2$, where $a_i^2 \propto X_i^{2\gamma}$ and γ is known.

8.4 When there is only a single supplementary variable, the design-based generalized regression estimator of $Y_{\bullet} = \sum_{i=1}^N Y_i$, (the population total of the survey variable values Y_i) simplifies to

$$\hat{Y}_{\bullet GREG} = \sum_{i=1}^N \delta_i Y_i \pi_i^{-1} + \left(X_{\bullet} - \sum_{i=1}^N \delta_i X_i \pi_i^{-1}\right)\hat{\boldsymbol{\beta}}_{GREG},$$

where δ_i is the sample inclusion indicator (taking the value 1 when the ith population unit is in sample and 0 otherwise), π_i is the inclusion probability of that ith population unit, X_i is the value of its supplementary variable, $X_{\bullet} = \sum_{i=1}^N X_i$, and $\hat{\boldsymbol{\beta}}_{GREG} = \sum_{i=1}^N \delta_i b_i Y_i$ is a sample estimator of $\boldsymbol{\beta}$ (the regression coefficient of Y_i on X_i) defined by the choices of the b_i. These b_i are typically functions of the X_i and π_i. Note that $\sum_{i=1}^N \delta_i Y_i \pi_i^{-1}$ and $\sum_{i=1}^N \delta_i X_i \pi_i^{-1}$ are the Horvitz–Thompson estimators of $Y_{\bullet}$ and $X_{\bullet}$ respectively.

Under model-based inference, the predictor (or prediction-based estimator) of $Y_{\bullet}$ is

$$\hat{Y}_{\bullet PRED} = \sum_{i=1}^N \delta_i Y_i + \left(X_{\bullet} - \sum_{i=1}^N \delta_i X_i\right)\hat{\boldsymbol{\beta}}_{PRED},$$

where $\hat{\beta}_{PRED}$ is an unbiased and consistent estimator (and ideally the best linear unbiased estimator) of β under a model such as

$$\xi: \quad Y_i = \beta X_i + U_i; \quad E_\xi U_i = 0; \quad E_\xi U_i^2 = \sigma_i^2;$$
$$E_\xi(U_i U_j) = 0 \qquad \text{for all} \quad i = 1, 2, \ldots, N.$$

In such circumstances $\hat{\boldsymbol{\beta}}_{PRED}$ takes the same functional form as $\hat{\boldsymbol{\beta}}_{GREG}$, namely $\sum_{i=1}^{N} \delta_i b_i Y_i$, but the b_i are generally different, and in pure prediction-based inference they do not depend on the π_i.

In order to arrive at an estimator supported by design-based and model-based inference simultaneously, it has been suggested that the conditions $\hat{Y}_{\bullet GREG} = \hat{Y}_{\bullet PRED} = \hat{Y}_{\bullet}$ and $\hat{\boldsymbol{\beta}}_{GREG} = \hat{\boldsymbol{\beta}}_{PRED} = \hat{\boldsymbol{\beta}}$ be imposed.

(a) Show that these two conditions lead to the requirement that

$$\hat{\beta} = \frac{\sum_{i=1}^{N} \delta_i Y_i (\pi_i^{-1} - 1)}{\sum_{i=1}^{N} \delta_i X_i (\pi_i^{-1} - 1)},$$

and therefore that $b_i \propto \pi_i^{-1} - 1$.

(b) Write the resulting GREG and PRED version of $\hat{Y}_{\bullet}$ in forms that enable the 'case weights' w_i, defined by the identity $\hat{Y}_{\bullet} \equiv \sum_{i=1}^{N} \delta_i w_i Y_i$, to be expressed in the GREG version as equal to π_i^{-1} plus a term proportional to $\pi_i^{-1} - 1$, and in the PRED version as equal to 1 plus a term proportional to $\pi_i^{-1} - 1$.

(c) What case weight do these forms imply for population units that are included in sample with certainty (and thefore have $\pi_i^{-1} = 1$)? Why might this case weight be considered particularly appropriate for units included in sample with certainty?

8.5 (a) Compare and contrast, using your own words, the main features of design-based (or randomization-based) inference on the one hand, and model-based (or prediction-based) inference on the other hand.

(b) Discuss whether, and if so in what way, it might be appropriate to combine both forms of inference in a single estimator.

Hint. Exercise 8.4 deals with an issue that you may find relevant here. Suggested length of answer is 300–400 words.

8.6 Discuss the pros and cons of using the estimated anticipated variance of a cosmetically calibrated estimator, instead of its estimated design variance, when the design of a future survey is being decided.

9

Short-Cut Variance Estimation for the Horvitz–Thompson and Generalized Regression Estimators

Report for Supervisor: Introduction 146
Some Approximate Formulae for the Design Variance of the Horvitz–Thompson Estimator 148
A Model–Assisted Check on the Usefulness of the Approximate Horvitz–Thompson Estimator Design Variance Formulae 154
Sample Estimators of the High-Entropy Anticipated Variance of the Horvitz–Thompson Estimator 156
Sample Estimators of the Design Variance of the Horvitz–Thompson Estimator Suitable for Use with Ordered Systematic Sampling 159
Adaptation to Estimating the Design Variance of a Generalized Regression Estimator 161
Some Empirical Results 163
Response from Supervisor 167
Postscripts 167
Exercises 172

Report for Supervisor: Introduction

9.1 You have set us quite a demanding task! Fortunately, however, we found an easily accessible set of papers from the Second International Conference on Establishment Surveys (ICES-II) which between them do very nearly what you ask. Brewer (2001) provides expressions that approximate the design variance of the Horvitz–Thompson estimator ‘in situations where the joint or second order inclusion probabilities, commonly denoted by π_{ij}, were not deliberately manipulated so as to change the design variance of the HTE from what might be regarded as its *natural* value’, and goes on to suggest ways of estimating that natural design variance. Aires (2001) notes that this natural level of design variance arises because the selection procedure used is one of ‘high entropy’, meaning that the resulting relationship between the population and the sample follows no particular pattern. Brewer and Gregoire (2001) test the validity and usefulness of these concepts, using a Monte Carlo experiment on forest data.

We also found some other high-entropy estimators that deserve mention. They appear to perform about as well in practice, but they do not have quite the same level of theoretical support.

9.2 First, however, we need to consider what 'high entropy' means. 'Entropy' is a measure of disorganization or randomness. If we put the units that constitute a large population into a random order, we can be reasonably confident of that ordering, and therefore also any systematic sample selected from it, having high entropy.

It is possible, but it would be rare, for a random ordering to have low entropy. There is, to take the extreme case, one chance in $10! = 3\,628\,800$ of a random ordering of a population of 10 different names being exactly in alphabetical order, and less than one chance in 2×10^{18} of that happening for a random ordering of a population of 20 names. Practically speaking, if we select a systematic sample from a randomized list of 1000 businesses, or even of 50 elephants, we can be reasonably confident that we are operating in a high-entropy situation. (There are also many other ways of selecting high-entropy samples with unequal probabilities without replacement, but none is nearly as simple operationally.)

If, however, we deliberately put a population into a meaningful order, such as geographical or size order, before making a systematic selection, we would be more sure of selecting a fair share of small units (and, of course, of large-ones too) than we would be if we were selecting systematically from a randomly ordered population. The low-entropy sample would therefore be a more representative sample and the estimates based on it would have lower variances, but the estimation of those variances would involve complications. That is an issue we intend to address in some detail before completing this report.

Besides the conference papers that we mentioned at the outset, there are several earlier studies that provide approximate formulae for the π_{ij} in high-entropy situations. The two that we believe to be most useful are those by Hartley and Rao (1962) and by Asok and Sukhatme (1976).

Hartley and Rao examined the case of systematic sampling from a randomly ordered population (Goodman and Kish, 1950). Asok and Sukhatme examined an entirely different method of selection devised by Sampford (1967). To order $O(n^3N^{-3})$, however, Asok and Sukhatme's formulae for the π_{ij} were identical to those found by Hartley and Rao. That would have been an incredible coincidence if the two very different procedures studied had not both been subject to the influences of high entropy.

The derivations are lengthy and will not be reproduced or even summarized here, but to order $O(n^3N^{-3})$ both these selection procedures yielded

$$\pi_{ij} \cong \frac{1}{2}\pi_i\pi_j(c_i + c_j), \tag{9.1}$$

where

$$c_i = n^{-1}(n-1)\left(1 - n^{-2}\sum_{k=1}^{N}\pi_k^2 + 2n^{-1}\pi_i\right). \tag{9.2}$$

(The c_i here should not be confused with the very different c_i in **8.13**!) It follows from (9.1) – without (9.2) – that

$$\pi_i\pi_j - \pi_{ij} \equiv \frac{1}{2}\pi_i\pi_j(2 - c_i - c_j), \tag{9.3}$$

and it will simplify our presentation if we stay with this more general case and allow ourselves a little freedom with the choice of c_i. We will, however, always choose expressions that explicitly contain the factor $n^{-1}(n-1)$, and for which the remaining factor exceeds unity only by terms of order $O(N^{-1})$.

So, with (9.3) as a convenient tool, we will next derive some useful approximations to the high-entropy variance of the HTE.

Some Approximate Formulae for the Design Variance of the Horvitz–Thompson Estimator

9.3 The population total of the item y for a finite population of N units may be written $Y_{\bullet} = \sum_{i=1}^{N} Y_i$. If a sample of n units is drawn from that population without replacement and with first-order inclusion probabilities π_i, the HTE of that total is $\hat{Y}_{\bullet HT} = \sum_{i=1}^{N} \delta_i Y_i \pi_i^{-1}$. For the important special case where the sample size n is fixed, Sen (1953) and Yates and Grundy (1953) showed independently that $\hat{Y}_{\bullet HT}$ had the design variance

$$\mathrm{V}\hat{Y}_{\bullet HT} = \frac{1}{2}\sum_{i=1}^{N}\sum_{j(\neq i)=1}^{N}(\pi_i\pi_j - \pi_{ij})\left(Y_i\pi_i^{-1} - Y_j\pi_j^{-1}\right)^2, \tag{9.4}$$

where π_{ij} is the second–order or joint inclusion probability of the ith and jth population units together in the same sample. Both therefore suggested the variance estimator

$$\hat{\mathrm{V}}_{SYG}\hat{Y}_{\bullet HT} = \frac{1}{2}\sum_{i=1}^{N}\sum_{j(\neq i)=1}^{N}\delta_i\delta_j\pi_{ij}^{-1}(\pi_i\pi_j - \pi_{ij})\left(Y_i\pi_i^{-1} - Y_j\pi_j^{-1}\right)^2. \tag{9.5}$$

This is usually unbiased over repeated sampling, as can be seen by taking the expectation of the right-hand side, that is, by replacing the product $\delta_i\delta_j$ by its expectation, π_{ij}. The exception occurs when one or more of the π_{ij} is zero, in which case a term or terms disappear from the expectation and the estimator is negatively biased.

For any fixed value of n, $\hat{\mathrm{V}}_{SYG}\hat{Y}_{\bullet HT}$ is known to perform better than an earlier variance estimator suggested by Horvitz and Thompson (1952), although the latter is also valid (and usually unbiased) for samples of random size. For both these variance estimators, however, their dependence on the π_{ij} has proved problematical (Särndal, 1996; Brewer, 1999b). Brewer's (2001) alternative formulation of (9.4), which was intended to circumvent the need to know the individual π_{ij}, is obtained as follows. We start with a small and obvious modification of (9.4) itself:

$$\begin{aligned}
\mathrm{V}\hat{Y}_{\bullet HT} &= \frac{1}{2}\sum_{i=1}^{N}\sum_{j(\neq i)=1}^{N}(\pi_i\pi_j - \pi_{ij})\left\{\left(Y_i\pi_i^{-1} - Y_{\bullet}n^{-1}\right) - \left(Y_j\pi_j^{-1} - Y_{\bullet}n^{-1}\right)\right\}^2 \\
&= \frac{1}{2}\sum_{i=1}^{N}\sum_{j(\neq i)=1}^{N}(\pi_i\pi_j - \pi_{ij})\left\{\left(Y_i\pi_i^{-1} - Y_{\bullet}n^{-1}\right)^2 + \left(Y_j\pi_j^{-1} - Y_{\bullet}n^{-1}\right)^2\right. \\
&\quad \left. - 2\left(Y_i\pi_i^{-1} - Y_{\bullet}n^{-1}\right)\left(Y_j\pi_j^{-1} - Y_{\bullet}n^{-1}\right)\right\} \\
&= \sum_{i=1}^{N}\sum_{j(\neq i)=1}^{N}(\pi_i\pi_j - \pi_{ij})\left(Y_i\pi_i^{-1} - Y_{\bullet}n^{-1}\right)^2 \\
&\quad - \sum_{i=1}^{N}\sum_{j(\neq i)=1}^{N}(\pi_i\pi_j - \pi_{ij})\left(Y_i\pi_i^{-1} - Y_{\bullet}n^{-1}\right)\left(Y_j\pi_j^{-1} - Y_{\bullet}n^{-1}\right). \qquad (9.6)
\end{aligned}$$

Using (4.7a) and (4.7c) we can rewrite the first term in (9.6) as

$$\begin{aligned}
&\sum_{i=1}^{N}\sum_{j(\neq i)=1}^{N}(\pi_i\pi_j - \pi_{ij})\left(Y_i\pi_i^{-1} - Y_{\bullet}n^{-1}\right)^2 \\
&= \sum_{i=1}^{N}\left(\sum_{j(\neq i)=1}^{N}\pi_j\right)\pi_i\left(Y_i\pi_i^{-1} - Y_{\bullet}n^{-1}\right)^2 \\
&\quad - \sum_{i=1}^{N}\left(\sum_{j(\neq i)=1}^{N}\pi_{ij}\right)\left(Y_i\pi_i^{-1} - Y_{\bullet}n^{-1}\right)^2 \\
&= \sum_{i=1}^{N}(n - \pi_i)\pi_i\left(Y_i\pi_i^{-1} - Y_{\bullet}n^{-1}\right)^2 - \sum_{i=1}^{N}\pi_i(n-1)\left(Y_i\pi_i^{-1} - Y_{\bullet}n^{-1}\right)^2 \\
&= \sum_{i=1}^{N}\pi_i(1 - \pi_i)\left(Y_i\pi_i^{-1} - Y_{\bullet}n^{-1}\right)^2 \\
&= \sum_{i=1}^{N}\pi_i\left(Y_i\pi_i^{-1} - Y_{\bullet}n^{-1}\right)^2 - \sum_{i=1}^{N}\pi_i^2\left(Y_i\pi_i^{-1} - Y_{\bullet}n^{-1}\right)^2. \qquad (9.7)
\end{aligned}$$

The first term in (9.7) is virtually the same as the with-replacement design variance of the Hansen–Hurwitz estimator, $\hat{Y}_{\bullet HH}$. The second term in (9.7) can then be interpreted as an approximation to the finite-population correction. These two terms together therefore plausibly constitute a first approximation to the entire 'natural' or 'high-entropy' design variance of the HTE and, importantly, neither of them depends on the π_{ij}. That in turn suggests that the second term in (9.6) – the only term in $\hat{Y}_{\bullet HT}$ that *does* depend on the π_{ij} – would be small compared with either of the terms in (9.7), and for high-entropy selection procedures this is indeed the case. The two terms in (9.7) are $O(n^{-1}N^2)$ and $O(N)$ respectively, but the second term in (9.6), as we shall see, is only $O(n^{-1}N)$ in high-entropy situations. So only about one Nth part of the high-entropy variance of the HTE is then dependent on the values of the π_{ij}. (In low-entropy situations, such as where selection is systematic from a meaningfully ordered population, that proportion can be much greater in absolute terms, and is typically negative.)

In the high-entropy situation we may use (9.3) to develop the second term in (9.6) as

$$
\begin{aligned}
&-\sum_{i=1}^{N}\sum_{j(\neq i)=1}^{N}(\pi_i\pi_j-\pi_{ij})\left(Y_i\pi_i^{-1}-Y_{\bullet}n^{-1}\right)\left(Y_j\pi_j^{-1}-Y_{\bullet}n^{-1}\right)\\
&\cong-\sum_{i=1}^{N}\sum_{j(\neq i)=1}^{N}\pi_i\pi_j\left\{\frac{1}{2}(2-c_i-c_j)\right\}\left(Y_i\pi_i^{-1}-Y_{\bullet}n^{-1}\right)\left(Y_j\pi_j^{-1}-Y_{\bullet}n^{-1}\right)\\
&=-\sum_{i=1}^{N}\sum_{j(\neq i)=1}^{N}\pi_i\pi_j\left(Y_i\pi_i^{-1}-Y_{\bullet}n^{-1}\right)\left(Y_j\pi_j^{-1}-Y_{\bullet}n^{-1}\right)\\
&\quad+\frac{1}{2}\sum_{i=1}^{N}\sum_{j(\neq i)=1}^{N}\pi_i\pi_jc_i\left(Y_i\pi_i^{-1}-Y_{\bullet}n^{-1}\right)\left(Y_j\pi_j^{-1}-Y_{\bullet}n^{-1}\right)\\
&\quad+\frac{1}{2}\sum_{i=1}^{N}\sum_{j(\neq i)=1}^{N}\pi_i\pi_jc_j\left(Y_i\pi_i^{-1}-Y_{\bullet}n^{-1}\right)\left(Y_j\pi_j^{-1}-Y_{\bullet}n^{-1}\right)\\
&=-\sum_{i=1}^{N}\sum_{j=1}^{N}\pi_i\pi_j\left(Y_i\pi_i^{-1}-Y_{\bullet}n^{-1}\right)\left(Y_j\pi_j^{-1}-Y_{\bullet}n^{-1}\right)\\
&\quad+\sum_{i=1}^{N}\pi_i^2\left(Y_i\pi_i^{-1}-Y_{\bullet}n^{-1}\right)^2\\
&\quad+\frac{1}{2}\sum_{i=1}^{N}\sum_{j=1}^{N}\pi_i\pi_jc_i\left(Y_i\pi_i^{-1}-Y_{\bullet}n^{-1}\right)\left(Y_j\pi_j^{-1}-Y_{\bullet}n^{-1}\right)\\
&\quad-\frac{1}{2}\sum_{i=1}^{N}\pi_i^2c_i\left(Y_i\pi_i^{-1}-Y_{\bullet}n^{-1}\right)^2\\
&\quad+\frac{1}{2}\sum_{i=1}^{N}\sum_{j=1}^{N}\pi_i\pi_jc_j\left(Y_i\pi_i^{-1}-Y_{\bullet}n^{-1}\right)\left(Y_j\pi_j^{-1}-Y_{\bullet}n^{-1}\right)\\
&\quad-\frac{1}{2}\sum_{j=1}^{N}\pi_j^2c_j\left(Y_j\pi_j^{-1}-Y_{\bullet}n^{-1}\right)^2
\end{aligned}
$$

$$
\begin{aligned}
&= -\left\{\sum_{i=1}^{N}\pi_i\left(Y_i\pi_i^{-1} - Y_{\bullet}n^{-1}\right)\right\}\left\{\sum_{j=1}^{N}\pi_j\left(Y_j\pi_j^{-1} - Y_{\bullet}n^{-1}\right)\right\} \\
&\quad + \sum_{i=1}^{N}\pi_i^2\left(Y_i\pi_i^{-1} - Y_{\bullet}n^{-1}\right)^2 \\
&\quad + \frac{1}{2}\left\{\sum_{i=1}^{N}\pi_i c_i\left(Y_i\pi_i^{-1} - Y_{\bullet}n^{-1}\right)\right\}\left\{\sum_{j=1}^{N}\pi_j\left(Y_j\pi_j^{-1} - Y_{\bullet}n^{-1}\right)\right\} \\
&\quad - \frac{1}{2}\sum_{i=1}^{N}\pi_i^2 c_i\left(Y_i\pi_i^{-1} - Y_{\bullet}n^{-1}\right)^2 \\
&\quad + \frac{1}{2}\left\{\sum_{i=1}^{N}\pi_i\left(Y_i\pi_i^{-1} - Y_{\bullet}n^{-1}\right)\right\}\left\{\sum_{j=1}^{N}\pi_j c_j\left(Y_j\pi_j^{-1} - Y_{\bullet}n^{-1}\right)\right\} \\
&\quad - \frac{1}{2}\sum_{i=1}^{N}\pi_i^2 c_i\left(Y_i\pi_i^{-1} - Y_{\bullet}n^{-1}\right)^2.
\end{aligned}
$$

However, both $\sum_{i=1}^{N}\pi_i\left(Y_i\pi_i^{-1} - Y_{\bullet}n^{-1}\right)$ and $\sum_{j=1}^{N}\pi_j\left(Y_j\pi_j^{-1} - Y_{\bullet}n^{-1}\right)$ are equal to zero, so that

$$
\begin{aligned}
&-\sum_{i=1}^{N}\sum_{j(\neq i)=1}^{N}(\pi_i\pi_j - \pi_{ij})\left(Y_i\pi_i^{-1} - Y_{\bullet}n^{-1}\right)\left(Y_j\pi_j^{-1} - Y_{\bullet}n^{-1}\right) \\
&\cong 0 + \sum_{i=1}^{N}\pi_i^2\left(Y_i\pi_i^{-1} - Y_{\bullet}n^{-1}\right)^2 + 0 - \frac{1}{2}\sum_{i=1}^{N}\pi_i^2 c_i\left(Y_i\pi_i^{-1} - Y_{\bullet}n^{-1}\right)^2 \\
&\quad + 0 - \frac{1}{2}\sum_{i=1}^{N}\pi_i^2 c_i\left(Y_i\pi_i^{-1} - Y_{\bullet}n^{-1}\right)^2 \\
&= \sum_{i=1}^{N}\pi_i^2(1 - c_i)\left(Y_i\pi_i^{-1} - Y_{\bullet}n^{-1}\right)^2. \qquad (9.8)
\end{aligned}
$$

Since, from (9.2), the high-entropy value of $1 - c_i$ is $O(n^{-1})$, the second term in (9.6) is, as foreshadowed, only $O(n^{-1}N)$, or about one Nth part of the total high-entropy variance.

Summing (9.7) and (9.8), the two terms of (9.6) combined amount to

$$
\begin{aligned}
\mathrm{V}\hat{Y}_{\bullet HT} &\cong \sum_{i=1}^{N}\pi_i\left(Y_i\pi_i^{-1} - Y_{\bullet}n^{-1}\right)^2 - \sum_{i=1}^{N}\pi_i^2\left(Y_i\pi_i^{-1} - Y_{\bullet}n^{-1}\right)^2 \\
&\quad + \sum_{i=1}^{N}\pi_i^2\left(Y_i\pi_i^{-1} - Y_{\bullet}n^{-1}\right)^2 - \sum_{i=1}^{N}\pi_i^2 c_i\left(Y_i\pi_i^{-1} - Y_{\bullet}n^{-1}\right)^2
\end{aligned}
$$

$$= \sum_{i=1}^{N} \pi_i \left(Y_i \pi_i^{-1} - Y_{\bullet} n^{-1} \right)^2 - \sum_{i=1}^{N} \pi_i^2 c_i \left(Y_i \pi_i^{-1} - Y_{\bullet} n^{-1} \right)^2$$

$$= \sum_{i=1}^{N} \pi_i (1 - c_i \pi_i) \left(Y_i \pi_i^{-1} - Y_{\bullet} n^{-1} \right)^2. \tag{9.9}$$

Substituting formula (9.2) for c_i in (9.9), we finally arrive at the specific approximation,

$$\tilde{V}\hat{Y}_{\bullet HT} = \sum_{i=1}^{N} \pi_i \left[1 - \pi_i \left\{ n^{-1}(n-1) \right\} \left(1 - n^{-2} \sum_{k=1}^{N} \pi_k^2 + 2n^{-1}\pi_i \right) \right] \times \left(Y_i \pi_i^{-1} - Y_{\bullet} n^{-1} \right)^2, \tag{9.10}$$

which, since it follows to $O(n^3 N^{-3})$ the high-entropy approximations to π_{ij} arrived at by Hartley and Rao (1962) and by Asok and Sukhatme (1976), is likely to be a good approximation to any high-entropy variance of the HTE.

However, when $\pi_i = nN^{-1}$ for all i, as is the case under *srswor*, (9.9) gives the correct expression for the *srswor* variance only if $c_i = n^{-1}(n-1)N(N-1)^{-1}$; whereas for (9.2), and therefore for (9.10), $c_i = n^{-1}(n-1)(N+1)N^{-1}$. In the next section we shall suggest what we believe to be a suitable way of avoiding this discrepancy.

9.4 Other formulae of the general form (9.9) but with somewhat different expressions for c_i were used in Brewer (2001) and in Brewer and Gregoire (2001). These are of interest not only because their c_i formulae guarantee the correct expression for the *srswor* variance, but also because they can be constructed using only (9.9) and (4.7), which equations happen to be valid whenever the sample size is a fixed number, regardless of whether the selection procedure used is of high entropy or not (although, admittedly, the way in which equations (4.7) are actually used implicitly *assumes* that the entropy is high).

Brewer (2001) pointed out that the relationship between (4.7b) and (4.7d) suggested the choice

$$c_i = c = \frac{n-1}{n - n^{-1} \sum_{k=1}^{N} \pi_k^2}. \tag{9.11}$$

This formula had earlier been suggested to him on other grounds by P.S. Kott in a private communication. Its attraction was that the c_i did not vary with i. A similar use of (4.7b) and (4.7d) had been made in equation (18) of Tillé (1996).

Brewer further conjectured, however, that the more specific relationship between (4.7a) and (4.7c), which instead suggested the choice

$$c_i = \frac{n-1}{n - \pi_i}, \tag{9.12}$$

would probably provide a more appropriate estimator; and the fact that (9.12) resembled (9.10), more closely than (9.11) did, tended to confirm his conjecture.

In addition, he suspected that a further improvement in accuracy might be attainable by using

$$c_i = \frac{(n-1)/n}{1 - 2n^{-1}\pi_i + n^{-2}\sum_{k=1}^{N} \pi_k^2}, \tag{9.13}$$

since that agreed with (9.2) to $O(N^{-1})$.

Now it happens that (9.11), (9.12) and (9.13) all return the correct variance formula when the sampling procedure is *srswor*, which is the reason why we now prefer to use them, rather than (9.2), with (9.9). We would use (9.11) if we wanted a c_i that did not vary with i, and (9.12) if we were after maximum simplicity, but we would use (9.13) if we wanted the greatest possible accuracy.

You should note that the papers of Hartley and Rao (1962) and of Asok and Sukhatme (1976) provide approximate formulae for $\mathrm{V}\hat{Y}_{\bullet HT}$ by the substitution of their π_{ij} approximations directly into the SYG variance formula (9.4). However, because of the large number of terms in the double summation, this is a considerably more tedious route to follow than the use of (9.9).

9.5 We mentioned in **9.1** that another family of approximate expressions for the HTE variance also merited consideration. That family uses the approximate formula for the π_{ij} that Hájek (1964) derived for another high-entropy selection procedure (which he called rejective sampling). That approximation is

$$\pi_{ij} \cong \pi_i \pi_j \left[1 - (1-\pi_i)(1-\pi_j) \left\{ \sum_{k=1}^{N} \pi_k (1-\pi_k) \right\}^{-1} \right], \tag{9.14}$$

and it implies that

$$\pi_i \pi_j - \pi_{ij} \cong \pi_i \pi_j (1-\pi_i)(1-\pi_j) \left\{ \sum_{k=1}^{N} \pi_k (1-\pi_k) \right\}^{-1}. \tag{9.15}$$

If we substitute (9.15) into the SYG variance formula (9.4), then after some simplification we obtain Hájek's approximation to the HTE variance, namely

$$\tilde{\mathrm{V}}_{HAJ} \hat{Y}_{\bullet HT} = \sum_{i=1}^{N} \pi_i (1-\pi_i) \left(Y_i \pi_i^{-1} - \tilde{Y}_{\bullet} n^{-1} \right)^2, \tag{9.16}$$

where $\tilde{Y}_{\bullet} = \sum_{i=1}^{N} a_i Y_i$ and $a_i = \left\{ \sum_{j=1}^{N} \pi_j (1-\pi_j) \right\}^{-1} n(1-\pi_i)$.

Formula (9.16), which looks like (9.9) with $\tilde{Y}_{\bullet}$ instead of $Y_{\bullet}$ and $c_i = 1$, is the starting point for this alternative family of variance approximations. Formula (4.2) of Rosén (1997b, p. 171) is one of several that Rosén has produced for high-entropy selection procedures. This one is for an order sampling selection procedure known as 'Pareto πps'. If we replace the target inclusion probabilities

λ_i in it with the actual inclusion probabilities, π_i, we obtain

$$\tilde{V}_{ROS}\hat{Y}_{\bullet HT} = N(N-1)^{-1}\sum_{i=1}^{N}\pi_i(1-\pi_i)\left(Y_i\pi_i^{-1} - \tilde{Y}_{\bullet}n^{-1}\right)^2. \tag{9.17}$$

This expression differs from (9.9) in the following three ways:

(i) The replacement of an unspecified c_i by the specific requirement $c_i = 1$.
(ii) Multiplication of the whole expression by the factor $N(N-1)^{-1}$, as in (9.17).
(iii) The replacement of $Y_{\bullet}$ by $\tilde{Y}_{\bullet}$.

All the approximations in the alternative family differ from (9.9) in one or more of those three ways. We shall now consider each of them in turn.

Difference (i) is suboptimal. The results in **9.2** indicate clearly that c_i has to be slightly larger than $(n-1)/n$. Choosing $c_i = 1$ decreases the approximate variance by a factor that under *srswor* amounts to $N^{-1}(N-1)$. Because of this, Rosén (1997a, p. 142) introduced the correction factor $N(N-1)^{-1}$ that we have already noted as difference (ii). Since the only part of the variance affected by the π_{ij} is the small second term in (9.6), it is inappropriate to apply a correction factor to the entire variance. Difference (i) signals a deficiency in the approximation (9.16), and difference (ii) is (to use Rosén's own description) an 'ad hoc' way of remedying it.

Difference (iii) is more difficult to assess. Under *srswor*, each of the a_i is equal to unity, so $\tilde{Y}_{\bullet}$ and $Y_{\bullet}$ are identical, and there is no call for a correction factor on that account. However, $Y_{\bullet}$ is unequivocally a simpler choice than $\tilde{Y}_{\bullet}$, so we consider the onus to be on those who favour using $\tilde{Y}_{\bullet}$ to make a convincing case for it. (The differences should show up well when some of the π_i are close to unity. This would be unlikely to correspond to any realistic situation, but it would probably provide a sensitive test.)

That much said, we should re-emphasize the fact that both Hájek's (9.16) and Rosén's (9.17) seem to perform well in practice, as do the variance estimators based on them. Deville (1999) is another who has used a variance estimator based on Hájek's approximation (9.14) to good effect. At present, the only claim we can make for the superiority of (9.9) (with values of c_i slightly in excess of $(n-1)/n$, of course) is a superiority in mathematical logic, but we will put these formulae to an empirical test if and when we get the opportunity.

A Model-Assisted Check on the Usefulness of the Approximate Horvitz–Thompson Estimator's Design Variance Formulae

9.6 Rather than leave the questions raised in **9.5** inadequately resolved, we decided to try another route towards obtaining a suitable approximation for the high-entropy variance. If the population follows a simple regression model, it automatically has high entropy, so we have no need to introduce it through the selection procedure.

Consider, then, the following ratio model as a possible description of the population being sampled:

$$\xi_\pi: \qquad Y_i = \beta\pi_i + U_i; \;\; \mathrm{E}_{\xi_\pi} U_i = 0; \;\; \mathrm{E}_{\xi_\pi} U_i^2 = \sigma_i^2; \;\; \mathrm{E}_{\xi_\pi}(U_i U_j) = 0, \quad j \neq i. \tag{9.18}$$

This is something of a shorthand model. It is intended to reflect the situation where the expected values of the Y_i are *intrinsically* proportional to the X_i, and then the inclusion probabilities π_i are *chosen* to be proportional to the X_i. It is, of course, impossible for the Y_i to be directly dependent on the inclusion probabilities as such, since those probabilities may be set quite arbitrarily by the person designing the sample. (It was such an arbitrary setting of the π_i that cost the circus statistician his job, you may remember!)

The ξ_π-expectation (or prediction expectation under ξ_π) of the approximate design variance given by (9.9) is

$$\begin{aligned}
\mathrm{E}_{\xi_\pi} \bar{\mathrm{V}}\hat{Y}_{\bullet HT} &= \mathrm{E}_{\xi_\pi} \sum_{i=1}^{N} \pi_i(1 - c_i\pi_i)\left(Y_i\pi_i^{-1} - Y_{\bullet}n^{-1}\right)^2 \\
&= \mathrm{E}_{\xi_\pi} \sum_{i=1}^{N} \pi_i(1 - c_i\pi_i)\left(U_i\pi_i^{-1} - U_{\bullet}n^{-1}\right)^2 \\
&= \mathrm{E}_{\xi_\pi} \sum_{i=1}^{N} \pi_i(1 - c_i\pi_i)\left\{U_i\left(\pi_i^{-1} - n^{-1}\right) - n^{-1} \sum_{j(\neq i)=1}^{N} U_j\right\}^2 \\
&= \sum_{i=1}^{N} \pi_i(1 - c_i\pi_i)\left\{\sigma_i^2\left(\pi_i^{-1} - n^{-1}\right)^2 + n^{-2} \sum_{j(\neq i)=1}^{N} \sigma_j^2\right\} \\
&= \sum_{i=1}^{N} \pi_i(1 - c_i\pi_i)\left\{\sigma_i^2\left(\pi_i^{-2} - 2\pi_i^{-1}n^{-1}\right) + n^{-2} \sum_{j=1}^{N} \sigma_j^2\right\} \\
&= \sum_{i=1}^{N} \left\{\sigma_i^2\left(\pi_i^{-1} - 2n^{-1}\right) + n^{-2}\pi_i \sum_{j=1}^{N} \sigma_j^2 \right. \\
&\qquad \left. - \sigma_i^2 c_i\left(1 - 2n^{-1}\pi_i\right) - n^{-2}c_i\pi_i^2 \sum_{j=1}^{N} \sigma_j^2\right\} \\
&= \sum_{i=1}^{N} \sigma_i^2\left(\pi_i^{-1} - 2n^{-1}\right) + n^{-1} \sum_{j=1}^{N} \sigma_j^2
\end{aligned}$$

$$- \sum_{i=1}^{N} \sigma_i^2 c_i \left(1 - 2n^{-1}\pi_i\right) - n^{-2} \left(\sum_{j=1}^{N} c_j \pi_j^2 \right) \sum_{j=1}^{N} \sigma_j^2$$

$$= \sum_{i=1}^{N} \sigma_i^2 \left\{ \pi_i^{-1} - n^{-1} - c_i\left(1 - 2n^{-1}\pi_i\right) - n^{-2} \sum_{j=1}^{N} c_j \pi_j^2 \right\}. \qquad (9.19)$$

Ideally, this should be equal to $\mathrm{E}_{\xi_\pi} \mathrm{V}\hat{Y}_{\bullet HT}$, which is $\sum_{i\propto 1}^{N} \sigma_i^2 \left(\pi_i^{-1} - 1\right)$ (Godambe, 1955; Godambe and Joshi, 1965). This leads to the implicit formula

$$c_i = \frac{1 - n^{-1} - n^{-2} \sum_{k=1}^{N} c_k \pi_k^2}{1 - 2n^{-1}\pi_i}. \qquad (9.20)$$

Equation (9.20) can be solved for c_i iteratively, starting with the trial value $c_i^{[1]} = 1 - n^{-1}$. To $O(N^{-1})$, this iterative solution is the same as both (9.2) and (9.13), the latter being the one of Brewer's three suggestions in **9.3** that most closely resembles (9.2).

Alternatively, a closed expression can be derived by putting (9.19) equal to $\sum_{i=1}^{N} \sigma_i^2 (\pi_i^{-1} - 1)$ and then requiring that $c_i = c$ for all i, in which case we obtain

$$c = \frac{\left(1 - n^{-1}\right) \sum_{i=1}^{N} \sigma_i^2}{\sum_{i=1}^{N} \sigma_i^2 - 2n^{-1} \sum_{i=1}^{N} \sigma_i^2 \pi_i + n^{-2} \sum_{i=1}^{N} \sigma_i^2 \sum_{j=1}^{N} \pi_j^2}. \qquad (9.21)$$

If this equation is substituted in (9.9), it also returns the exact variance formula for *srswor*. Even without *srswor*, substituting $\sigma^2 \pi_i$ for σ_i^2 in (9.21) returns (9.11) for c. We found it reassuring that the two analyses, one purely design-based and the other model-assisted, led to so nearly the same expressions for the 'natural' or high-entropy design variance of the HTE.

Sample Estimators of the High-Entropy Anticipated Variance of the Horvitz–Thompson Estimator

9.7 A plausible sample estimator of the approximate design variance of the HTE given in (9.9), and one that can be constructed so as to be exactly design-unbiased under *srswor*, is

$$\hat{\mathrm{V}}\hat{Y}_{\bullet HT} = \sum_{i=1}^{N} \delta_i \left(c_i^{-1} - \pi_i\right) \left(Y_i \pi_i^{-1} - \hat{Y}_{\bullet HT} n^{-1}\right)^2. \qquad (9.22)$$

The choice of the c_i is, as we have seen, somewhat flexible, but if they are defined by (9.11), then (9.22) is the estimator used by Brewer and Gregoire (2001) in their empirical investigations; and the tables at the end of this chapter are based on it. Any choice of c_i that satisfies $c_i = n^{-1}(n-1)N(N-1)^{-1}$ when $\pi_i = nN^{-1}$ for all i will, as we have seen, satisfy the requirement that (9.22) is design-unbiased under *srswor*. However, its properties under the more general case of *πpswor* are not easily evaluated, so it seems sensible to consider its properties as an estimator of the anticipated variance instead, as we did for certain other variance estimators in Chapter 5.

The ξ_π-expectation of an HTE variance estimator would ideally be $\sum_{i=1}^N \delta_i \sigma_i^2 \pi_i^{-1}(\pi_i^{-1} - 1)$, because this in turn has design expectation $\sum_{i=1}^N \sigma_i^2(\pi_i^{-1} - 1)$, which is the lower bound for the anticipated variance of any unbiased estimator (Godambe, 1955; Godambe and Joshi, 1965). Unfortunately, if the model ξ_π of (9.18) is substituted into (9.22), its ξ_π-expectation differs from $\sum_{i=1}^N \delta_i \sigma_i^2 \pi_i^{-1}(\pi_i^{-1} - 1)$ by terms of order $O(Nn^{-1})$. Although these terms have opposite signs and therefore tend to cancel, they are not entirely negligible, being only $O(N^{-1})$ smaller than the variance itself.

To improve on (9.22), we used the following strategy. We aimed to estimate the HTE's anticipated variance by $\hat{\mathrm{V}}_1 \hat{Y}_{\bullet HT} = \sum_{i=1}^N \delta_i (A - F\pi_i)(Y_i \pi_i^{-1} - \hat{Y}_{\bullet HT} n^{-1})^2$, where A and F were chosen so as to ensure that $\mathrm{E}\mathrm{E}_{\xi_\pi} \hat{\mathrm{V}}_1 \hat{Y}_{\bullet HT}$ was as close to $\sum_{i=1}^N (\pi_i^{-1} - 1)\sigma_i^2$ as possible. We therefore required:

$$\mathrm{E}\mathrm{E}_{\xi_\pi} \sum_{i=1}^N \delta_i (A - F\pi_i)(Y_i \pi_i^{-1} - \hat{Y}_{\bullet HT} n^{-1})^2 \cong \mathrm{E}_{\xi_\pi} \mathrm{V} \hat{Y}_{\bullet HT} = \sum_{i=1}^N \sigma_i^2 (\pi_i^{-1} - 1). \tag{9.23}$$

To that end, we derived expressions for $\mathrm{E}_{\xi_\pi} \sum_{i=1}^N \delta_i (Y_i \pi_i^{-1} - \hat{Y}_{\bullet HT} n^{-1})^2$ and $\mathrm{E}_{\xi_\pi} \sum_{i=1}^N \delta_i \pi_i (Y_i \pi_i^{-1} - \hat{Y}_{\bullet HT} n^{-1})^2$, equated the coefficients of $\sum_{i=1}^N \sigma_i^2 \pi_i^{-1}$ and $\sum_{i=1}^N \sigma_i^2$, and then solved for A and F. The algebra required was tedious and will be omitted, but the final equating of coefficients (after omitting some terms of negligible order) led to $An^{-1}(n-1) - Fn^{-2}\sum_{i=1}^N \pi_i^2 \cong 1$ and $Fn^{-2}(n-1)^2 \cong 1$. Solving, we obtained $F \cong n^2(n-1)^{-2}$ and $A \cong n(n-1)^{-1}\{1 + (n-1)^{-2}\sum_{i=1}^N \pi_i^2\}$, so our approximately unbiased estimator of $\mathrm{V}\hat{Y}_{\bullet HT}$ was

$$\hat{\mathrm{V}}_1 \hat{Y}_{\bullet HT} = n(n-1)^{-1} \sum_{i=1}^N \delta_i \left\{ 1 + (n-1)^{-2} \sum_{k=1}^N \pi_k^2 - n(n-1)^{-1}\pi_i \right\} \times (Y_i \pi_i^{-1} - \hat{Y}_{\bullet HT} n^{-1})^2. \tag{9.24}$$

This looked superficially reasonable, but we noted that putting $\pi_i = nN^{-1}$ for all i did not quite return the *srswor* variance. After making a small adjustment, we found an expression that did attain this value under *srswor*. That expression was

$$\hat{\mathrm{V}}_2 \hat{Y}_{\bullet HT} = n(n-1)^{-1} \sum_{i=1}^N \delta_i \left\{ 1 + (n-1)^{-1} n^{-1} \sum_{k=1}^N \pi_k^2 - n(n-1)^{-1}\pi_i \right\} \times (Y_i \pi_i^{-1} - \hat{Y}_{\bullet HT} n^{-1})^2. \tag{9.25}$$

We must acknowledge, of course, that this adjustment is arbitrary in the same way as the introduction of the factor $N(N-1)^{-1}$ into (9.15) was arbitrary, but this time it is applied to a small and relevant term. Moreover, if we define c_i by (9.13), then (9.25) is close to (9.22). In fact, if we equate (9.25) to (9.22) we arrive at

$$c_i = \frac{(n-1)/n}{1-(2n-1)(n-1)^{-1}n^{-1}\pi_i + (n-1)^{-1}n^{-1}\sum_{k=1}^{N}\pi_k^2}, \tag{9.26}$$

which is close to (9.13), being just a trifle in the opposite direction to (9.12).

The design expectation of the expression in (9.25) still differs from the anticipated variance of the HTE, but only by a single term of order $O(Nn^{-2})$ – which is therefore smaller than the anticipated variance by a factor of order $O(N^{-1}n^{-1})$ – and by other terms that are of smaller magnitude still. These results confirm our conviction that (9.22) with c_i defined by (9.26) yields about as accurate an estimator of the high-entropy variance of the HTE as could reasonably be expected, at least without undue complication.

The fact that (9.26) delivers a value of c_i that satisfies $c_i = n^{-1}(n-1)N(N-1)^{-1}$ when $\pi_i = nN^{-1}$ is of considerable significance. The estimator (9.22) in itself is purely design based. Putting the condition on the c_i does no more than narrow down the class of design-based estimators to those that deliver an exactly unbiased estimator under *srswor*. In optimizing the estimator of the anticipated variance within a quite differently defined class, namely of those estimators that are linear combinations of $\sum_{i=1}^{N}\delta_i(Y_i\pi_i^{-1} - \hat{Y}_{.HT}n^{-1})^2$ and $\sum_{i=1}^{N}\delta_i\pi_i(Y_i\pi_i^{-1} - \hat{Y}_{.HT}n^{-1})^2$, and arriving (however fortuitously) at an estimator within the narrowed-down version of the original class, we have done no more than move from purely design-based inference to model-assisted sampling inference.

But the similarities between the two approaches do not stop there. The estimator (9.26) is not merely within the narrowed-down version of the original class; it is almost identical with the particular case '(9.22) with c_i defined by (9.13)' which we have already described as the one 'we would use … if we wanted the greatest possible accuracy'. We were pleased when, in **9.6**, the variance formulae arrived at by purely design-based inference and model-assisted inference were nearly coincident. Now we find the same thing happening when it comes to the sample estimation of that variance.

9.8 The form which (9.25) takes when $n = 2$ is of particular interest This is partly because many instances occur where only two units are selected from every stratum, particularly in multistage sampling (Chapters 10 and 11). It is also of interest, however, because the choice of this smallest possible sample size puts the asymptotics used in its derivation to a very severe test. Substituting $n = 2$ into (9.25) and using subscripts 1 and 2 to denote the two units selected (but continuing to allow $\sum_{k=1}^{N}\pi_k^2$ to denote the sum of the π_k^2 over all the N population units), we obtain:

$$\begin{aligned}
\hat{\hat{\mathrm{V}}}_2\hat{Y}_{\bullet HT} &= 2\left(1+\frac{1}{2}\sum_{k=1}^{N}\pi_k^2-2\pi_1\right)\left\{Y_1\pi_1^{-1}-\frac{1}{2}\left(Y_1\pi_1^{-1}+Y_2\pi_2^{-1}\right)\right\}^2\\
&\quad+2\left(1+\frac{1}{2}\sum_{k=1}^{N}\pi_k^2-2\pi_2\right)\left\{Y_2\pi_2^{-1}-\frac{1}{2}\left(Y_1\pi_1^{-1}+Y_2\pi_2^{-1}\right)\right\}^2\\
&= 2\sum_{i=1}^{2}\left(2+\sum_{k=1}^{N}\pi_k^2-2\pi_1-2\pi_2\right)\times\frac{1}{4}\left(Y_1\pi_1^{-1}-Y_2\pi_2^{-1}\right)^2\\
&= \left\{1-\left(\pi_1+\pi_2-\frac{1}{2}\sum_{k=1}^{N}\pi_k^2\right)\right\}\left(Y_1\pi_1^{-1}-Y_2\pi_2^{-1}\right)^2. \qquad (9.27)
\end{aligned}$$

Had selection been with replacement, the design-unbiased variance estimator would have been simply $\left(Y_1\pi_1^{-1}-Y_2\pi_2^{-1}\right)^2$, so (9.27) has an implied finite-population correction factor which is the average of $1-\left(2\pi_1-\frac{1}{2}\sum_{k=1}^{N}\pi_k^2\right)$ and $1-\left(2\pi_2-\frac{1}{2}\sum_{k=1}^{N}\pi_k^2\right)$. With $n=2$, all three of π_1, π_2 and $\frac{1}{2}\sum_{k=1}^{N}\pi_k^2$ are $O(2/N)$, which is also $O(n/N)$, so the finite-population correction *term*, $\pi_1+\pi_2-\frac{1}{2}\sum_{k=1}^{N}\pi_k^2$, or equivalently $\pi_1+\pi_2-\sum_{k=1}^{N}\pi_k^2/n$, is also $O(n/N)$, which is intuitively what we would expect.

In summary, the $\hat{\mathrm{V}}_2\hat{Y}_{\bullet HT}$ of (9.25) appears to be a good estimator on three grounds:

(i) Its double expectation differs from the anticipated variance of $\hat{Y}_{\bullet HT}$ under the model ξ_π of (9.18) by a term that is only $O(Nn^{-2})$, or $O(N^{-1}n^{-1})$ times the anticipated variance itself.
(ii) Under *srswor* it is exactly equal to the standard unbiased *srswor* variance estimator.
(iii) It provides an intuitively sound estimator when $n=2$.

Sample Estimators of the Design Variance of the Horvitz–Thompson Estimator Suitable for Use with Ordered Systematic Sampling

9.9 Meaningfully ordered systematic sampling is clearly not a procedure for which (9.25) could be expected to provide a convenient or adequate estimator of the HT design variance. An estimator that used only the differences between consecutive observations would have a better chance of being useful.

Consider the situation where an even number of units, $n=2m$, has been selected using ordered systematic sampling. We divide the population into m notional strata. These strata are of equal 'size', not in terms of numbers of units but in terms of the measure of size that is used to determine inclusion probabilities.

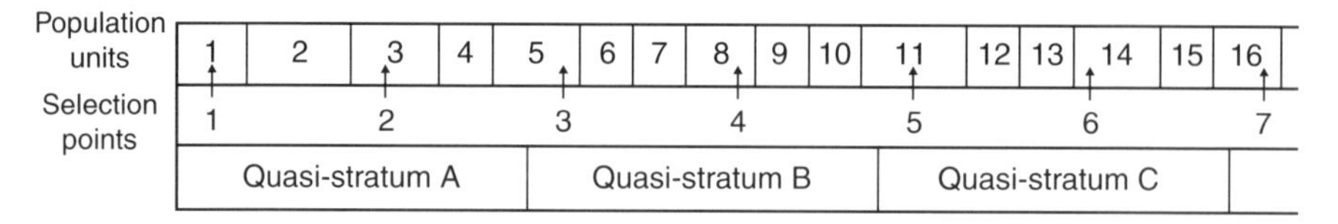

Figure 9.1 Selecting a systematic sample from an ordered population.

Consequently, these notional strata are not in general composed of whole units. If a unit straddles two notional strata (as unit 5 straddles strata A and B in Figure 9.1) and if it is selected because it contains a selection point for one of them, then the whole of that unit is regarded as one of the two representing that stratum, regardless of the fact that part of it is actually in another notional stratum.

We shall next estimate the m stratum totals and add them to obtain an estimate of the entire population. We shall also form estimates of the m stratum design variances and add them to estimate the design variance of the estimate of the entire population. Then we shall modify that estimator so as to make use also of the $m-1$ differences between neighbouring sample units in different but contiguous strata. Finally, we shall produce a suitable formula to cover the case where n is odd.

First then, consider the case where there is only a single stratum, and $n = 2$. By the definition of the notional or quasi-strata, the non-sample units within a quasi-stratum are not clearly defined, so it is advisable to choose a variance estimator that does not depend on the $\sum_{k=1}^{N} \pi_k^2$. For that reason, Brewer and Gregoire (2001) chose (9.22) with c_i defined by (9.12) as their estimator of the anticipated variance. This led them to the variance estimator:

$$\hat{\mathrm{V}}\hat{Y}_{\bullet HT} = 2\left\{\frac{1}{4}(1-\pi_1)\left(Y_1\pi_1^{-1} - Y_2\pi_2^{-1}\right)^2 + \frac{1}{4}(1-\pi_2)\left(Y_2\pi_2^{-1} - Y_1\pi_1^{-1}\right)^2\right\}$$
$$= \frac{1}{2}(2-\pi_1-\pi_2)\left(Y_1\pi_1^{-1} - Y_2\pi_2^{-1}\right)^2, \qquad (9.28)$$

where the subscripts 1 and 2 refer again to the two selected units. This is about as good an estimator as we can construct in the circumstances, for even if we were to try to stay with (9.27) and replace $\sum_{k=1}^{N} \pi_k^2$ by its HTE, that HTE would be $\pi_1 + \pi_2$, and that would send us back to (9.28).

As already noted in **9.5**, the expression $\left(Y_1\pi_1^{-1} - Y_2\pi_2^{-1}\right)^2$ by itself is the design-unbiased estimator of variance for *srswr*, while $\frac{1}{2}(2-\pi_1-\pi_2)$ under *srswor* takes the value $1 - nN^{-1}$ when $n = 2$. The estimator (9.28) therefore carries some intuitive appeal, and seems unlikely to be seriously misleading. (Also, in the circumstances, we do not have very much choice!)

Continuing, therefore, to use (9.28) as our tentative variance estimator for a single stratum, the estimator of variance for the m strata is

$$\hat{\mathrm{V}}\hat{Y}_{\bullet HT} = \sum_{h=1}^{m} \frac{1}{2}(2-\pi_{h1}-\pi_{h2})\left(Y_{h1}\pi_{h1}^{-1} - Y_{h2}\pi_{h2}^{-1}\right)^2.$$

This is the appropriate formula if there are m pairs of units providing squared differences. If, however, we now abolish the notional strata and consider all $n-1$ squared differences from pairs of neighbouring sampling units, our sum will have $n-1$ terms instead of m, so to keep to the same expectation we will need to use

$$\hat{\mathrm{V}}\hat{Y}_{\bullet HT} = m(n-1)^{-1}\sum_{k=1}^{n-1}\frac{1}{2}(2-\pi_k-\pi_{k+1})\left(Y_k\pi_k^{-1}-Y_{k+1}\pi_{k+1}^{-1}\right)^2.$$

Finally if there is an odd number of sample units selected (and we are of course assuming here that the selection is carried out in such a fashion that the number of sample units is predetermined) the value m must be replaced by the value it takes when n is even, namely $n/2$, so our tentative estimator in this context becomes

$$\hat{\mathrm{V}}\hat{Y}_{\bullet HT} = n\{2(n-1)\}^{-1}\sum_{k=1}^{n-1}\frac{1}{2}(2-\pi_k-\pi_{k+1})\left(Y_k\pi_k^{-1}-Y_{k+1}\pi_{k+1}^{-1}\right)^2, \tag{9.29}$$

regardless of whether n is odd or even.

Adaptation to Estimating the Design Variance of a Generalized Regression Estimator

9.10 The GREG estimator of total was defined in **8.7** as

$$\hat{Y}_{\bullet GREG} = \mathbf{1}_n'\boldsymbol{\pi}_s^{-1}\mathbf{y}_s + \left(\mathbf{1}_N'\mathbf{X} - \mathbf{1}_n'\boldsymbol{\pi}_s^{-1}\mathbf{X}_s\right)\hat{\boldsymbol{\beta}}_{GREG} \tag{8.17}$$

$$= \mathbf{1}_N'\mathbf{X}\hat{\boldsymbol{\beta}}_{GREG} + \mathbf{1}_n'\boldsymbol{\pi}_s^{-1}(\mathbf{y}_s - \mathbf{X}_s\hat{\boldsymbol{\beta}}_{GREG}). \tag{9.30}$$

Note that $\mathbf{1}_n'\boldsymbol{\pi}_s^{-1}\mathbf{y}_s$ is the HTE of $Y_{\bullet} = \mathbf{1}_N'\mathbf{y}$ and $\mathbf{1}_n'\boldsymbol{\pi}_s^{-1}\mathbf{X}_s$ is the HTE of $\mathbf{1}_N'\mathbf{X}$.

It is common practice (Särndal *et al.*, 1992, Section 6.6) to estimate the design variance of (9.30) by using its asymptotic equivalence to the difference estimator

$$\hat{Y}_{\bullet DIFF} = \mathbf{1}_n'\boldsymbol{\pi}_s^{-1}\mathbf{y}_s + \left(\mathbf{1}_N'\mathbf{X} - \mathbf{1}_n'\boldsymbol{\pi}_s^{-1}\mathbf{X}_s\right)\boldsymbol{\beta}$$

$$= \mathbf{1}_N'\mathbf{X}\boldsymbol{\beta} + \mathbf{1}_n'\boldsymbol{\pi}_s^{-1}(\mathbf{y}_s - \mathbf{X}_s\boldsymbol{\beta}). \tag{9.31}$$

In (9.31), the principal term, $\mathbf{1}_N'\mathbf{X}\boldsymbol{\beta}$, is free from sampling error and the expression $\mathbf{1}_n'\boldsymbol{\pi}_s^{-1}(\mathbf{y}_s - \mathbf{X}_s\boldsymbol{\beta})$ is the HTE of $\mathbf{1}_N'(\mathbf{y} - \mathbf{X}\boldsymbol{\beta})$. Särndal *et al.* therefore estimate the design variance of $\hat{Y}_{\bullet DIFF}$ using the Sen–Yates–Grundy estimator of the design variance of $\mathbf{1}_n'\boldsymbol{\pi}_s^{-1}(\mathbf{y}_s - \mathbf{X}_s\boldsymbol{\beta})$, or at least they do so in principle; but of course $\boldsymbol{\beta}$ is not known exactly, so in practice they estimate the design variance of $\hat{Y}_{\bullet GREG}$ using the Sen–Yates–Grundy estimator of the design variance of $\mathbf{1}_n'\boldsymbol{\pi}_s^{-1}(\mathbf{y}_s - \mathbf{X}_s\hat{\boldsymbol{\beta}}_{GREG})$. This results in an underestimation, because $\mathbf{1}'\mathbf{X}\hat{\boldsymbol{\beta}}_{GREG}$ is not free from sampling error in the same way as $\mathbf{1}'\mathbf{X}\boldsymbol{\beta}$ is. However, the design variance of $\mathbf{1}_n'\boldsymbol{\pi}_s^{-1}(\mathbf{y}_s - \mathbf{X}_s\hat{\boldsymbol{\beta}}_{GREG})$ is $O(N^2n^{-1})$, while that of $\mathbf{1}'\mathbf{X}\hat{\boldsymbol{\beta}}_{GREG}$ is only $O(N^2n^{-2})$, so for large samples the approximation is reasonable.

We will adopt the approximation described in principle above, but rather than use the Sen–Yates–Grundy formula to estimate the design variance of $\mathbf{1}'_n\boldsymbol{\pi}_s^{-1}(\mathbf{y}_s - \mathbf{X}_s\hat{\boldsymbol{\beta}}_{GREG})$, which depends on knowledge of the sample π_{ij}, we will instead modify expression (9.22) so as to make it appropriate for estimating the design variance of $\mathbf{1}'_n\boldsymbol{\pi}_s^{-1}(\mathbf{y}_s - \mathbf{X}_s\hat{\boldsymbol{\beta}}_{GREG})$ rather than that of $\hat{Y}_{\bullet HT} = \mathbf{1}'_n\boldsymbol{\pi}_s^{-1}\mathbf{y}_s$.

To make this modification, we introduce the notation $\hat{\bar{Y}}_i = \mathbf{X}'_i\hat{\boldsymbol{\beta}}_{GREG}$, where $\mathbf{X}'_i$ is the row vector of the supplementary variables matrix $\mathbf{X}$ for unit i, and in consequence $\hat{\bar{Y}}_i$ is the sample estimator of the underlying prediction expectation of Y_i, namely $\bar{Y}_i = \mathbf{X}'_i\boldsymbol{\beta}$. We then replace every (explicit and implicit) appearance of Y_i in (9.22) by $Y_i - \hat{\bar{Y}}_i$.

In addition, we follow Brewer and Gregoire in introducing the factor $n/(n-p)$ into the estimator, to compensate for the loss of p degrees of freedom when estimating $\boldsymbol{\beta}$. This is a rather crude adjustment, since $\hat{\boldsymbol{\beta}}_{GREG}$ is not arrived at by according each observation equal weight, but it is almost certainly preferable to not making any adjustment at all. The approximate design variance of the GREG estimator of total can therefore be tentatively estimated by

$$\hat{\hat{V}}\hat{Y}_{\bullet GREG} = n(n-p)^{-1}\sum_{i=1}^{N}\delta_i(c_i^{-1} - \pi_i)\pi_i^{-2}\left(Y_i - \hat{\bar{Y}}_i\right)^2, \qquad (9.32)$$

c_i being defined by (9.11), (9.12), (9.13) or (9.26).

This estimator is also appropriate for the anticipated variance defined by Isaki and Fuller (1982). For the prediction variance, however, the factor $\pi_i^{-2}\left(c^{-1} - \pi_i\right)$ or $\pi_i^{-2}\left(c_i^{-1} - \pi_i\right)$ should be replaced by the near equivalent $w_i(w_i - 1)$, where w_i is the sample weight or case weight (see Chapter 8).

Finally, if the sample design is (meaningfully) ordered systematic sampling, the parameter $\boldsymbol{\beta}$ must be estimated across the notional strata. If the estimation is across all n observations, the crude bias correction factor is $n/(n-p)$ and the resulting estimator of design variance is

$$\hat{\hat{V}}\hat{Y}_{\bullet GREG} = n\{2(n-1)\}^{-1}n(n-p)^{-1}\sum_{k=1}^{n-1}\frac{1}{2}(2 - \pi_k - \pi_{k+1}) \times \left\{(Y_k - \hat{\bar{Y}}_k)\pi_k^{-1} - (Y_{k+1} - \hat{\bar{Y}}_{k+1})\pi_{k+1}^{-1}\right\}^2. \qquad (9.33)$$

Remark 9.10.1 A better way of allowing for the 'loss of p degrees of freedom' would be to use the unbiased estimation theory of **8.14** to estimate the individual σ_i^2 in the relevant prediction model. These estimates, denoted by $\tilde{\sigma}_i^2$ in (8.32) and (8.33), could then be used to estimate either the prediction variance or the anticipated variance, or both. However, this involves the solution of $p(p+1)/2$ simultaneous equations, or equivalently inverting a matrix of order $p(p+1)/2$. Brewer and Gregoire became aware of this option during the last two weeks prior to presenting their conference paper, but did not then have time to use it.

Some Empirical Results

9.11 The empirical results presented in this section are taken from Brewer and Gregoire (2001). As indicated in **9.1**, they test the validity and usefulness of the concepts described in this report, using a Monte Carlo experiment on forest data. The forest in question consisted of 14 443 loblolly pine trees in Alabama. The survey variable Y_i was volume of timber, and the supplementary variables $\mathbf{X}_i'$ were basal area and height.

The primary purpose of their investigation was to discover whether their estimators – (9.22) and (9.32) in this report – could be applied in circumstances where the selection procedure resulted in samples of random rather than fixed size, by the expedient of treating any actual sample as though it had been deliberately selected to have the sample size n that actually eventuated. In other words, these formulae were used after conditioning each sample on its achieved size, and in order to perform this conditioning, the inclusion probabilities were multiplied by the ratio of the achieved sample size to the expected or target sample size. The estimated design variances of the 'HT' estimates they obtained using these adjusted sizes in (9.22) were compared with the actual Monte Carlo variances observed across their estimated totals of timber volume.

Various combinations of basal area and height were also used to produce GREG estimates of these totals, and the estimated design variances of these GREG estimates were similarly compared with their Monte Carlo design variances. The most accurate GREG estimates were obtained when basal area and height were multiplied together to obtain a single supplementary variable (actually expressed as diameter squared times height or D^2H). Regression on basal area alone (A) was also important, however, because height, which is normally 'measured' by eye estimates, is substantially less useful than basal area, and often not collected at all. When A was used alone an intercept variable was introduced, but it proved counter-productive to use it with D^2H. Both GREG estimators were cosmetically calibrated (see Chapter 8) so as to have prediction inference as well as randomization inference to back them.

The reason for these investigators' interest in samples of random size was that the most common selection procedure used to sample trees in forests is Poisson sampling, which (as noted in Chapter 4) does indeed result in such randomly sized samples. The samples of principal interest for their study were therefore those selected using that method, but important comparisons were made with samples selected systematically, both from the population randomly ordered and from it arranged in order of tree size. (The nature of their data did not permit them to use a geographical ordering.) The systematic samples from randomly ordered populations provided them with a direct test of the usefulness of their formulae (9.22) and (9.32) for samples of fixed size. Those drawn from the population arranged in size order also permitted them to test the estimators (9.29) and (9.33).

A single run of 100 000 samples was used for each sample size for each procedure separately. Each of the systematically selected samples drawn from a random ordering of the population was drawn from a different random ordering.

Rows 1 and 2 in each section of Table 9.1 show the percentage biases of the unconstrained and constrained HTEs, respectively. Following long-standing forestry usage, the constrained HTE is labelled '$3P7$'. Rows 3 and 4 show the corresponding biases for the two best GREG estimators for samples of (expected) size 144, 48 and 24. Only the GREG estimator based on basal area and an intercept term displayed any appreciable bias. A small non-zero bias is shown for the HTE

Table 9.1 Observed Monte Carlo percentage biases in estimators of total timber volume

Estimator	Poisson sampling	Systematic sampling (population in random orderings)	Systematic sampling (population in size order)
Expected sample size 144			
Uncond. HT ($\hat{Y}_{\bullet HT}$)	0.02	0.00	0.00
Cond. HT ($\hat{Y}_{\bullet 3P7}$)	0.00	0.00	0.00
GREG (1,A)	−0.07	−0.07	0.00
GREG (D^2H)	−0.01	0.00	−0.01
Expected sample size 48			
Uncond. HT ($\hat{Y}_{\bullet HT}$)	0.02	−0.03	0.00
Cond. HT ($\hat{Y}_{\bullet 3P7}$)	−0.02	−0.03	0.00
GREG (1,A)	−0.27	−0.28	−0.05
GREG (D^2H)	−0.03	−0.03	0.00
Expected sample size 24			
Uncond. HT ($\hat{Y}_{\bullet HT}$)	0.01	0.00	−0.01
Cond. HT ($\hat{Y}_{\bullet 3P7}$)	−0.01	0.00	−0.01
GREG (1,A)	−0.59	−0.59	−0.16
GREG (D^2H)	−0.03	−0.03	0.04

Table 9.2 Observed Monte Carlo percentage RMSEs for estimators of total timber volume

Estimator	Poisson sampling	Systematic sampling (population in random orderings)	Systematic sampling (population in size order)
Expected sample size 144			
Uncond. HT ($\hat{Y}_{\bullet HT}$)	8.72	2.87	2.12
Cond. HT ($\hat{Y}_{\bullet 3P7}$)	2.87	2.87	2.12
GREG (1,A)	2.26	2.26	2.15
GREG (D^2H)	1.42	1.41	1.48
Expected sample size 48			
Uncond. HT ($\hat{Y}_{\bullet HT}$)	15.07	5.00	3.74
Cond. HT ($\hat{Y}_{\bullet 3P7}$)	5.04	5.00	3.74
GREG (1,A)	4.01	3.97	3.67
GREG (D^2H)	2.50	2.50	2.49
Expected sample size 24			
Uncond. HT ($\hat{Y}_{\bullet HT}$)	21.47	7.07	5.36
Cond. HT ($\hat{Y}_{\bullet 3P7}$)	7.22	7.07	5.36
GREG (1,A)	5.91	5.79	5.21
GREG (D^2H)	3.63	3.54	3.41

under Poisson sampling. Since the HTE is strictly unbiased, this non-zero value is actually a measurement error contingent on the finite size of the Monte Carlo experiment.

Table 9.2 shows the percentage root mean squared errors for the same four estimators. The relatively large values for the unconstrained HTE under Poisson sampling are due to the variability in the achieved sample size. Arranging the population in size order before systematic selection is seen to reduce the design variances substantially. These are not 'high-entropy' variances, and therefore should not be estimated using (9.22) or (9.32).

The first row in each section of Table 9.3 shows the observed biases in the estimates of design variance for the constrained HTE ($3P7$), using (9.22) for Poisson and randomly ordered systematic sampling and (9.29) for size-ordered systematic sampling. The second row shows the observed biases for the cosmetically calibrated GREG estimator using (9.32) for Poisson and randomly ordered systematic sampling and (9.33) for size-ordered systematic sampling. Only (9.33) displays any serious levels of bias, but it is unfortunate that Brewer and Gregoire did not examine the variability of these estimates as well as their biases.

Tables 9.4 and 9.5 deal with the question as to how appropriate (9.22) and (9.32) are for estimating the design variance of the constrained HTE and GREG estimator respectively, using Poisson samples for which the achieved sample size varies appreciably from the expected or target sample size. Once again the biases in the estimators of total are trivial, and both (9.22) and (9.32) perform remarkably well in reflecting the manner in which the observed Monte Carlo variances change with the achieved sample size. Once again, however, there is no information available as to the stability of these variance estimators. It is to be hoped that Brewer and Gregoire will remedy this deficiency before too long. In the meantime our intuition assures us that (9.22) is likely to perform at least as well as the corresponding with-replacement variance estimator, and we do not have any serious misgivings about (9.32). The estimators for size-ordered (or any other meaningfully ordered) systematic sampling remain, however, in considerable need of further investigation.

Table 9.3 Observed percentage biases of variance estimators for estimates of total timber volume

Estimator	Poisson sampling	Systematic sampling (population in random orderings)	Systematic sampling (population in size order)
Expected sample size 144			
Cond. HT ($\hat{Y}_{\bullet 3P7}$)	0.4	−0.3	2.1
GREG (D^2H)	0.1	0.0	−6.7
Expected sample size 48			
Cond. ($\hat{Y}_{\bullet 3P7}$)	0.4	−0.3	3.2
GREG (D^2H)	0.1	0.1	1.7
Expected sample size 24			
Cond. HT ($\hat{Y}_{\bullet 3P7}$)	0.2	−0.2	2.8
GREG (D^2H)	−0.4	0.8	9.3

Table 9.4 Performance of variance estimators $\hat{V}\hat{Y}_{\bullet 3P7}$ for conditional HT estimates of total timber volume by increasing quintile of achieved sample size

Quintile	Average sample size	Observed bias (%)	Observed SE (%)	Observed RMSE (%)	Estimated SE (%)
Expected sample size 144					
1	127.6	0.04	3.04	3.04	3.05
2	137.6	0.03	2.93	2.93	2.93
3	143.9	0.00	2.87	2.87	2.87
4	150.2	−0.02	2.78	2.78	2.78
5	160.9	−0.03	2.72	2.72	2.71
Expected sample size 48					
1	38.6	−0.03	5.55	5.55	5.60
2	44.2	0.03	5.18	5.18	5.20
3	47.8	−0.02	5.05	5.05	5.01
4	51.6	−0.02	4.79	4.79	4.82
5	57.8	−0.04	4.55	4.55	4.56
Expected sample size 24					
1	17.4	0.05	8.39	8.39	8.35
2	21.3	0.02	7.46	7.46	7.51
3	23.9	0.01	7.08	7.08	7.10
4	26.5	−0.02	6.80	6.80	6.75
5	31.0	−0.03	6.19	6.19	6.24

Table 9.5 Performance of variance estimators $\hat{V}\hat{Y}_{\bullet GREG(D^2H)}$ for cosmetically calibrated GREG estimates of total timber volume by increasing quintile of achieved sample size

Quintile	Average sample size	Observed bias (%)	Observed SE (%)	Observed RMSE (%)	Estimated SE (%)
Expected sample size 144					
1	127.6	−0.01	1.53	1.53	1.53
2	137.6	−0.01	1.47	1.47	1.47
3	143.9	−0.01	1.44	1.44	1.43
4	150.2	−0.02	1.40	1.40	1.40
5	160.9	0.00	1.36	1.36	1.36
Expected sample size 48					
1	38.6	−0.05	2.78	2.78	2.80
2	44.2	−0.03	2.68	2.68	2.66
3	47.8	−0.03	2.53	2.53	2.51
4	51.6	−0.03	2.41	2.41	2.41
5	57.8	−0.04	4.55	4.55	4.56
Expected sample size 24					
1	17.4	−0.04	4.24	4.24	4.19
2	21.3	−0.04	3.76	3.76	3.77
3	23.9	−0.02	3.53	3.53	3.55
4	26.5	−0.02	3.39	3.39	3.37
5	31.0	−0.04	3.11	3.11	3.12

Response from Supervisor

9.12 This is most encouraging. At present we appear to have insufficient evidence to be sure, but it certainly looks as though we will soon be able to estimate the design variance of the HT and related estimators (including the GREG) accurately enough for most purposes without having to evaluate those tiresome second-order inclusion probabilities.

But sampling with unequal probabilities is usually encountered in the context of multistage area sampling designs for household surveys, and there it has been common to use selection *with* replacement, not only because the estimation of the HT design variance is so awkward in itself, but also because the design variance estimation procedure for *any* multistage sampling estimator is simpler and more convenient when selection is made with replacement at each stage – except perhaps the last. Can you advise me how much extra complexity is necessarily incurred as the result of selecting a multistage sample without replacement rather than with replacement? It would be convenient for training purposes if you wrote me two reports on multistage sampling, one using sampling with replacement and the other using sampling without replacement.

Postscripts

9.13 After completing the above report we received two private communications from M.E. Donadio that compare the various estimators described in our report with two others, one used by Rosén and one by Deville, that belong to the Hájek family. Hájek's (1964) own variance estimator, also used by Rosén, is

$$\hat{\hat{\mathrm{V}}}_{HAJ}\hat{Y}_{\bullet HT} = (n-1)^{-1}n\sum_{i=1}^{N}\delta_i(1-\pi_i)\big(Y_i\pi_i^{-1} - \hat{\hat{Y}}_{\bullet}n^{-1}\big)^2, \tag{9.34a}$$

where

$$\hat{\hat{Y}}_{\bullet} = \sum_{i=1}^{N}\delta_i\pi_i^{-1}\breve{a}_iY_i \tag{9.34b}$$

and

$$\breve{a}_i = \left\{\sum_{j=1}^{N}\delta_j(1-\pi_j)\right\}^{-1} n(1-\pi_i). \tag{9.34c}$$

The other, used by Deville (1999) replaces the $(n-1)^{-1}n$ in (9.34a) by the more elaborate factor $\left\{1 - n^{-2}\sum_{i=1}^{N}\delta_i\breve{a}_i^2\right\}^{-1}$, but is otherwise identical. It will be denoted by $\hat{\hat{\mathrm{V}}}_{DEV}\hat{Y}_{\bullet HT}$.

The earlier Donadio communication used the following model to generate an artificial population of size $N = 100$: $X_k = k$, $Y_k = X_k + 2Z_kX_k^{0.5}$, where Z_k is $N(0,1), k = 1,2,\ldots,N$. He then selected 10 000 independent samples of each of three different sizes, $n = 10$, 20 and 40, using the high-entropy Pareto πps selection procedure (already referred to in **9.4**) with selection probabilities $\pi_k \propto X_k$. He then calculated the means and coefficients of variation of the resulting HTEs of $Y_{\bullet} = \sum_{k=1}^{N} Y_k$. Unsurprisingly, the means coincided closely with the true value of $Y_{\bullet}$, which was 5134. The coefficients of variation of $\hat{Y}_{\bullet HT}$ were 8.66% for $n = 10$, 5.73% for $n = 20$ and 3.61% for $n = 40$. The corresponding variances, 197 874, 86 533, and 34 352, respectively, were approximated by (9.9) with (9.11), with empirical or Monte Carlo biases of −0.77%, 1.59% and −2.12%, respectively. Replacing (9.11) by (9.12) or (9.13) made little difference. Using the $\tilde{V}_{HAJ}\hat{Y}_{\bullet HT}$ of (9.16), the same biases were not appreciably different at −0.85% , 1.52% and −2.26%, respectively.

In Table 9.6, following Donadio, we summarize the performances of the empirical variance estimates of ten variance estimators. Their symbols have been simplified for this tabular presentation as follows. $\hat{V}_{HAJ}$ is the $\hat{\hat{V}}_{HAJ}\hat{Y}_{\bullet HT}$ of (9.34a). $\hat{V}_{DEV}$ is Deville's modification, just described, of $\hat{V}_{HAJ}$. $\hat{V}_{9.11}$, $\hat{V}_{9.12}$, $\hat{V}_{9.13}$ and $\hat{V}_{9.26}$ are the variance estimators formed by taking (9.22) with c_i defined by (9.11), (9.12), (9.13) and (9.26), respectively. $\hat{V}_{HR}$ and $\hat{V}_{AS}$ are the estimators formed by substituting the full Hartley and Rao (1962) and Asok and Sukhatme (1976) approximations for π_{ij}, respectively, into the SYG variance estimator (9.4).

$\hat{V}_{JKWR}$ is capable of two interpretations. It is the estimator that would have been unbiased had sampling been *ppswr* and the Hansen–Hurwitz estimator of total used with it. It is also, as it happens, equivalent to the delete-one jackknife estimator if used without adjustment for the fact that sampling was actually $\pi pswor$. $\hat{V}_{JKWOR}$ is the same estimator reduced by the factor $N^{-1}(N - n)$ to allow (rather crudely) for the sampling being without replacement. $\hat{V}_{BS}$ is an estimator arrived at by using the bootstrap rather than the jackknife. The jackknife and the bootstrap are resampling methods of estimation about which we shall eventually have to write you a short note, mainly to tell you why we are not that keen about using

Table 9.6 Relative bias and relative MSE of variance estimators for a randomly generated population (Pareto πps selection)

Variance estimator	Relative bias (%)			Relative MSE (%)		
	$n = 10$	$n = 20$	$n = 40$	$n = 10$	$n = 20$	$n = 40$
$\hat{V}_{HAJ}$	0.42	0.40	−2.90	92	68	60
$\hat{V}_{DEV}$	0.46	0.49	−2.50	92	69	60
$\hat{V}_{9.11}$	0.10	0.13	−2.64	91	68	60
$\hat{V}_{9.12}$	0.49	0.58	−2.05	92	69	61
$\hat{V}_{9.13}$	0.88	1.02	−1.45	93	70	62
$\hat{V}_{HR}$	0.93	1.01	−1.44	94	70	63
$\hat{V}_{AS}$	0.93	0.98	−1.58	94	70	63
$\hat{V}_{JKWR}$	11.33	24.78	58.30	96	76	87
$\hat{V}_{JKWOR}$	0.19	−0.18	−5.02	85	58	39
$\hat{V}_{BS}$	−8.50	−3.63	−4.27	84	66	59

them. And, by the way, in case you think we cannot add up to 11, you will not find $\hat{V}_{9.26}$ in Table 9.6, but you will find it in Table 9.7. It was just easier to introduce it here rather than later.

One thing that Table 9.6 illustrates, though it was never intended to, is the danger of basing comparisons on a single population, whether real, or (as in the case of Table 9.6) generated from a model. Donadio's population is, we believe, just atypical enough to be slightly misleading. If he had generated 100 randomized samples from each of 100 realizations of his model (instead of 10 000 samples from one realization) we are sure that $\hat{V}_{9.11}$ would not have had the lowest bias for $n = 10$ and $n = 20$. $\hat{V}_{HR}$ and $\hat{V}_{AS}$ would, no doubt, have taken first and second place for that honour, either beating the other in a photo finish. What one should first look for in Table 9.6, we decided, was which of the other more tractable estimators comes closest to them in the Bias Stakes.

In the absence of $\hat{V}_{9.26}$ (which had not been invented when Donadio sent this earlier communication) we were pleased to see that award go to $\hat{V}_{9.13}$. That is where we would have placed our money. $\hat{V}_{9.12}$ is a clear second, so we would even have won the quinella, but alas, the trifecta would have eluded us, for $\hat{V}_{DEV}$ is undeniably a short head in front of $\hat{V}_{9.11}$. That placing does not greatly surprise us, however, for when $n = 2$ we have noted that $\hat{V}_{DEV}$ and $\hat{V}_{9.12}$ are actually equivalent. Where $\hat{V}_{DEV}$ is, $\hat{V}_{HAJ}$ can hardly be far behind, and that leaves the resampling methods as the also-rans.

After looking at the biases, we tried to make some sense of the relative MSEs. That was difficult, partly no doubt because the results for the biases had come out in very much the way we were expecting, and the relative MSEs were so different. What was one to make, for instance, of the dazzling form of $\hat{V}_{JKWOR}$ for the Relative MSE Stakes, particularly for the case $n = 40$, when it had done so poorly there in the Bias? After looking at the individual data, which contained at least one and possibly up to three influential and extreme observations (large π_i^{-1} coupled with large positive Z_i), we were on the point of declaring the track dangerous and cancelling the race. But fortunately we were able to check with Donadio, who informed us that the resampling estimators for this population

Table 9.7 Performance of HT variance estimators for a population of 20 blocks in Ames, Iowa

Variance estimator	Random systematic		Pareto πps	
	Relative bias (%)	Relative MSE (%)	Relative bias (%)	Relative MSE (%)
$\hat{V}_{HAJ}$	1.90	136.6	1.20	134.9
$\hat{V}_{9.11}$	2.56	138.3	1.85	136.6
$\hat{V}_{9.12}, \hat{V}_{DEV}$	2.01	136.8	1.31	135.1
$\hat{V}_{9.13}$	1.46	135.2	0.77	133.6
$\hat{V}_{9.26}$	0.91	133.8	0.23	132.2
$\hat{V}_{HR}$	0.92	133.7	0.24	132.1
$\hat{V}_{JKWR}$	16.53	156.9	15.71	155.0

were more biased than the direct ones, but also more stable. So evidently there is a trade-off there. For small domains variance dominates bias, so the resampling estimators would be useful; but for large domains (including domains stretching over many strata with $n = 2$ in each) bias would be more important and the direct estimators would be preferable.

Table 9.7 comes from Donadio's second communication and is based on the population of 20 blocks in Ames, Iowa, provided in Horvitz and Thompson (1952). It contains results for both systematic sampling from a randomly ordered population and for Pareto πps. The comparisons are similar to those in Table 9.6.

The list of estimators used for these two tables is, however, somewhat different from that in Table 9.6. $\hat{V}_{9.26}$ is included, but the only resampling method this time is the one that corresponds to the use of *ppswr*. Donadio omitted $\hat{V}_{AS}$, perhaps because he expected it to be close to $\hat{V}_{HR}$.

In Table 9.7 there is no discrepancy whatever between performance in bias and in relative MSE. The orderings are chiefly remarkable for the close approach of $\hat{V}_{9.26}$ to $\hat{V}_{HR}$, which in these tables comes very near to achieving the smallest bias and smallest relative MSE to which its pedigree entitles it. It is no surprise to see $\hat{V}_{9.13}$ in third place or, now, to see $\hat{V}_{HAJ}$ edging out $\hat{V}_{9.12}$ (wearing $\hat{V}_{DEV}$'s colours) into fifth place. We are perhaps a little sad to see $\hat{V}_{9.11}$ (which we had once strongly fancied) finishing second last, but with the exception of $\hat{V}_{JKWR}$, it was a strong field. As we pointed out back in **9.4**, Hájek's stable held some strong competitors, and they might be said to have lost these close races primarily on handicap.

There is insufficient information about the resampling methods here to decide whether they might have been more stable than the direct ones for this population also.

9.14 We have just received a third private communication, this time from Brewer and Donadio jointly. It appears that the Brewer and Gregoire (2001) high-entropy variance estimator, numbered (9.32) in this chapter, needed rather more improvement than we had suggested in Remark **9.10.1**. The resulting improved version of (9.32) also helps to tie the variance estimators of Chapters 8 and 9 together in an easily memorable format. (Unfortunately it appears that the corresponding low-entropy variance estimator, (9.33), is more difficult to improve upon.)

When c_i is defined by (9.12), we find that

$$c_i^{-1} - \pi_i = \{(n - \pi_i)/(n - 1)\} - \pi_i = \{n/(n - 1)\}(1 - \pi_i). \qquad (9.35)$$

Substituting (9.35) in (9.32), the latter then contains an adjustment factor $n^2/\{(n - p)(n - 1)\}$ in a situation where $n/(n - p)$ appears to be more appropriate. The unwanted factor, $n/(n - 1)$, actually comes from the approximate formula for the variance of the HT estimator, (9.9), via (9.12) and (9.35). But the HT estimator is itself that special case of the GREG in which the regressor values X_i are proportional to the inclusion probabilities π_i. This fact is not immediately obvious, because in that situation $\hat{X}_{\bullet HT} = X_{\bullet}$, in consequence of which the calibration term $(X_{\bullet} - \hat{X}_{\bullet HT})\hat{\beta}$ takes the value zero, with the end result that it seldom or never appears explicitly in the HTE formula. Nevertheless, the Y_i are effectively being regressed on the X_i, so that $p = 1$, which accounts for the presence of the factor $n/(n - 1)$ in (9.35).

It follows that a better variance estimator than (9.32) would have been

$$\hat{\hat{\mathrm{V}}}\hat{Y}_{.GREG} = \{n/(n - p)\} \sum_{i=1}^{N} \delta_i \pi_i^{-1} \left(\pi_i^{-1} - 1\right)\left(Y_i - \hat{\hat{Y}}\right)^2. \qquad (9.36)$$

This closely resembles the 'selected units only' version of the estimator of the anticipated variance of a Cosmetically Calibrated Estimator (CCE), as described in Section **8.11**; however, given the results in Section **8.14**, a better and asymptotically unbiased estimator, both of the design variance itself and of this anticipated variance, would be that suggested in Remark **9.10.1**, namely

$$\mathrm{E}_{\xi_{REG}} \hat{\hat{\mathrm{V}}}\hat{Y}_{.C} = \sum_{i=1}^{N} \delta_i \pi_i^{-1} \left(\pi_i^{-1} - 1\right) \tilde{\sigma}_i^2. \qquad (9.37)$$

(There is something of a logical problem here if the GREG is not itself a CCE, but it must be remembered that the design variance of the GREG is always estimated on the basis that it is asymptotically the same as the design variance of the HTE of the GREG's estimated residuals. Also, the HTE is itself both a GREG and a CCE. We will therefore proceed on the basis that the design variance of any GREG is close to and asymptotically equal to the design variance of its nearest cosmetically calibrated counterpart.)

So we now have the situation where the design variance and the anticipated variance can both be estimated by the same expression, namely the right hand side of (9.37). But that is not all. The prediction variance of $(\hat{Y}_{.C} - Y_.)$ can be estimated by the leading term in equations (8.28) and (8.29), with σ_i^2 replaced by its unbiased estimator $\tilde{\sigma}_i^2$, i.e.

$$\hat{\mathrm{V}}_{\xi_{REG}}(\hat{Y}_{.C} - Y_.) = \sum_{i=1}^{N} \delta_i w_i (w_i - 1) \tilde{\sigma}_i^2. \qquad (9.38)$$

The only difference between the right hand sides of (9.37) and (9.38) is that the π_i^{-1} in the former are replaced by w_i in the latter, and we know that the w_i tend asymptotically to π_i^{-1}. Moreover, there is a good reason why there should be such a difference between the prediction variance on the one hand and the design and anticipated variances on the other; namely that each sample has its own prediction variance, whilst the design and anticipated variances both involve taking averages over all samples permitted by the relevant sampling procedure.

9.15 There will, however, be a problem in applying the formulae (9.37) and (9.38) when the sample sizes are very small. In Section **5.5** we found that we could not use Theorem **5.3.1** to estimate the individual σ_i^2 for the sample bulls, because there were only two bulls in that sample. It seems probable that an analogous problem would arise with the use of (9.37) and (9.38) if the sample size were smaller than or equal to $p + 1$.

In Section **5.5** we got round this problem by modelling the variance function as $\sigma_i^2 = \sigma^2 X_i^{2\gamma}$, and we could do the same here. Moreover, in Section **5.5** we only used this model to estimate the sample σ_i^2, but we could have used it to estimate the nonsample σ_i^2 as well, and – provided we had chosen a sensible value for γ – we would probably have ended up with a more precise estimate of the prediction variance, because we would then have been using additional information, namely the known values of the individual nonsample X_i. These two options are always available, regardless of the size of the sample, large or small. The corresponding estimation formulae are

$$\mathrm{E}_{\xi REG} \hat{\hat{\mathrm{V}}} \hat{Y}_{\bullet C} = \sum_{i=1}^{N} (\pi_i^{-1} - 1)\tilde{\sigma}_i^2 \tag{9.39}$$

for the design and anticipated variances and

$$\hat{\mathrm{V}}_{\xi REG}(\hat{Y}_{\bullet C} - Y_{\bullet}) = \sum_{i=1}^{N} (w_i - 1)\tilde{\sigma}_i^2 \tag{9.40}$$

for the prediction variance.

We hope you will excuse us for pushing yet again what has now become our favourite barrow, but we cannot resist the temptation to point out that the simplicity, similarities and appealing logic behind the estimators in equations (9.37)–(9.40) could only have been obtained by using the randomization based and prediction based inferential approaches simultaneously. It is something like our using both eyes together instead of just one at a time, and discovering to our surprise that we then have depth of vision!

Exercises

9.1 In Section **4.7**, the consultants gave up the attempt to estimate the conditional design variances of their HTE for the cows' stratum because of the ambiguities regarding the joint probabilities of inclusion of the sample elephants. But there is no ambiguity about the first-order inclusion probabilities if they are conditioned on the achieved sample size, $n = 3$. In addition, equation (9.22) is now available, with a choice between equations (9.11), (9.12), (9.23) and (9.26) for defining c_i.

(a) Using (9.12) to define c_i, estimate the variance of the HTE for the cows' stratum.

(b) Is (9.22) with (9.12) the best available choice of design-variance estimator when $n = 2$? Give reasons why it is or is not, and estimate the corresponding variance for the bulls' stratum using whatever method you consider most appropriate.

(c) Work out whether the consultants would then be able to satisfy the circus owner's stated requirement (estimating the total weight of the 50 elephants within 10% with 99% confidence) using only design-based inference and assuming a t distribution for your estimator of variance. Describe carefully how you arrive at the number of degrees of freedom appropriate for that estimator.

9.2 (a) Prove that the prediction expectation of the variance estimator given in (9.25) is identically equal to $\sum_{i=1}^{N} \delta_i \sigma_i^2 \pi_i^{-1}(\pi_i^{-1} - 1)$ under *srswor*.

(b) Also prove that it still has the same prediction expectation $\sum_{i=1}^{N} \delta_i \sigma_i^2 \pi_i^{-1}(\pi_i^{-1})$, whatever the selection procedure, provided $n \geq 3$.

9.3 (a) Starting with an estimator of the form $\hat{\mathrm{V}}_1 \hat{Y}_{\bullet HT} = \sum_{i=1}^{N} \delta_i (A - F\pi_i)\left(Y_i \pi_i^{-1} - \hat{Y}_{\bullet HT} n^{-1}\right)^2$, optimize the expressions for A and F by equating coefficients down to order $n^{-1}N$ to obtain equation (9.24).

(b) Show that (9.24) does not generally yield the correct numerical value under *srswor*. Comment on the suggestion that the alternative estimator (9.25) might therefore be preferable. Is it possible to optimize the estimator subject to the condition that it must yield the correct numerical value under *srswor*?

10

Multistage Area Sampling for Household Surveys: Sampling with Replacement

Report for Supervisor: Introduction 174
How a Multistage Equal Probability Sample Can Be Selected 177
Selecting Persons Associated with Dwellings: Eligibility and Coverage 183
Survey Coverage and Survey Scope 185
The Self-Weighting Nature of an Equal Probability Multistage Sample 186
Estimation Formulae for Multistage Samples 188
Variance Estimation Formulae for Multistage Samples 191
Estimating the Total Variance 196
Estimating the Individual Stages of Variance 197
Optimal Levels of Clustering 199
The Variance Components Reconsidered 199
The Cost Parameters 203
Equations for Optimum Clustering 204
A Quick Fix 205
Acknowledgement from Supervisor 208
Exercises 208

Report for Supervisor: Introduction

10.1 This report has been prepared in response to your request for a briefing on multistage area sampling in household surveys. By this we mean the selection first of large geographical areas such as counties, then of smaller areas within the selected counties, then of still smaller areas within them if necessary, until eventually one ends up with a sample of individual dwellings and of the people who live in them.

There are two principal reasons for using multistage sampling with its concomitant clustering of the sample dwellings. The first is that simple random samples spread over large geographical areas are unrealistically costly to enumerate by personal contact. If mail or telephone (or perhaps, in the future, electronic contact) is used instead, the need for multistage sampling is less compelling, but if personal contact is still used to follow up non-respondents and/or non-contacts, it could still be economical to use a multistage clustered sample for this reason alone.

The second reason relates to the construction of the sample frame. Realistically, this involves having, at some point, one or more lists of dwellings or households.

Although it is possible to construct a sample frame for a telephone survey using random-digit dialling, such a task involves detailed knowledge of the way in which telephone numbers are allocated (for instance, between households and businesses) and the acquisition of this knowledge has almost become a speciality in itself.

Putting these two reasons together, the need to know how to construct a multistage sample of persons or dwellings remains quite compelling.

In this report, we concentrate on the problem of constructing a multistage sample of private dwellings. It should not be forgotten that an appreciable proportion of many human populations is likely to live in non-private dwellings, including (amongst other categories) hotels, boarding houses, boarding schools, aged persons' homes, hospitals, barracks and prisons. Each type of non-private dwelling has its own challenge for the survey investigator, but many surveys of persons are legitimately limited to those who live in private dwellings, and this sector is well worth considering on its own.

10.2 As you have intimated, the analysis of multistage area samples is considerably simpler if selections are made with replacement rather than without. That fact has not prevented survey statisticians from selecting multistage samples without replacement, but it does seem to have inhibited the use of the appropriate variance estimation formulae.

If we were only interested in estimating the overall variance, the use of rather approximate formulae would not matter all that much. Ignoring the finite-population correction factor can overestimate that variance by a moderate amount, but most of us do not mind erring a little on the safe side. The more serious consequence is that these approximations distort the estimation of variance components, and therefore make it difficult to design samples with appropriate levels of clustering.

Even when sampling with replacement is deliberately used in order to arrive at realistic estimates of variance components, traps can still be encountered. We know, for instance, that back in the 1950s, when the Australian Labour Force Survey was still at the design stage, a great deal of effort was put into estimating the components of variance from pilot surveys. Hand-designed forms, which would in these computer-oriented times be regarded as of lunatic size and complexity, were laboriously filled in with a view to designing the world's most efficient household survey. For simplicity, selection was carried out with replacement at every stage but the last. That final stage was the selection of dwellings within sample blocks. Since this was carried out using equal probabilities, no need was felt to select with replacement. Selecting *srswor* would actually have been suitable, but selection was in fact made systematically from a geographically ordered list.

The results were almost heartbreakingly disappointing. Apparently sensible estimates of the final-stage component of variance were soon obtained, but the estimates for the second last stage (which involved subtraction of the final-stage estimates) were in every case negative, and the ambitious project had to be all but abandoned. The use of systematic sampling from a geographically ordered list at the last stage decreased the actual variance, and evidently quite substantially, but (as so often happens) this decrease in variance was accompanied by a small increase in the estimated variance. When this inflated estimate of final-stage variance was subtracted from a realistic estimate of the variance for the last two stages combined, the difference was negative.

The project did not have to be completely abandoned. The problem did not affect the higher stages of sampling, and it was possible to salvage something even from the two lowest stages. When people work so closely with their data as those people did back in the 1950s, they often develop an intuitive feel for what the actual parameters might be. They were able to establish a consistent set of figures which they reckoned could not be too far from the true situation, and designed their survey sample accordingly. It might not have been the most efficient multistage design in the world at the time, but it was almost certainly far better than they would have been able to arrive at by mere guesswork. (Eventually that intuitive feeling developed into an imputation procedure. It is described in **10.25** below.)

This historical preamble may seem rather peripheral to the business of describing the selection procedures and summarizing the formulae relevant to multistage sampling, but we believe it carries a serious moral all the same. Ken Foreman often used to say that it never hurt to get your hands dirty with X_{ij}s. (Conventions change. These days he would have had to say Y_{ij}s.)

10.3 You were therefore quite right in suggesting that the presentation should start with a description of multistage sampling *with* replacement. Although the time must be fast approaching, if it has not already arrived, when the increment in complexity will be regarded as insufficiently important to inhibit the use of multistage sampling without replacement, the latter topic will still be easier to follow if the with-replacement theory has been outlined and understood first.

The actual process of sampling with replacement is, however, somewhat the more awkward to describe, on account of the fact that the expected number of appearances of a population unit in sample is not the same as the probability of its inclusion in sample. (Logic requires that in general it has to be somewhat greater.) Following the precedent set by Hansen *et al.* (1953) we will here regard the results of sampling with replacement as 'approximations to those for sampling without replacement where the sampling fractions are not too large' (Vol. I, p. 142). In that spirit we will further take the liberty of referring to the expected number of appearances of the ith population unit in sample somewhat imprecisely as its 'probability of selection'. This wording has the advantage of being close to but still readily distinguishable from 'its probability of inclusion in sample'. The latter wording, and its notational equivalent π_i, will be reserved for use when the sampling is strictly without replacement.

Using these conventions about wording and notation, we can now say that the type of multistage sample considered in this report is one in which each last-stage sample unit (in our case, each dwelling) has the same 'probability of selection' as any other; say, one in a hundred, or more generally one in g, where g (the *sampling interval*, or reciprocal of the *sampling fraction*) is any integer. Such a sampling procedure is called an *equal probability selection method* or *epsem*, and a sample drawn in that fashion is called an *epsem* sample.

How a Multistage Equal Probability Sample Can Be Selected

10.4 Sampling from a finite population typically starts with the finding or compiling of a *sample frame* – a list of population units that are also potential sampling units. When the population of interest is all the people that live in a particular country, or even a particular city, it can never be the case that any available list of these people is completely up to date. Nevertheless, lists can mostly be found that are useful in providing measures of size for selection purposes. Such lists include electoral registers, as in the UK or Australia, and the Village Books, once maintained by the Department of Native Affairs in the then Territory of Papua and New Guinea, that provided the sampling frame for that Territory's first comprehensive population census in 1966.

It is somewhat easier to deal with lists of dwellings than with lists of people. Even here, however, it is usually necessary to use two, three or even four stages of sampling. The number of stages required increases with the sparseness of the population. In Australia, for instance, three stages are sufficient in urban areas, and also in the more densely populated rural areas, but four stages are needed in most of the rural and all the remote areas. What follows here is a modified and somewhat simplified version of the selection procedures used for private dwellings in Australia, with particular attention being paid to the four-stage procedure used in thinly populated rural areas. Since the Australian Bureau of Statistics (ABS) no longer uses selection with replacement, the description that follows will resemble what used to be done once, rather than what is done now.

In Australia, lists of local government areas (LGAs) by state are readily available, and the largest LGAs – notably Brisbane and the Australian Capital Territory – are already divided into areas of more convenient size. Conversely, some remote LGAs have very few inhabitants, and it is appropriate to combine such LGAs into more suitable areas. We then have a list of what are known as *primary sampling units* (PSUs). Many of these PSUs are sufficiently densely populated for the first stage of selection to be omitted. Such PSUs are described as *self-representing areas* (SRAs).

In the worked example that follows, we will be making considerable use of unpublished training materials (Australian Bureau of Statistics, 2000), but we have simplified their design, and otherwise modified them to suit our own purposes. We will limit our description to the manner in which the full four stages are selected in rural areas. The three stages of selection used in the self-representing PSUs correspond to the second, third and fourth of these, so it is preferable to describe these three stages of sampling as the second, third and fourth – even in SRAs – rather than describe the same types of sample units as being (say) second-stage sample units in one part of the country and third-stage units in the remainder. The first stage of selection in SRAs is therefore called a *dummy stage*.

Wherever the first stage of selection is a real one, groups of similar and often contiguous PSUs are formed into strata. (See Chapter 2 for a discussion of the advantages of stratification when sampling with equal probabilities. The same arguments apply with little modification to more complex sample designs.) A sample of two PSUs is then selected from each stratum, two being the smallest number for which variances can be estimated unbiasedly. (If any larger number were to be selected, some of the advantages of stratification would be surrendered to no effect.) Since we are interested in using randomization-based as well as prediction-based inference, we will be selecting the sample PSUs with known inclusion probabilities, and we will shortly demonstrate that it is convenient to select them with probabilities proportional to size. The most recent Census population would be an appropriate and accessible measure of size for that purpose, but 'number of private dwellings', from the same Census source, is even more appropriate and just as easily accessible.

10.5 Table 10.1 shows how PSUs can be selected within a given stratum using *ppswr*. Column 1 contains the number by which the PSU is identified within this Stratum. Column 2 indicates the numbers of private dwellings in each PSU as taken from the most recently available Census publication, the total being 9651. The overall sample fraction in this particular State is one in 147, and we wish to select two PSUs from it, so we need to divide the stratum up into $2 \times 147 = 294$ clusters. The required cluster size is therefore $9651/294 \cong 32.8$ dwellings.

Dividing each of the dwelling figures in column 2 by 32.8 and rounding, we obtain the numbers of clusters in column 3. These originally summed to 293, so the 19 clusters in PSU 10 were increased to 20, yielding the required 294. (639/32.8 is actually 19.48, so the amount of 'forcing' required was trivial.)

The numbers of clusters in column 3 are cumulated in column 4. It is useful to imagine PSU 1 as holding 47 lottery tickets with the numbers 1–47 inclusive, PSU 2 as holding the 28 tickets numbered 48–75 inclusive and so on. The last numbered ticket is then of course 294.

Next we need to select two of these PSUs to be in sample. For this purpose we select two random numbers in the range 1–294 independently. Strictly speaking, that means that we need to select two numbers between 1 and 294 *with*

Table 10.1 Example of PSU selection

Sample fraction 1/147 Number of sample PSUs 2 Cluster size 32.8

PSU no.	No. of dwellings	No. of clusters	Cumulated clusters	Selection no.	Within-PSU sample fraction
1	1550	47	47		
2	911	28	75		
3	1153	35	110	100	1/35
4	1457	44	154	148	1/44
5	1055	32	186		
6	553	17	203		
7	728	22	225		
8	873	27	252		
9	732	22	274		
10	639	20	294		
Total	9651	294			

replacement, so there is a small chance that we might select the same number twice. If we hadn't liked that idea, we could have fudged things a little and selected those numbers without replacement, but then we would have needed to use a somewhat more complicated variance estimator (Sánchez-Crespo, 1997). Hence we do in fact select those numbers with replacement. The two numbers we select are 100 and 148, and the selected PSUs are the ones holding the lottery tickets with those numbers. PSU 3 holds ticket number 100 and PSU 4 holds number 148, so these are the two PSUs that appear in column 5. Since one cluster is to be selected from each sample PSU, the within-PSU sampling fraction is the reciprocal of the number of clusters in it, as indicated in column 6.

10.6 Having selected a sample of PSUs, we can proceed to the second stage of selection by forming and then selecting *secondary sample units* (SSUs) within the selected PSUs only. This cuts down the effort of constructing an adequate sample frame quite considerably. The most appropriate choice for the SSU in Australia is the Census Collector's District (CD). Numbers of dwellings are readily available for them, they are conveniently sized (five or ten of them to a typical PSU) and no CD crosses any LGA boundary. Note that, in a number of instances, the CD sizes are very small and some amalgamation is required to form a secondary sample unit (SSU) of appropriate size. For convenience we will still refer to such amalgamations as CDs. Two or more CDs are then selected from each sample PSU. The actual number is determined by finding the optimal amount of clustering, given estimates of the population variances relevant to each stage of sampling. This operation will be described later in the report (**10.23**ff.).

Table 10.2 shows how four CDs could be selected within PSU 4, again using *ppswr*. Column 1 contains the number by which the CD is identified within PSU 4. Column 2 indicates the numbers of private dwellings in each of these CDs as taken from the most recently available Census publication, the total being 1457 (as in Table 10.1). The sample fraction in this PSU is one in 44, that being the number of first-stage clusters it contains. We will be selecting four CDs from it, so we need to divide the stratum up into 4 × 44 = 176 second-stage clusters.

Table 10.2 Example of SSU selection from PSU 4

Sample fraction 1/44 Number of sample SSUs 4 Cluster size 8.28

CD no.	No. of dwellings	No. of clusters	Cumulated clusters	Selection numbers	Within-PSU sample fraction
1	220	27	27		
2	198	24	51		
3	217	26	77		
4	280	34	111	78, 96	2/34
5	282	34	145	133, 130	2/34
6, 7, 8	260	31	176		
Total	1457	176			

The required second-stage cluster size is therefore $1457/176 \cong 8.28$ dwellings. This is slightly larger than a quarter of the first-stage cluster size used for selecting PSUs in Table 10.1, which was 32.8, but the only reason for the difference is rounding.

Dividing each of the dwelling figures in column 2 by 8.28 and rounding, we obtain the numbers of clusters in column 3. These sum to 176, so no adjustment is necessary.

The numbers of clusters in column 3 are cumulated in column 4. We now imagine CD 1 as holding 27 second-stage lottery tickets with the numbers 1–27 inclusive, CD 2 as holding the 24 tickets numbered 28–51 inclusive and so on. The last numbered ticket is then of course 176.

Next we need to select four of these CDs to be in sample. For this purpose we select four random numbers in the range 1–176 independently; that is, we need to select four numbers between 1 and 176 with replacement. The relevant random numbers in this case happen to be 78, 96, 133 and 130, and these appear in column 5. We have not selected any number twice, but we have selected two of the CDs twice, because CD 4 holds the 34 second-stage lottery tickets numbered 78–111 (both 78 and 96 falling in that range) and CD 5 holds the 34 tickets numbered 112–145 (both 133 and 130 falling in that range). Had any CD been selected only once, we would have been required to select a single third-stage sample from it. Since, however, we have selected both CD 4 and CD 5 twice, we will need to select *two* third-stage samples from each of them. This doubles the sampling fraction in column 6 from 1/34 to 1/17 for both the sample CDs.

10.7 The third-stage or *tertiary sample unit* (TSU) is typically the 'Block' – an area with clearly visible boundaries, ideally streets or roads. In rural areas, some blocks may need to be defined in the field. Blocks do not come with Census measures of size, so it is necessary to find some other source of dwelling counts within each selected CD in order to be able to carry out a selection of blocks with probabilities proportional to size. Administrative records can usually be found that make block counts possible – for instance, from bodies that supply water, electricity or telephones, or alternatively from the LGA that collects rates. Failing everything else, it may be necessary to do the block counting in the field. (This would have been an impossibly large task had there been no selections of PSUs and CDs first.)

Table 10.3 shows how three blocks could be selected within CD 4, again using *ppswr*. Column 1 contains the number by which the block is identified within this CD. Column 2 indicates the numbers of private dwellings in each block. Regardless of the source, there will be the possibility that the total number of dwellings arrived at for the CD will differ from the Census count. If the discrepancy is very large, this is likely to be because the area is one of rapid development, and it may even be felt necessary to disregard the Census figures and restart the selection procedure at the PSU level. Fortunately, such occurrences are rare. It is more often the case that the survey investigators will accept that the sample in this particular area needs to be substantially larger or smaller than planned, in order to retain its representative nature.

Table 10.3 Example of block selection from CD 4

Sample fraction 2/34				Number of sample blocks 6 (3 from each of 2 samples)		Anticipated cluster size 2.76 Actual cluster size 2.97	
				Selection		Within-CD sampling fractions	
Block no.	No. of dwellings	No. of clusters	Cumulated clusters	1st Sample	2nd Sample	1st Sample	2nd Sample
1	34	12	12				
2	27	9	21	14		1/9	
3	65	22	43	36	34, 40	1/22	2/22
4	87	29	72				
5	90	30	102	95	74	1/30	1/30
Total	303	102					

In our example, we have only a small discrepancy, 280 dwellings in the Census and 303 from LGA records, so the increase in the expected sample size is only 8%. In such a case we retain the sampling fraction at 2/34 and allow the expected cluster size to rise from 2.76 to 2.97. With this size of cluster we initially obtain only 101 clusters in total, whereas we need $3 \times 34 = 102$, so once again we change the number of clusters where that change causes the least distortion, in this case increasing the number of clusters for block 1 from 11 to 12, and forcing the total to 102.

Next, we need to select three of the Blocks to be in each of the two third-stage samples. The first three numbers selected are shown in column 5 as 14, 95 and 36, so the first sample consists of Blocks 2, 5 and 3. The next three are those in column 6; 34, 74 and 40, so the second sample consists of Block 3 twice and Block 5 once. The within-block sampling fractions for the first sample are as shown in column 7 and those for the second are in column 8.

10.8 The fourth and last stage of selection is that of dwellings within a selected block. For that purpose it is necessary to make an actual list of the dwellings in that block and identify them in such a fashion that they are readily recognizable for the survey interviewer.

Table 10.4 is an example of such a list as might be compiled on the fringe of a built-up area where house numbers are not exhibited in the immediate vicinity of every dwelling. The descriptions relate to features that are likely to remain identifiable or visible on a reasonably permanent basis. House colours can easily be changed, and even trees can be removed, so neither of these features is a suitable descriptor. There is a further potential discrepancy now; between the fairly up-to-date count based on LGA records and what is visible in the field.

In fact, two additional dwellings are found. There are two plausible conjectures that can be made in such circumstances. These may be dwellings only very recently under construction, or two existing dwellings may have been missing from LGA records. In the latter instance, other similar dwellings may have been missed elsewhere in the CD, and an investigation along these lines should be considered.

Block 2 contains 29 listed dwellings, from which nine clusters are to be formed. This last stage of selection is *epsem* – that is, the probabilities of selection in sample are all the same – and in consequence there is no need to sample with

Table 10.4 An example field list for Block 2 in CD 4 of PSU 4

Dwelling serial no.	Street name	Street no.	Further details
1	Kiaer St	17	
2	Kiaer St	15	
3	Kiaer St	13	
4	Kiaer St	11	
5	Kiaer St	9	
6	Kiaer St	7	
7	Kiaer St	5	
8	Kiaer St	3	
9	Kiaer St	1	
10	Bowley St	24	
11	Bowley St	26	
12	Bowley St	28	
13	Bowley St	30	
14	Bowley St	32	
15	Bowley St	34	
16	Bowley St	36	
17	Bowley St	38	
18	Bowley St	40	
20	Neyman St	U/C*	Bl 8/Sec 20, adjacent 40 Bowley St
21	Neyman St	U/C	Bl 7/Sec 20
22	Neyman St	U/C	Bl 6/Sec 20
23	Neyman St	U/C	Bl 5/Sec 20
24	Neyman St	U/C	Bl 4/Sec 20
25	Neyman St	U/C	Bl 3/Sec 20
26	Neyman St	U/C	Bl 2/Sec 20
27	Neyman St	U/C	Bl 1/Sec 20
28	Hansen's Way		Two storey half-timbered building with thatched roof. Living quarters above shop.
29	Hansen's Way		Single storey stone cottage, end 15 metre drive. Slate roof, one window either side front door.

*U/C: under construction.

replacement. Sampling without replacement is not only easier but also clearly more efficient, so we will use it. Two of the nine clusters will consist of four dwellings and each of the remaining seven will each consist of three. It has been mentioned before, however, that if we are interested in working out an optimal multistage design, we will need to be able to estimate the components of variance at each stage unbiasedly. This fact prevents us from selecting systematically from an ordered list (such as that shown in Table 10.4). Hence we will need to form two clusters of four dwellings and seven clusters of three dwellings in a totally random fashion.

Note that these 'clusters' will not, in general, consist of neighbouring dwellings. Had we been forming the clusters systematically, dwellings in the same cluster would only rarely have been neighbours. (As an example of when they would, suppose every third dwelling was being selected out of seven in a circle, and that the random start was 1. Then the selected dwellings would be 1, 4, and 7; and 7 and 1 would be adjoining.)

Without loss of generality, we can decide that Clusters 1 and 2 shall consist of four dwellings and that each of Clusters 3–9 shall consist of three. Using a table of random numbers, we can arrange the integers 1–29 in random order. Cluster 1 can then be defined as the first four of these 29 in that random order, Cluster 2 as the next four, Cluster 3 the next three, Cluster 4 the next three, ... and Cluster 9 the last three. Going back to Table 10.3, we see that we need only one of these clusters to be selected for the first sample within CD 4, and none for the second sample. We randomly select a number from 1 to 9 for this purpose, and it turns out to be Cluster 5, which of course consists of three dwellings randomly selected without replacement from Block 2.

The selection procedure is only slightly more complicated when we come to select from blocks like Block 3 that have been selected more than once. Block 3 has to be divided into 22 clusters. Suppose the Census count of 65 dwellings is still correct. Then one of those clusters will consist of two dwellings, and each of the remaining 21 will consist of three. Without loss of generality, we describe the cluster consisting of two dwellings only as Cluster 1. We next arrange the 65 dwellings in random order. The first two in that order are Cluster 1, the next three are Cluster 2, ... and the last three are Cluster 22. From Table 10.3 we need to select two of these 22 clusters for the first sample and one for the second sample.

(Strictly speaking, there would be no need to randomly order either the 65 dwellings in Block 3 or the 29 in Block 2, if only a one-off sample were required. Only the three dwellings in the sample cluster would need to be randomly assigned. But if the sample is to be rotated from cluster to cluster over time, and most such samples are, it will be convenient to have all the clusters defined exactly from the beginning.)

Selecting Persons Associated with Dwellings: Eligibility and Coverage

10.9 Sections **10.4–10.8** contain a fairly complete description of how a four-stage sample can be selected from a stratum containing nearly 10 000 dwellings, but usually the persons associated with the selected dwellings are more relevant to the survey than the dwellings are themselves. This might seem to imply the need for yet another stage of selection, but in fact this potential fifth stage is rarely required. Usually either one person is selected from each sample dwelling, or else all persons in that dwelling regarded as eligible are included in the sample. For a Labour Force Survey most persons aged 15 and over would be considered eligible, but there are likely to be certain necessary exclusions.

Some of the difficult categories that need to be considered when devising eligibility rules are these:

- foreign diplomats, their dependants and the dwellings that they occupy;
- persons normally resident in another country; and
- permanent members of the country's defence forces.

If only one eligible person is selected, the apparent fifth stage of selection is only a dummy stage. In effect, *persons* are already being selected at the *fourth* stage. True, these persons are being selected with unequal probabilities; for instance, one of four eligible people in a selected dwelling has only a quarter of the probability of inclusion in sample as person who is living alone in another dwelling in the same cluster. But this does not mean that there is an extra stage of selection, only that selection at the fourth stage is taking place with unequal inclusion probabilities.

If, instead, all eligible people in a sample dwelling are automatically in sample themselves, there is not even that dummy stage of selection. Both the dwelling and all eligible people within it are being selected at the fourth stage, and it would be misleading to describe the deliberate choice of all people having a certain characteristic as a fifth stage. To be a genuine fifth stage, something must be done that is intermediate between taking all the eligible persons in a sample dwelling, and taking only one of them.

Finally, unambiguous *coverage rules* are needed to eliminate the under-enumeration of some persons and double-counting of others. If persons are to be associated with sample dwellings at all, it is absolutely necessary to ensure that each eligible person encountered during a survey operation can be associated with one identifiable dwelling and with that dwelling only. That dwelling may be a private one, or a non-private dwelling such as a hotel, hospital or boarding school. (A person associated with a non-private dwelling would be omitted from a survey limited to private dwellings, even if present when the interviewer called.) Some of the difficult categories that need to be considered when devising coverage rules are:

- children from a dwelling's household that are away in boarding schools or camps;
- other usual residents of the household who are temporarily away;
- visitors whose own home is temporarily unoccupied;
- people who have two homes; and
- homeless people.

In the case of a homeless person, the 'dwelling' referred to would of course need to be some kind of dwelling substitute where the person stands the best chance of being contacted. In the case of persons temporarily absent from their usual place of residence, the most important considerations are usually whether they have come from a non-private dwelling or from another private dwelling, how long have they been absent from it, and whether that dwelling is currently occupied or not. A useful check on the suitability of a set of coverage rules is to think of a number of potentially ambiguous situations, and then to work out for each such situation whether there is any possibility of the person concerned being wrongly excluded or counted more than once.

No one set of coverage rules is likely to be suitable for all survey purposes, but every survey needs its own unambiguous set of coverage rules that associates each eligible person encountered in the survey with one dwelling only.

The eligibility and coverage rules used by the ABS (2001, p. 192), for example, are as follows:

> The Labour Force Survey includes all usual residents of Australia aged 15 and over except:
>
> - members of the permanent defence forces;
> - certain diplomatic personnel of overseas governments, customarily excluded from census and estimated population counts;
> - overseas residents in Australia; and
> - members of non-Australian defence forces (and their dependants) stationed in Australia.
>
> In the Labour Force Survey coverage rules are applied which aim to ensure that each person is associated with only one dwelling, and hence has only one chance of selection. The chance of a person being enumerated at two separate dwellings in the one survey is considered to be negligible. Persons who are away from their usual residence for six weeks or less at the time of interview are enumerated at their usual residence (relevant information may be obtained from other usual residents present at the time of the survey).

Note that the coverage rules for visitors who are staying overnight at a selected dwelling do not appear to be easily accessible from official ABS documentation, but we have it on reliable authority that they are included in the coverage if any one of the following conditions applies: they usually live in a special dwelling; they usually live in a private dwelling where neither the visitor nor any other of the usual residents is staying that week; or they usually live in a private dwelling where at least one of the other usual residents is staying that week, but the visitor will be away from that dwelling for more than six weeks. The last condition complements the 'six weeks or less' rule quoted above from the official documentation. The two rules combined ensure that people away from their usual private dwellings retain their fair chance of being selected for enumeration, regardless of how long they remain absent.

Finally, there is a potential ambiguity about the word 'dwelling'. So far we have used it to denote a structure that has the potential to be lived in. (Some dwellings are under construction. Others are complete but unoccupied.) But at least in Australia, the Census definition of 'dwelling' does not permit it to contain more than one 'household', a *household* being a group of people that share at least some of their meals on a regular basis. So what is a single dwelling for sample frame and sample selection purposes can sometimes contain two or even more Census dwellings. Such dwellings lack at least one physical boundary and appear in the Census as 'share(s) of flat' or 'share(s) of private house'. Since this is only a potential ambiguity, however, we will continue to use the word 'dwelling' to denote exclusively a recognizable structure suitable for sample frame and sample selection purposes.

Survey Coverage and Survey Scope

10.10 It is also worth mentioning here that the word 'coverage' is sometimes used to mean the types of information collected in a survey as well as (or even instead of) the extent of the population from which that information has been collected. In the relevant United Nations guidelines, however, the *coverage* of a survey is defined by 'the geographic region(s), social groups or other constituent parts of a population covered by the census or survey' (Turner, 1996). (This includes what we have termed 'eligibility' above, as well as 'coverage' proper.) In the context of the present report, those 'constituent parts' are specified types of dwelling or specified types of person, or both, in a defined geographical area.

Another term used to describe the nature of the information collected in the survey (as defined by the questions that appear in the survey's schedules or questionnaires) is 'the survey *scope*'. We clearly remember having seen 'scope' used with this connotation in another closely related UN publication, but we have not as yet been able to trace it.

Incidentally, today's UN guidelines are still closely based on those compiled mid-century by a committee that originally included W.E. Deming, R.A. Fisher, P.C. Mahalanobis and F. Yates (see United Nations Statistical Office, 1964). They are well worth referring to when preparing a sample survey report in almost any context.

The Self-Weighting Nature of an Equal Probability Multistage Sample

10.11 There are several related issues here. Do the sample selection procedures described in **10.4–10.8** above truly constitute an *epsem*? Is an *epsem* sample necessarily self-weighting? If not, is this sample self-weighting?

The fact that the procedures of **10.4–10.8** do constitute an *epsem* is readily demonstrable. Consider the probability of any dwelling in Block 2 of CD 4 of PSU 4 being selected in sample. Two PSUs were selected, so the unconditional 'probability of selection' of PSU 4 was $2 \times 44/294$. The conditional 'probability of selection' of CD 4 within PSU 4 given that PSU 4 had been selected was $4 \times 34/176$. The conditional 'probability of selection' of Block 2 within CD 4 within PSU 4 given that CD 4 had been selected was $3 \times 9/102$. The conditional inclusion probability for any dwelling in Block 2 within CD 4 within PSU 4 given that Block 2 had been selected was 1/9. Hence the unconditional inclusion probability for any dwelling in Block 2 within CD 4 within PSU 4 was

$$\frac{1}{9} \cdot \frac{3 \times 9}{3 \times 34} \cdot \frac{4 \times 34}{4 \times 44} \cdot \frac{2 \times 44}{2 \times 147} \equiv \frac{1}{147}, \tag{10.1}$$

and the same figure of 1/147 would be obtained regardless of the block chosen. Equation (10.1) is, in fact, simply a special case of the general identity

$$\frac{1}{g_{ijk}} \cdot \frac{qg_{ijk}}{qg_{ij}} \cdot \frac{ng_{ij}}{ng_i} \cdot \frac{mg_i}{mg} \equiv \frac{1}{g}, \tag{10.2}$$

where m is the number of sample PSUs within a stratum, n is the number of sample CDs within sample PSUs, q is the number of sample blocks within sample CDs,

g is (as before) the overall sampling interval, g_i is the sampling interval within the ith sample PSU, g_{ij} is the sampling interval within the ijth sample CD, and g_{ijk} is the sampling interval within the ijkth sample block. These sampling intervals are those used when selecting PSUs, CDs and blocks in Tables 10.1–10.3. Multiplying by the sampling interval g converts the *sample take* or sample sum over the entire survey to an estimate of the population total, but the influence of the other sampling intervals is a little more subtle. It is easiest here to work backwards.

Multiplying by g_{ijk} converts the sample take within the ijkth sample block to an estimate of the population total within that block. That is straightforward. Multiplying by g_{ij}, however, converts the *sum* of the estimated block totals for *all* q sample blocks in the ijth sample CD to an estimate of the total within that CD. Consequently, multiplying a single estimated block total by g_{ij} converts it into one of the q contributions that make up that estimated total for the CD, one for each sample block. Hence it is not g_{ij} alone, but the operator $g_{ij} \sum_{k=1}^{q} g_{ijk}^{-1}$ that converts the estimated block total for the ijkth sample block into an estimate of the population total for the ijth sample CD.

Correspondingly, it is the operator $g_i \sum_{j=1}^{n} g_{ij}^{-1}$ that converts the estimated CD total for the ijth sample CD into an estimate of the population total for the ith sample PSU, and the operator $g \sum_{i=1}^{m} g_i^{-1}$ that converts the estimated PSU total for the ith sample PSU into an estimate of the population total for the entire survey.

Note that P_i, the probability of selecting the ith PSU at a single draw, is equal to g_i/mg, and therefore that PSU's 'probability of selection' is g_i/g.

Note also that no subscript is used here to denote stratum. In practice there will almost always be more than a single stratum, but each stratum can for the most part be considered independently of every other stratum, so the extra subscript is not needed.

10.12 Translating (10.2) into prose, 'the unconditional "probability of selection" for a dwelling located within any block is equal to the overall sampling fraction' or, equivalently, 'the sampling procedure described in Sections **10.4–10.8** above is an *epsem*'.

If a sampling procedure is an *epsem*, does it necessarily follow that the procedure is also self-weighting? Ideally it does, and the obvious weight to choose is the inverse of the inclusion probability, that inverse being g for every dwelling included in sample. In practice, however, it is usual for other considerations to arise that cause the sample weights to differ from one sample dwelling to another.

One obvious consideration would be sample non-response. Response to a household survey is usually high, especially if conducted by personal interview and backed up by legislation that makes it compulsory, as many government surveys are in Australia. It could, however, be (say) 93% in one stratum and 97% in another. The simplest way to allow for this is to multiply the sampling interval for the first stratum by 100/93 and that for the second by 100/97. If that is done, the sample is still self-weighting within each stratum separately.

There may, however, be categories of interviewees within a stratum that have higher response rates than others, and then this simple adjustment can be improved upon. For instance, it is usual for young males to have lower contact rates and elderly females to have lower response rates than the remainder of the population. If these differentials are also taken into account, the selection procedure will not be exactly self-weighting, within a geographical stratum, though it will usually be nearly so.

The same kind of consideration may enter even in the absence of non-response. If, for example, the proportions of the population in various age–sex classifications are known, these proportions can be used as benchmarks, that is, the sample weights can be modified in such a way that the sample estimates reflect these known population proportions exactly. So whether non-response is present or not, it may be considered better to surrender the self-weighting property of the sampling procedure than to adhere to it.

Would this matter? Well, it certainly would matter in one respect. Any difference in weight from sample unit to sample unit, however small, must mean that the estimation procedure is more complex than it would be without that differential. But in these days when so much calculation can safely be left to the computer and its programming, such complications can be taken in one's stride. What is of far greater potential importance is the loss in efficiency if some parts of the sample are considerably more highly weighted than others.

That is where it pays for the sample to have been designed to be self-weighting in the first instance. Provided the overall response level is reasonably high, the loss in efficiency is then almost always tolerable. One way of looking at this consequence is to recognize that optimal allocations throughout survey sampling tend to be flat. It is possible to depart quite substantially from the precisely optimal allocation and still achieve an efficiency of 80% or even 90% (and this is more true of household surveys than of business surveys, because one household tends to resemble another to a much greater extent than one business resembles another).

So surveys of households should be designed as self-weighting on two grounds: first, because a sample designed that way is simple to handle; and secondly, because such a design is likely to result in a nearly optimal set of sampling weights, even after such considerations as non-response and the knowledge of benchmarks (totals of supplementary variables) have been taken into account.

We can now therefore answer the three questions posed at the start of **10.11**. First, the sample selection procedures described in **10.4–10.8** do constitute an *epsem*. Secondly, an *epsem* sample is not necessarily self-weighting, but it can be so provided response is complete and no adjustment is made for known population totals (other than the dwelling counts used when selecting). Finally, the sample here could be self-weighting, but again only if response is complete, and then it's up to the survey designer.

Estimation Formulae for Multistage Samples

10.13 Suppose for the moment that response is indeed complete and that we choose to make the sample weights in every case equal to the overall sampling interval, g. Then a design-unbiased estimator of the total number of final-stage sample units (dwellings) in the population at the time of a survey is gn, where n is the number of sample dwellings. (Note that it is unlikely this total will be known exactly, and so the estimator gn may be quite a useful one to have.)

However, since sampling with replacement is used at all stages except the last, and since *different* lower-stage samples are selected whenever a unit at a given stage is selected more than once, we cannot employ the notation we used earlier, in **1.9–1.10**, where ν_i denoted the number of times the ith population unit was selected in sample. We will instead use a notation introduced in **1.6**, and widely used in survey sampling, where the subscript i attached to a *lower*-case roman letter denotes the unit selected at the ith draw.

The notation $\delta_{ijkl}y_{ijkl}$ will be retained for a unit included in sample at the final stage of sampling, because – at that stage – selection is without replacement; but it must be understood that this is a hybrid notation and that y_{ijkl} is the value of y observable on the lth of *all* the dwellings listed within the ijkth *sample* block. The value of δ_{ijkl} is unity if that lth dwelling is included in the fourth-stage sample, and zero otherwise.

The notation y_{ijkl} is used in preference to the notation Y_{ijkl} because all the subscripts except the last refer to the sample units rather than to all the units in the population. In addition, sampling at the final stage is always without replacement, so there is no need to indicate the order in which the final-stage units have been selected. The notation y_{ijkl}, if not particularly elegant, is at least unambiguous.

10.14 Armed with this notation, we may define the estimator $\hat{y}_{ijk\bullet}$, of the total $y_{ijk\bullet}$ for the ijkth sample block, by $\hat{y}_{ijk\bullet} = g_{ijk} \sum_{l=1}^{T^*_{ijk}} \delta_{ijkl}y_{ijkl}$, where T^*_{ijk} is the current number of dwellings *listed* in the ijkth sample block as opposed to T_{ijk}, the number used for block selection purposes. We can similarly write the estimator $\hat{y}_{ij\bullet\bullet}$ of the total for the ijth sample CD as $\hat{y}_{ij\bullet\bullet} = g_{ij} \sum_{k=1}^{q} (\hat{y}_{ijk\bullet}/g_{ijk})$, the estimator $\hat{y}_{i\bullet\bullet\bullet}$ of the total for the ith sample PSU as $\hat{y}_{i\bullet\bullet\bullet} = g_i \sum_{j=1}^{n} (\hat{y}_{ij\bullet\bullet}/g_{ij})$, and the estimator $\hat{Y}_{\bullet\bullet\bullet\bullet}$ of the whole stratum total as

$$\begin{aligned}\hat{Y}_{\bullet\bullet\bullet\bullet} - g &\sum_{i=1}^{m} \frac{\hat{y}_{i\bullet\bullet\bullet}}{g_i} \\ = g &\sum_{i=1}^{m} \sum_{j=1}^{n} \sum_{k=1}^{q} \sum_{l=1}^{T^*_{ijk}} \delta_{ijkl}y_{ijkl}, \end{aligned} \tag{10.3}$$

the intermediate sample intervals, g_i etc., cancelling with their corresponding reciprocals, g_i^{-1} etc., throughout the entire expression.

At first sight, formula (10.3) does not appear to be telling us anything that is not already obvious – namely, that self-weighting samples are self-weighting. On closer inspection, however, it supplies a useful clue as to why sample designers are prepared to sacrifice this self-weighting property rather readily. There is an attractive alternative to (10.3),

$$\hat{Y}^*_{\bullet\bullet\bullet\bullet} = g \sum_{i=1}^{m} \sum_{j=1}^{n} \sum_{k=1}^{q} g_{ijk}^{-1} \frac{T^*_{ijk}}{t_{ijk}} \sum_{l=1}^{T^*_{ijk}} \delta_{ijkl}y_{ijkl}, \tag{10.4}$$

where t_{ijk} is the number of dwellings actually included in the fourth stage sample within the ijkth block, as opposed to the *a priori* expected number, which is $g_{ijk}^{-1}T_{ijk}$. The estimator (10.4) is conditioned on the achieved values of the t_{ijk}, that is to say, it treats the t_{ijk}, which are really random variables, as though they had been fixed in advance.

10.15 There are two reasons why t_{ijk} can differ from $g_{ijk}^{-1}T_{ijk}$. The first is the possible difference between T_{ijk} and T_{ijk}^*, and the second is the *end-effect*, which can come into play even if the dwellings that make up T_{ijk} and T_{ijk}^* are identical. Unless $(g_{ijk}/g_{ij})T_{ijk}$ is an integer, t_{ijk} will not be the same as $g_{ijk}^{-1}T_{ijk}$, but it will never differ from $g_{ijk}^{-1}T_{ijk}^*$ by as much as a whole unit. In practice, very small geographical blocks are combined to make up survey 'blocks' of a minimum size or greater, so the value of $g_{ijk}^{-1}T_{ijk}^*$ will usually be large enough for the end-effect not to matter a great deal, although it will always be present.

There are in fact at least three advantages in using (10.4) rather than (10.3) as our estimator of total, and we describe them below. The first two depend on the possible difference between T_{ijk} and T_{ijk}^*, and on the end-effect; but the third is always there, no matter how ideal the sampling process might have been.

1. Since the final-stage clusters do not generally contain equal numbers of dwellings, using (10.3) can contribute appreciably to the final-stage variance of the estimate. For instance, the estimator (10.4) is clearly more accurate than (10.3) for the item 'number of dwellings', and consequently also for items highly correlated with 'number of dwellings', some of which, such as 'number of persons', can also be quite important.
2. When deriving a formula for the variance of (10.3), we need to acknowledge that the real fourth-stage sample units were not the dwellings themselves but the clusters of dwellings described in **10.8**. Using the differences between these cluster values, rather than those between the individual dwelling values, makes a proper allowance for the addition to variance caused by the end-effect, but it complicates both the notation and the derivation itself quite considerably. By contrast, the substitution of $w_{ijk} = (g/g_{ijk})(T_{ijk}^*/t_{ijk})$ for the original weight, g, when estimating the variance of (10.4), removes the influence of the end-effect automatically.
3. To estimate the last-stage variance of (10.3) unbiasedly, we would need at least two clusters of dwellings in sample within every sample block, instead of only one.

One practical point must be borne in mind, however, when using (10.4) as an alternative to (10.3). If the survey interviewer finds in the field that T_{ijk}^* differs from T_{ijk} (or from any earlier value of T_{ijk}^*), the numbers of dwellings within each of the g_{ijk} clusters must be adjusted by randomly allocating any new dwellings among them in a suitable fashion. If, in addition, dwellings already allocated to a cluster have disappeared, one of two options must be followed. Either a dwelling once allocated to a cluster must always remain within it, in which case the numbers of dwellings in a cluster may end up differing from the average by more than one; or else the survey interviewer must know how to reallocate any updated set of dwellings to clusters in a more optimal fashion.

The latter is not a particularly difficult problem, but it is not completely trivial either. If sampling at the last stage is ever carried out with replacement, then ensuring that interviewers know what to do with the clustering when dwellings 'are born' and/or 'die' must be a small but essential part of their training If, however, sampling at the last stage is without replacement, interviewers have no need to know how to allocate additional dwellings to clusters. Systematic sampling at the last stage makes their lives that much simpler.

Variance Estimation Formulae for Multistage Samples

10.16 The simplicity of the estimation formulae in **10.13–10.15** makes multistage sampling rather attractive, and self-weighting designs particularly attractive. Unfortunately, not all this simplicity carries over into the formulation and estimation of variance. We will therefore switch here to the discussion of a two-stage design, as that will cover all the concepts needed for writing down the formulae for a three- or four-stage sample design in a more lengthy but still straightforward fashion.

For a two-stage design, identity (10.2) reduces to

$$\frac{1}{g_i} \cdot \frac{mg_i}{mg} \equiv \frac{1}{g}, \tag{10.5}$$

where g is still the overall sampling interval, but now over two stages rather than four. Equation (10.3) similarly simplified would naturally become

$$\hat{Y}_{\bullet\bullet} = g \sum_{l=1}^{m} \sum_{l=1}^{T_i} \delta_{il} y_{il} \tag{10.6}$$

$$= \sum_{i=1}^{m} \left(\frac{g}{g_i} \right) \hat{y}_{i\bullet}, \tag{10.7}$$

where

$$\hat{y}_{i\bullet} = g_i \sum_{l=1}^{T_i} \delta_{il} y_{il}. \tag{10.8}$$

The estimator (10.6)–(10.7) is both strictly design-unbiased and self-weighting. Although the estimator we will eventually be using is neither of these, it will be easier to develop the variance of (10.6)–(10.7) first, and make adjustments later, than to attack the more complicated problem head on.

10.17 In particular, there is an important theorem much used in multistage sampling, the proof of which requires the estimator in question to be design-unbiased.

Theorem 10.17.1 The variance of the $\hat{Y}_{..}$ defined by (10.6)–(10.7) is separable into two components, one from each stage of sampling.

Proof. For the $\hat{Y}_{..}$ defined by (10.7) we have

$$\begin{aligned}
\mathrm{V}(\hat{Y}_{..}) &\equiv \mathrm{E}(\hat{Y}_{..} - Y_{..})^2 \\
&= \mathrm{E}\left[\sum_{i=1}^{m}\{(g/g_i)\hat{y}_{i.} - m^{-1}Y_{..}\}\right]^2 \\
&= \mathrm{E}_{[1]}\mathrm{E}_{[2]}\left[\sum_{i=1}^{m}\{(g/g_i)y_{i.} - m^{-1}Y_{..}\} + \left\{\sum_{i=1}^{m}(g/g_i)(\hat{y}_{i.} - y_{i.})\right\}\right]^2,
\end{aligned} \tag{10.9}$$

where $y_{i.}$ is the (unknown) population total for the PSU selected at the ith draw, $\mathrm{E}_{[1]}$ denotes the expectation over all possible first-stage samples and $\mathrm{E}_{[2]}$ denotes the expectation over all possible final-stage samples, holding the first-stage sample fixed. Squaring out (10.9) we have,

$$\begin{aligned}
\mathrm{V}(\hat{Y}_{..}) = {} & \mathrm{E}_{[1]}\sum_{i=1}^{m}\{(g/g_i)y_{i.} - m^{-1}Y_{..}\}^2 + 0 \\
& + 2\mathrm{E}_{[1]}\left[\sum_{i=1}^{m}\{(g/g_i)y_{i.} - m^{-1}Y_{..}\}\sum_{i=1}^{m}(g/g_i)\mathrm{E}_{[2]}(\hat{y}_{i.} - y_{i.})\right] \\
& + \mathrm{E}_{[1]}\left\{\sum_{i=1}^{m}(g/g_i)^2\mathrm{E}_{[2]}(\hat{y}_{i.} - y_{i.})^2\right\} \\
& + 2\mathrm{E}_{[1]}\left[\sum_{i=1}^{m-1}\sum_{i'>i}^{m}(g/g_i)(g/g_{i'})\mathrm{E}_{[2]}\{(\hat{y}_{i.} - y_{i.})(\hat{y}_{i'.} - y_{i'.})\}\right].
\end{aligned} \tag{10.10}$$

The zero in the first line of (10.10) stands for the cross product terms from the first stage of sampling, which are zero because the first stage draws are made independently of each other. In addition $\mathrm{E}_{[2]}(\hat{y}_{i.} - y_{i.}) \equiv 0$ for all i, so the second line in (10.10) also disappears. Further, the final-stage sampling within in any first-stage draw is carried out independently of the final-stage sampling within any other first-stage draw (even if both are selected from the same PSU). Hence the cross products in the fourth line each have final-stage expectation zero and we are left only with

$$\mathrm{V}(\hat{Y}_{..}) = \mathrm{V}_{[1]}(\hat{Y}_{..}) + \mathrm{V}_{[2]}(\hat{Y}_{..}) \tag{10.11}$$

where

$$\mathrm{V}_{[1]}\hat{Y}_{..} = \mathrm{E}_{[1]}\sum_{i=1}^{m}\{(g/g_i)y_{i.} - m^{-1}Y_{..}\}^2 \tag{10.12}$$

is the *first-stage (component of) variance* and

$$\mathrm{V}_{[2]}\hat{Y}_{\bullet\bullet} = \mathrm{E}_{[1]}\left\{\sum_{i=1}^{m}(g/g_i)^2\mathrm{E}_{[2]}(\hat{y}_{i\bullet} - y_{i\bullet})^2\right\} \tag{10.13}$$

is the *final-stage (component of) variance.* ◇

Remark 10.17.1 When there are more than two stages of sampling, expression (10.13) encompasses the variance components for all stages other than the first.

Remark 10.17.2 Theorem 10.17.1, and its proof, are valid regardless of whether sampling is with replacement (*ppswr*) as in this chapter or without replacement (π*pswor*) as in the next.

10.18 Expressions (10.12) and (10.13) are capable of further development.

For (10.12) we have the first-stage expectation of m terms but, since the first stage of selection is carried out with each draw both identical with and independent of every other draw, the cross-product terms disappear and each of the resulting m terms has the same expectation. We may therefore write,

$$\mathrm{V}_{[1]}\hat{Y}_{\bullet\bullet} = \mathrm{E}_{[1]}\sum_{i=1}^{m}\{(g/g_i)y_{i\bullet} - m^{-1}Y_{\bullet\bullet}\}^2 \tag{10.12}$$

$$= m\mathrm{E}_{[1]}\{(g/g_i)y_{i\bullet} - m^{-1}Y_{\bullet\bullet}\}^2$$

$$= m^{-1}\mathrm{E}_{[1]}\{(mg/g_i)y_{i\bullet} - Y_{\bullet\bullet}\}^2 \tag{10.14}$$

$$= m^{-1}\sum_{i=1}^{M}(g_i/mg)\{(mg/g_i)y_{i\bullet} - Y_{\bullet\bullet}\}^2. \tag{10.15}$$

In (10.14), g_i/mg corresponds to the p_i in the 'second Proof' of Theorem 4.6.2, and in (10.15) it corresponds to the P_i used throughout the discussion of *ppswr* selection in Chapter 4. In fact, the variance expression in (10.15) is precisely parallel to that in (4.4), but in (10.15) it is placed in a multistage context.

This also provides us with the reassurance that (10.15) is of the right order of magnitude – a useful check to make when deriving expressions of this or greater complexity.

10.19 Development of the final-stage variance, (10.13), is also straightforward, provided we treat the dwellings rather than the clusters as the effective final-stage units.

Replacing the operator $\mathrm{E}_{[1]} \sum_{i=1}^{m}$ in (10.13) by $m \sum_{i=1}^{M} P_i$, or equivalently by $m \sum_{i=1}^{M} g_i/mg$, leads to

$$\begin{aligned}
\mathrm{V}_{[2]} \hat{Y}_{\bullet\bullet} &= m \sum_{i=1}^{M} \{g_i/(mg)\}\{(g/g_i)^2 \mathrm{E}_{[2]}(\hat{y}_{i\bullet} - y_{i\bullet})^2\} \\
&= \sum_{i=1}^{M} (g/g_i) \mathrm{E}_{[2]}(\hat{y}_{i\bullet} - y_{i\bullet})^2 \\
&= \sum_{i=1}^{M} (g/g_i) \mathrm{V}_{[2]} \hat{y}_{i\bullet}. \qquad (10.16)
\end{aligned}$$

An explicit expression for $\mathrm{V}_{[2]}\hat{y}_{i\bullet}$ cannot be written down without introducing additional notation relating to cluster totals, but in any case the $\mathrm{V}_{[2]}\hat{Y}_{\bullet\bullet}$ of (10.16) is somewhat different from the final-stage variance of the estimator of $Y_{\bullet\bullet}$ conditioned on the selection at the second or final stage. By analogy with (10.4), this conditioned estimator is

$$\hat{Y}^*_{\bullet\bullet} = g \sum_{i=1}^{m} g_i^{-1} \hat{y}^*_{i\bullet}, \qquad (10.17)$$

where

$$\hat{y}^*_{i\bullet} = \frac{T_i^*}{t_i} \sum_{l=1}^{T_i^*} \delta_{il} y_{il}. \qquad (10.18)$$

The second- or final-stage variance of $\hat{y}^*_{i\bullet}$ may be seen from the *srswor* theory of Chapter 1 to be

$$\mathrm{V}_{[2]}\hat{y}^*_{i\bullet} = T_i(T_i - t_i)t_i^{-1}(T_i - 1)^{-1} \sum_{l=1}^{T_i} \left(y_{il} - y_{i\bullet}T_i^{-1}\right)^2, \qquad (10.19)$$

and, from (10.16), the second- or final-stage variance of $\hat{Y}^*_{\bullet\bullet}$ is correspondingly

$$\mathrm{V}_{[2]}\hat{Y}^*_{\bullet\bullet} = \sum_{i=1}^{M} (g/g_i) T_i(T_i - t_i)t_i^{-1}(T_i - 1)^{-1} \sum_{l=1}^{T_i} \left(y_{il} - y_{i\bullet}T_i^{-1}\right)^2, \qquad (10.20)$$

which seems a reasonable variance to estimate for a conditioned analysis.

We may now wish to check whether (10.16) and (10.20) are of the right order of magnitude for the final stage of variance. The summation $\sum_{i=1}^{M}$ supplies an order M and the expression $g/g_i = (mP_i)^{-1}$ supplies a further order M/m. $\mathrm{E}_{[2]}(\hat{y}_{i\bullet} - y_{i\bullet})^2$, the variance within any first-stage selection, is of order $\bar{T}^2/\bar{t}$, where the bars indicate averages over the entire sample design. Thus (10.16) is of order $(M\bar{T})^2/m\bar{t}$. Here $M\bar{T}$ is the number of final-stage units in total and $m\bar{t}$ is the number of final stage units in sample. This is indeed the right order of magnitude for the final-stage component of variance. Expression (10.20) may be checked for order of magnitude in a similar fashion. $\sum_{i=1}^{M}(g/g_i)$ supplies the M^2/m and the remainder of the expression supplies the $\bar{T}^2/\bar{t}$.

Remark 10.19.1 In order to obtain (10.13), we had to run the risk that the same cluster might be selected up to m times in a PSU selected m times. In such a case the relevant sample dwellings would be subject (multiplicatively) to a further weight, which might be any integer up to m. Even the possibility of this further weighting increases the design-based variance automatically. The prediction-based variance is only affected if these double or multiple selections occur *in fact*, but (if they do happen) the increase in that variance can be quite severe. Either way, there is a price paid, in terms of the accuracy of the estimate of total, in order to be able to use simple variance formulae!

10.20 With (10.17), we relaxed the condition that the two-stage estimator of total must be strictly design-unbiased, and started to work in terms of something more realistic, namely the two-stage estimator corresponding to the four-stage (10.4). Substituting (10.18) in (10.17),

$$\hat{Y}^*_{\bullet\bullet} = g\sum_{i=1}^{m}(T_i^*/g_i t_i)\sum_{l=1}^{T_i^*}\delta_{il}Y_{il} \tag{10.21}$$

$$= \sum_{i=1}^{m} w_i \sum_{l=1}^{T_i^*}\delta_{il}Y_{il}, \tag{10.22}$$

where

$$w_i = \frac{g}{g_i} \times \frac{T_i^*}{t_i}. \tag{10.23}$$

The estimator defined by (10.21)–(10.23) is not quite design-unbiased, but in practice it is usually sufficiently close to being design-unbiased to justify invoking Theorem 10.17.1 when estimating variance. In addition, it is usually close enough to being self-weighting for the loss in efficiency due to the application of unequal weights to be negligible – unless, of course, the inequalities arise from multiple selections of PSUs!

Comparing (10.21)–(10.22) with (10.6)–(10.7), it is seen that the only difference between $\hat{Y}^*_{\bullet\bullet}$ and $\hat{Y}_{\bullet\bullet}$ lies in the definition of the second-stage estimator of $y_{i\bullet}$, either $\hat{y}^*_{i\bullet} = (T_i^*/t_i)\sum_{l=1}^{T_i^*}\delta_{il}y_{il}$ from (10.18), or $\hat{y}_{i\bullet} = g_i\sum_{l=1}^{T_i}\delta_{il}y_{il}$ following (10.8). Hence the only adjustment required to the variance formula is one that changes the second-stage variance from its unconditional value in (10.16) to its value conditioned on the T_i^* in (10.20). (Note, however, that the unconditonal variance was not spelled out in full in (10.16), in order to avoid the introduction of additional notation.)

Estimating the Total Variance

10.21 A particularly pleasing feature of multistage sampling with replacement is the ease with which the total variance, and even the components of that total variance, can be estimated, regardless of how many stages are involved in the sampling. In the remainder of this report, we will continue to use just two stages of selection, but the second stage should be understood as playing a role in which it represents all stages other than the first.

For the next theorem we once again revert temporarily to the design-unbiased estimator $\hat{Y}_{\bullet\bullet}$ of (10.6)–(10.7), because the result is then exact and we can approximate later. We will also need some additional notation. Let $\tilde{y}_{i\bullet} = (g/g_i)y_{i\bullet}$ and $\hat{\tilde{y}}_{i\bullet} = (g/g_i)\hat{y}_{i\bullet}$. Then $\hat{\tilde{y}}_{i\bullet}$ can be regarded as an estimator of one mth part of $Y_{\bullet\bullet}$, based on the ith first-stage sample draw and the sampling within it. Further, $\tilde{y}_{i\bullet}$ can usefully be thought of the value that $\hat{\tilde{y}}_{i\bullet}$ would have taken had there been no sampling at the second (or any later) stage. We may then write

$$\hat{Y}_{\bullet\bullet} = \sum_{i=1}^{m} \hat{\tilde{y}}_{i\bullet} = \sum_{i=1}^{m} \frac{g}{g_i}\hat{y}_{i\bullet}. \tag{10.24}$$

Finally, we will denote the value that $\hat{Y}_{\bullet\bullet}$ itself would have taken had there been no sampling at the second stage by

$$\hat{Y}_{\bullet\bullet[1]} = \sum_{i=1}^{m} \tilde{y}_{i\bullet} = \sum_{i=1}^{m} \frac{g}{g_i}y_{i\bullet}. \tag{10.25}$$

Theorem 10.21.1 When sampling is *ppswr* at the first stage, $\hat{\mathrm{V}}\hat{Y}_{\bullet\bullet} = m(m-1)^{-1}\sum_{i=1}^{m}(\hat{\tilde{y}}_{i\bullet} - m^{-1}\hat{Y}_{\bullet\bullet})^2$ is a design-unbiased estimator of the total variance, that is, of $\mathrm{V}\hat{Y}_{\bullet\bullet} = \mathrm{E}(\hat{Y}_{\bullet\bullet} - Y_{\bullet\bullet})^2$.

Proof.

$$\begin{aligned}
\mathrm{E}\hat{\mathrm{V}}\hat{Y}_{\bullet\bullet} &= \mathrm{E}m(m-1)^{-1}\sum_{i=1}^{m}(\hat{\tilde{y}}_{i\bullet} - m^{-1}\hat{Y}_{\bullet\bullet})^2 \\
&= m(m-1)^{-1}\mathrm{E}\sum_{i=1}^{m}\left[\{\tilde{y}_{i\bullet} + (\hat{\tilde{y}}_{i\bullet} - \tilde{y}_{i\bullet})\} - m^{-1}\left\{\hat{Y}_{\bullet\bullet[1]} + (\hat{Y}_{\bullet\bullet} - \hat{Y}_{\bullet\bullet[1]})\right\}\right]^2 \\
&= m(m-1)^{-1}\mathrm{E}\sum_{i=1}^{m}[\{\tilde{y}_{i\bullet} - m^{-1}\hat{Y}_{\bullet\bullet[1]}\} + \{(\hat{\tilde{y}}_{i\bullet} - \tilde{y}_{i\bullet}) - m^{-1}(\hat{Y}_{\bullet\bullet} - \hat{Y}_{\bullet\bullet[1]})\}]^2 \\
&= m(m-1)^{-1}\mathrm{E}\sum_{i=1}^{m}[\{\tilde{y}_{i\bullet} - m^{-1}\hat{Y}_{\bullet\bullet[1]}\}^2 + \{(\hat{\tilde{y}}_{i\bullet} - \tilde{y}_{i\bullet}) - m^{-1}(\hat{Y}_{\bullet\bullet} - \hat{Y}_{\bullet\bullet[1]})\}^2 \\
&\quad + 2\{\tilde{y}_{i\bullet} - m^{-1}\hat{Y}_{\bullet\bullet[1]}\}\{(\hat{\tilde{y}}_{i\bullet} - \tilde{y}_{i\bullet}) - m^{-1}(\hat{Y}_{\bullet\bullet} - \hat{Y}_{\bullet\bullet[1]})\}].
\end{aligned} \tag{10.26}$$

Now $\tilde{y}_{i\bullet} - m^{-1}\hat{Y}_{\bullet\bullet[1]}$ is a zero-expectation difference that depends only on the sampling at the first stage, and $(\hat{\tilde{y}}_{i\bullet} - \tilde{y}_{i\bullet}) - m^{-1}(\hat{Y}_{\bullet\bullet} - \hat{Y}_{\bullet\bullet[1]})$ is a zero-expectation difference that depends only on sampling at the second stage. Since these two differences are independent of each other, the expectation of their product is zero for all i, and the cross-product term in (10.26) vanishes. Hence,

$$\mathrm{E}\hat{\mathrm{V}}\hat{Y}_{\bullet\bullet} = m(m-1)^{-1}\left[\mathrm{E}_{[1]}\sum_{i=1}^{m}(\tilde{y}_{i\bullet} - m^{-1}\hat{Y}_{\bullet\bullet[1]})^2 + \mathrm{E}_{[2]}\sum_{i=1}^{m}\{(\hat{\tilde{y}}_{i\bullet} - \tilde{y}_{i\bullet}) - m^{-1}(\hat{Y}_{\bullet\bullet} - \hat{Y}_{\bullet\bullet[1]})\}^2\right]. \tag{10.27}$$

But from the *ppswr* theory of Chapter 4,

$$\begin{aligned}\mathrm{E}_{[1]}\sum_{i=1}^{m}(\tilde{y}_{i\bullet} - m^{-1}\hat{Y}_{\bullet\bullet[1]})^2 &= m^{-1}(m-1)(m\mathrm{V}_{[1]}\tilde{y}_{i\bullet})\\ &= (m-1)\mathrm{V}_{[1]}\tilde{y}_{i\bullet}\\ &= m^{-1}(m-1)\mathrm{V}_{[1]}\hat{Y}_{\bullet\bullet}.\end{aligned} \tag{10.28}$$

Correspondingly,

$$\begin{aligned}\mathrm{E}_{[2]}\sum_{i=1}^{m}\{(\hat{\tilde{y}}_{i\bullet} - \tilde{y}_{i\bullet}) - m^{-1}(\hat{Y}_{\bullet\bullet} - \hat{Y}_{\bullet\bullet[1]})\}^2 &= m^{-1}(m-1)\,m\mathrm{E}_{[2]}(\hat{\tilde{y}}_{i\bullet} - \tilde{y}_{i\bullet})^2\\ &= (m-1)\mathrm{V}_{[2]}\hat{\tilde{y}}_{i\bullet}\\ &= m^{-1}(m-1)\mathrm{V}_{[2]}\hat{Y}_{\bullet\bullet}.\end{aligned} \tag{10.29}$$

The proof of the theorem follows immediately when (10.28) and (10.29) are substituted into (10.27). ◇

Remark 10.21.1 The variance estimator $m(m-1)^{-1}\sum_{i=1}^{m}(\hat{\tilde{y}}_{i\bullet} - m^{-1}\hat{Y}_{\bullet\bullet})^2$ takes a simple and easily memorable form when $m = 2$, as is often the case with stratified multistage sampling. We then have two half-stratum estimates, $\hat{\tilde{y}}_{1\bullet}$ and $\hat{\tilde{y}}_{2\bullet}$. The sum of the two provides an unbiased estimate of the stratum total, and the squared difference between them, $(\hat{\tilde{y}}_{1\bullet} - \hat{\tilde{y}}_{2\bullet})^2$, is an unbiased estimator of the variance of that estimate.

Estimating the Individual Stages of Variance

10.22 The results (10.27)–(10.29) may be summarized in prose as follows. Provided the first-stage sample units in a multistage design are drawn independently (i.e. 'with replacement'), and the estimators of total used at every stage including the first are design-unbiased, then an estimator of total variance calculated using the convenient fiction 'that the totals of the first-stage units have been measured without error' is also design-unbiased.

Conversely, should we wish to estimate the variance at the first stage only, we will need to subtract an estimate of the variance arising from the remaining stages of sampling. In the special case of two-stage sampling, all that need be subtracted is an estimate of the second-stage variance.

If we use the strictly unbiased estimator $\hat{Y}_{\bullet\bullet}$ of (10.6)–(10.7), Theorem 10.17.1 holds exactly but there is a large component in the second stage of variance due to variability in cluster size. If we condition on the achieved cluster size and use the estimator $\hat{Y}^*_{\bullet\bullet}$ of (10.17) or (10.21), this 'cluster-size' component of variance virtually disappears and is reflected neither in the expectation of $\hat{V}\hat{Y}^*_{\bullet\bullet}$ itself nor in the direct estimate of second-stage variance that we would need to subtract from $\hat{V}\hat{Y}^*_{\bullet\bullet}$ if we wished to estimate the first stage of variance only. Although Theorem 10.17.1 no longer holds exactly, it is common practice to assume that it still holds sufficiently well to justify using it, and we know of no instance where its use has led to any problem.

The expression for the second-stage variance of the estimator conditioned on the achieved sample sizes within each selected PSU is (10.20). An unbiased estimator for this expression, based on the convenient fiction that the second-stage sample size was fixed at the achieved t_i, is

$$\begin{aligned}\hat{V}_{[2]}\hat{Y}_{\bullet\bullet} &= \sum_{i=1}^{M} \frac{g}{g_i} T_i^*(T_i^* - t_i)t_i^{-1}(t_i - 1)^{-1} \sum_{l=1}^{T_i^*} \delta_{il} \left\{ y_{il} - \frac{\hat{y}^*_{i\bullet}}{T_i^*} \right\}^2 \\ &= \sum_{i=1}^{M} \frac{g}{g_i} T_i^*(T_i^* - t_i)t_i^{-1}(t_i - 1)^{-1} \\ &\quad \times \sum_{l=1}^{T_i^*} \delta_{il} \left[y_{il} - \left\{ \frac{\sum_{l'=1}^{T_i^*} \delta_{il'} y_{il'}}{t_i} \right\} \right]^2 . \end{aligned} \tag{10.30}$$

As foreshadowed at the start of **10.16**, in deriving the variance component formulae for a two-stage design, we have had to cover all the concepts needed for a more general multistage design. The generalization to three stages is straightforward and not particularly lengthy. That for four stages is still conceptually straightforward, but it does require considerable time and patience to write it down!

The results (10.27)–(10.29) may be generalized to the estimation of variance from any stage as follows. Provided the sample units for any stage in a multistage design are drawn independently within the sample units drawn at the next higher stage, then an estimator of variance calculated on the assumption 'that the totals of the sample units for the stage in question have been measured without error' is a design-unbiased estimator of the variance for that stage, together with the variances from all the lower stages.

Optimal Levels of Clustering

10.23 The construction of a good multistage sample design includes most importantly the choice of the sample sizes at the various stages. For a two-stage design with a given overall sample size of t dwellings, the only relevant parameter to be chosen is m, and the target sample size within each of the m first-stage draws is then t/m. (Note that we say 'm first-stage draws' rather than 'm PSUs' – this is because one or more of the PSUs may be selected more than once.) For a four-stage sample the parameters to be specified are m, n and q, the target sample size within each of the block selections then being $\bar{t} = t/mnq$.

The first reason why multistage sampling was necessary (given in **10.1**) was that simple random samples spread over large geographical areas were unrealistically costly to enumerate by personal contact. This implied that the optimally clustered multistage sample would involve a compromise between a completely unclustered simple random sample (minimizing the variance for a fixed number of sample dwellings, $mnq\bar{t}$) and a completely clustered sample containing exactly that same number of contiguous dwellings (minimizing the cost of enumeration). In order to choose the clustering parameters, m, n and q with full optimality, it is necessary to know two things: the components of variance from each stage of sampling; and the way in which the costs of enumeration depend on the parameters m, n and q.

The Variance Components Reconsidered

10.24 Consider again the components of variance. For two-stage sampling the first- and final-stage variances are given by equations (10.15) and (10.20), respectively. For more complex multistage samples (10.15) is still valid, and it is a straightforward process to find the formulae for the lower-stage components of variance.

In favourable circumstances, it may be possible to evaluate the higher stages of variance directly using data from a census of population and dwellings. In Australia, for instance, Census data are available down to the level of CDs. It may not be possible to evaluate them for the survey variable of critical importance, but it may still be possible to choose a variable that is reasonably closely correlated with it. Suppose, for instance, that the survey in question is one dealing with household expenditure. If the bureau conducting the census publishes average household income for LGAs (from which the PSUs are constructed) and is further prepared to negotiate the release of similar data at the CD level for legitimate enquirers, it would be possible to optimize the clustering down to the CD level using household income as a proxy for household expenditure. That would unquestionably be good enough for practical purposes, because the optima relating to sample design are typically very flat, so all that is needed are figures of the right order of magnitude.

That still leaves open the question as to what to do about the two lower stages of variance, those for blocks and dwellings. One possibility is to use sample estimates of these variance components. Indeed, sample estimates could be used for all the variance components, and in the absence of suitable census data it may be necessary to take this option. Suppose for simplicity that we have a two-stage sample of blocks and dwellings, and that no census data are available at either level. Instead of the true last-stage (between-dwelling) variance given by (10.20), we could use the sample estimator of it given by (10.30). Also, instead of the true first-stage (between-block) variance given by (10.15), we could use the sample estimator of total variance given in the statement of Theorem 10.21.1 minus the sample estimator of last-stage variance – again given by (10.30).

Here, however, one would need to be careful. The sample used for this parameter estimation would need to be reasonably large (not less, say, than 100 blocks and 500 dwellings) before the resulting estimates of variance components – and, more particularly, of the between-block component – could be regarded as giving a useful indication.

10.25 Failing the possibility of finding useful estimates of variance components from the sample, we could fall back on imputation. We have already used a model of how population variances depend on unit size, albeit in another context, in Chapter 5. An appropriate modification of that model to relate to M sampling units at any stage, the ith of which contains T_i dwellings, is:

$$\xi_R: \quad Y_i = \beta T_i + U_i; \quad \mathrm{E}_{\xi_R} U_i = 0; \quad \mathrm{E}_{\xi_R} U_i^2 = \sigma_i^2; \quad \mathrm{E}_{\xi_R}(U_i U_j) = 0, \quad j \neq i;$$
$$i,j = 1,2,\ldots,M, \quad \text{where} \quad \sigma_i^2 = \sigma^2 T_i^{2\gamma} \quad \text{and} \quad 0.5 \leq \gamma \leq 1. \tag{10.31}$$

Although the subscript i here may be considered as applying to a sample unit defined at any stage, in order to avoid complications we will consider only a two-stage sample of blocks and dwellings. Then at the final or dwellings stage we have $T_i \equiv 1$ by definition. Also, since the blocks are the PSUs, we can legitimately denote their number by M.

The constant σ^2 may be estimated directly from the samples of dwellings within those blocks. Since it relates to individual dwellings, each being regarded as having unit size, it is the model parameter that corresponds to the design-based population variance within blocks. If we confine our attention to the ith block, that population variance is strictly speaking defined by $T_i^{*-1} \sum_{l=1}^{T_i^*} \{Y_{il} - Y_{i.} T_i^{*-1}\}^2$. However, when dealing with *srswor* (in Chapter 1) we found it convenient to estimate $(T_i^* - 1)^{-1} \sum_{l=1}^{T_i^*} \{Y_{il} - Y_{i.} T_i^{*-1}\}^2$ instead, an expression that has already been used in this report to arrive at (10.20). To estimate the model parameter σ^2 we would need to take a weighted mean of these expressions over the entire population, and the appropriate weight for the ith block would be $T_i^* - 1$.

The inequality $0.5 \leq \gamma \leq 1$ in model (10.31) implies three assumptions regarding the manner in which the population variances of the sample units vary with size, namely $\gamma > 0$, $\gamma \geq 0.5$ and $\gamma \leq 1$. All three of these model assumptions are in accordance with empirical observation; estimates of γ obtained from large populations are indeed typically greater than ½, and they seldom significantly exceed 1.

All three are also in accordance with intuition. First, the inequality $\gamma > 0$ implies that in absolute terms the population variances of these idealized sample units increase with size. This is clearly in accordance with common sense. Remember that we are dealing here with totals, not averages. It would be counter-intuitive if (say) the sums of unemployed persons in blocks of 25 or 50 dwellings were no more variable than the numbers of unemployed persons in individual dwellings.

Secondly, the stronger inequality $\gamma \geq 0.5$ implies that the rate of increase of those population variances is at least as great as the rate at which it would increase if those units were formed not on the basis of similarity or geographical contiguity, but simply by random aggregation. This inequalty is almost as intuitive as the first. If the blocks of 50 dwellings were actually random aggregations, the population variance of the block totals would be greater than that of the individual dwellings by a factor of 50. The model equations $E_{\xi_R} U_i^2 = \sigma_i^2$ and $\sigma_i^2 = \sigma^2 X_i^{2\gamma}$ imply that when $\gamma = ½$ the σ_i^2 grow at exactly that rate. And with $\gamma \geq 0.5$, the σ_i^2 have to grow at least as fast as that.

Finally, $\gamma \leq 1$ implies that the largest units are no more variable proportionally than the smaller ones are. When $\gamma = 1$, the standard deviations of the sample units increase linearly with size, which would be the case if all the dwellings within any given unit were identical. A standard deviation that increased more than proportionately with size can be imagined in theory, but would hardly be expected to appear in real life.

A little more surprisingly, but very fortunately, the estimates of γ obtained for a given variable, but using unit sizes falling into different ranges, are reasonably similar. This approximate constancy in γ over size ranges allows us to impute values of population variances for sample units of different sizes, even where the imputation involves extrapolation beyond the size ranges actually observed.

Suppose, for example, that in an idealized situation the PSUs each contain 3200 dwellings, that the PSU standard deviation for numbers of unemployed persons is 64, that the CDs each contain 200 dwellings, and that the CD standard deviation for numbers of unemployed persons is 8. The corresponding estimate of γ is then given by $64/8 = (3200/200)^{\hat{\gamma}}$, so the estimate $\hat{\gamma} = ¾$. If the blocks have an average size of 25 dwellings, the imputed population standard deviation for blocks is then $8 \times (25/200)^{3/4} \cong 1.68$, or equivalently $64 \times (25/3200)^{3/4} \cong 1.68$. The dwellings have size 1 by definition, so their imputed population standard deviation is $8 \times (1/200)^{3/4} \cong 0.15$ or $64 \times (1/3200)^{3/4} \cong 0.15$.

10.26 We showed in **10.25** how population variances for the various stages of sampling could be imputed using an estimated or assumed value of the heteroscedasticity parameter γ. We also intimated that it might be possible to use estimates of the population variances for some stages to estimate a value for γ, and then use that estimate, $\hat{\gamma}$, to impute population variances for the remaining stages. There is a problem here, however. The population variance for any given stage can only be estimated using population units that are widely different in size, but the resulting estimate is interpreted as relating to units that are all of the same size. The same problem also appears in reverse if and when we later impute population variances using the model (10.31), which treats all units at a given stage as being of the same size, when in fact they are of widely different sizes.

In fact, however, we are able to circumvent these two problems by using a formula for a generalized population variance that allows the block totals (and estimates of them) to be compared in an appropriate fashion. In order to show this without undue complications, we will once again assume that there are only two stages of selection: PSUs (which in this case are not LGAs but blocks) and dwellings. We will write the number of PSUs in the population as M and the number of dwellings in the population as T, T_i of them being in the ith PSU.

Consider again the expression $\sum_{i=1}^{M} P_i(Y_{i.}P_i^{-1} - Y_{..})^2$ that we last quoted in **10.18**, recognizing there its correspondence with (10.15). When sampling is *srswr*, $P_i = M^{-1}$ and

$$\sum_{i=1}^{M} P_i\left(Y_{i.}P_i^{-1} - Y_{..}\right)^2 = M^{-1}\sum_{i=1}^{M}(MY_{i.} - Y_{..})^2$$

$$= M^2M^{-1}\sum_{i=1}^{M}(Y_{i.} - M^{-1}Y_{..})^2, \qquad (10.32)$$

so $\sum_{i=1}^{M} P_i(Y_{i.}P_i^{-1} - Y_{..})^2$ is simply M^2 times the population variance, as traditionally defined. Thus if we take $M^{-2}\sum_{i=1}^{M} P_i(Y_{i.}P_i^{-1} - Y_{..})^2$, which is of order M^0, to define our generalization of population variance, we have an expression that agrees exactly with the traditional definition when sampling is *srswr*.

This expression, $M^{-2}\sum_{i=1}^{M} P_i(Y_{i.}P_i^{-1} - Y_{..})^2$, can be evaluated directly when using census data, or it can be design-unbiasedly estimated by $M^{-2}(m - 1)^{-1}\sum_{i=1}^{m}(Y_{i.}p_i^{-1} - \hat{Y}_{..})^2$ when using survey data. Suppose, first, that we evaluate these generalized population variances directly from census data. We are already committed to the model (10.31), so, substituting it into $M^{-2}\sum_{i=1}^{M} P_i(Y_{i.}P_i^{-1} - Y_{..})^2$ and writing $\sum_{i=1}^{M} U_i = U_.$, we obtain

$$\mathrm{E}_{\xi_R}M^{-2}\sum_{i=1}^{M} P_i(Y_{i.}P_i^{-1} - Y_{..})^2 = M^{-2}\sum_{i=1}^{M} P_i\mathrm{E}_{\xi_R}\left(U_iP_i^{-1} - U_.\right)^2$$

$$= M^{-2}\sum_{i=1}^{M} P_i\mathrm{E}_{\xi_R}\left(U_i^2P_i^{-2} - 2U_iP_i^{-1}U_. + U_.^2\right)$$

$$= M^{-2}\sum_{i=1}^{M} P_i\left(\sigma_i^2P_i^{-2} - 2\sigma_i^2P_i^{-1} + \sum_{j=1}^{M}\sigma_j^2\right)$$

$$= M^{-2}\left(\sum_{i=1}^{M}\sigma_i^2P_i^{-1} - 2\sum_{i=1}^{M}\sigma_i^2 + \sum_{j=1}^{M}\sigma_j^2\right)$$

$$= M^{-2}\left(\sum_{i=1}^{M} \sigma_i^2 P_i^{-1} - \sum_{i=1}^{M} \sigma_i^2\right)$$

$$= \sigma^2 M^{-2} \sum_{i=1}^{M} T_i^{2\gamma}(P_i^{-1} - 1). \qquad (10.33)$$

Note that the order of magnitude of this expression is $\sigma^2 \bar{T}^{2\gamma}$ where $\bar{T}$ is any measure of central tendency for the T_i. This is what we should expect from model (10.31), and reassures us that the generalized measure of population variance for blocks is meaningful. We can even take this kind of reasoning a stage further. For the ith PSU, $P_i = T_i T^{-1}$, and for the PSU of average size $P_i = (T/M)T^{-1} = M^{-1}$, which is the *srswr* value. It seems sensible, therefore, to take the arithmetic mean of the T_i as the best measure of central tendency, and therefore as the preferred measure of size for the PSUs.

If we already had an estimate of σ^2 from the sample dwellings, we could substitute that in the last line of (10.33), equate the result to $M^{-2}\sum_{i=1}^{M} P_i(Y_{i\bullet}P_i^{-1} - Y_{\bullet\bullet})^2$ and solve numerically for the estimate, $\hat{\gamma}$, of γ. That estimate might prove to be directly useful later, but its only immediate use would be as a check on the credibility of the estimate of the generalized population variance. If $\hat{\gamma}$ fell outside the range [0.5, 1], the population from which the estimate had been obtained would probably have been too small to be useful.

Alternatively, if no estimate of σ^2 is available from the sample dwellings, an estimate of it could be obtained from (10.33) by assuming a value of γ somewhere in the acceptable range. In the absence of any other information we would be inclined to take the value 0.75. In a large population of trees, however (14 443 loblolly pines in Alabama), Brewer and Gregoire (2001) found $\hat{\gamma}$ to be close to unity, and we understand that this is quite usual for tree populations.

When the relevant census information is not available, it is necessary to use the sample data instead and $M^{-2}(m-1)^{-1}\sum_{i=1}^{m}(Y_{i\bullet}p_i^{-1} - \hat{Y}_{\bullet\bullet})^2$ as the estimator of the generalized population variance. But since the design expectation of this expression is the same $M^{-2}\sum_{i=1}^{M} P_i(Y_{i\bullet}P_i^{-1} - Y_{\bullet\bullet})^2$ as we used when the census data *were* available, there is no substantial difference in the line of reasoning to be followed.

The Cost Parameters

10.27 Hansen *et al.* (1953) suggest several different cost functions, but they all follow the same pattern. For a two-stage design the more general of their two cost equations may be written $C = C_0 m^{1/2} + C_1 m + C_2 m\bar{t}$, where $\bar{t}$ is the average number of sample dwellings selected within each of the m first-stage sample draws. Of the three terms in this equation, the first relates to travel costs between sample PSUs, these being modelled as proportional to the distance travelled along a path linking them. The second term relates to costs that are proportional to the number of PSUs selected and the third to costs that are proportional to the number of dwellings selected overall. (Their cost equations omit any reference to survey overheads, since these have no impact on the optimality of the design.)

There is usually one *item* (a term used interchangeably with *survey variable*) that is especially important or especially difficult to measure, so that optimizing the sample design for that item ensures that the remaining items will also be satisfactorily estimated. Choosing that item to be our y, the optimum sample design minimizes the cost C subject to a given variance for $\hat{Y}_{\bullet\bullet}$, or alternatively minimizes the variance of $\hat{Y}_{\bullet\bullet}$ for a given cost C. This optimization may be carried out using Lagrange's method of undetermined multipliers.

Equations for Optimum Clustering

10.28 By way of illustration, consider the special case obtained by dropping the term in m from the Hansen *et al.* cost equation used in **10.27**, thereby reducing it to $C = C_0 m^{1/2} + C_2 m\bar{t}$. This is not an unreasonable approximation, since the principal cost associated with the first stage of sampling is that incurred for travel, and, as the authors explained, this tends to be proportional to $m^{1/2}$. The Lagrangian then is

$$L = B^2 m^{-1} + W^2 m^{-1}\bar{t}^{-1} - 2\lambda\left(C - C_0 m^{1/2} - C_2 m\bar{t}\right). \tag{10.34}$$

In this expression, the term $B^2 m^{-1}$ is the first stage of variance, identical with the $V_{[1]}\hat{Y}_{\bullet\bullet}$ of (10.15) and $W^2 m^{-1}\bar{t}^{-1}$ is the second stage of variance, which is the $V_{[2]}\hat{Y}_{\bullet\bullet}$ of (10.16) and is written out in full in (10.20). These equations provide implicit definitions of B^2 and W^2, respectively. (These are not identical to the B^2 and W^2 used by Hansen *et al.* (1953) in this context, but they serve much the same purpose.) The optimum values of m and $\bar{t}$ are then specified by

$$\frac{\partial L}{\partial m} = -B^2 m^{-2} - W^2 m^{-2}\bar{t}^{-1} + \lambda\left(C_0 m^{-1/2} + 2C_2\bar{t}\right) = 0 \tag{10.35}$$

and

$$\frac{\partial L}{\partial \bar{t}} = -W^2 m^{-1}\bar{t}^{-2} + 2\lambda C_2 m = 0. \tag{10.36}$$

From (10.35),

$$\lambda = \frac{m^{-2}(B^2 + W^2\bar{t}^{-1})}{C_0 m^{-1/2} + 2C_2\bar{t}}. \tag{10.37}$$

From (10.36),

$$\lambda = \frac{W^2}{2C_2 m^2\bar{t}^2}. \tag{10.38}$$

Equating (10.37) and (10.38) and cross-multiplying,

$$m^{-2}(B^2 + W^2\bar{t}^{-1})(2C_2 m^2\bar{t}^2) = W^2\left(C_0 m^{-1/2} + 2C_2\bar{t}\right), \tag{10.39}$$

which simplifies to

$$\bar{t} = m^{-1/4}\left(\frac{W^2 C_0}{2B^2 C_2}\right)^{1/2}. \tag{10.40}$$

Substituting (10.39) for $\bar{t}$ in the cost equation, we obtain

$$C = C_0 m^{1/2} + C_2 m\bar{t} = C_0^{1/2} m^{1/2} \left(C_0^{1/2} + C_2^{1/2} \frac{W m^{1/4}}{2^{1/2} B} \right), \tag{10.41}$$

which may be solved for m numerically.

The conclusions that can be inferred directly from (10.41) are that, other things being equal, a decrease in C_0 or C_2 or an increase in B^2/W^2 will lead to an increase in m. All these results are in accordance with intuition.

If there are more than two stages of sampling and/or more than two terms in the cost equation, the equations for the optimal levels of clustering become progressively more complex. If the occasion arises where such equations need to be derived, the second half of Chapter 9 (Sections 7–12) in Volume 2 of Hansen *et al*. (1953) may be found useful.

A Quick Fix

10.29 If it proves unduly difficult, or even simply too expensive, to spend the time and effort involved in calculating an optimal level of clustering for any particular sample survey, it may well be legitimate to take advantage of the 'flatness' or 'breadth' of the optimum and use the pattern of clustering already used by some reputable organization already experienced in the conduct of household surveys.

There is in any case a strong argument for using a small value for m. The US Bureau of the Census (USBC) uses $m = 1$ and the ABS mostly uses $m = 2$. The USBC strategy extracts the maximum efficiency out of stratification. Each sample PSU represents a small homogeneous and usually geographically contiguous stratum. Increasing the value of m would require that the strata be larger, and almost inevitably less homogeneous.

There is, however, a penalty to pay for choosing a value of m as small as one. There is then no way to estimate the variance of a stratum total in an unbiased fashion. The USBC collapses strata into pairs for this purpose, but this leads to an upwardly biased estimate of variance for each stratum pair. The ABS prefers to use $m = 2$ for this reason.

Logically, the same argument would lead to stratifying within each selected PSU and choosing $n = 1$ or $n = 2$ within each such stratum. However, this would not necessarily do away with the need to optimize the number of CDs selected within each PSU. Since second- and lower-stage strata can be formed within selected PSUs, the choice $n = 1$ or $n = 2$ only alters the problem to one of optimizing the sizes of the strata to be used at the second and lower stages of selection.

In practice, however, stratification is seldom (and may never have been) employed at stages other than the first. Perhaps it is considered to be too time-consuming an activity. Deliberate 'serpentine' geographical orderings of the CDs and of other lower-stage units are used instead of stratification, and the selection is systematic within those orderings. (Figure 10.1 gives an example as to how the 50 states of the USA could be ordered in a serpentine fashion.)

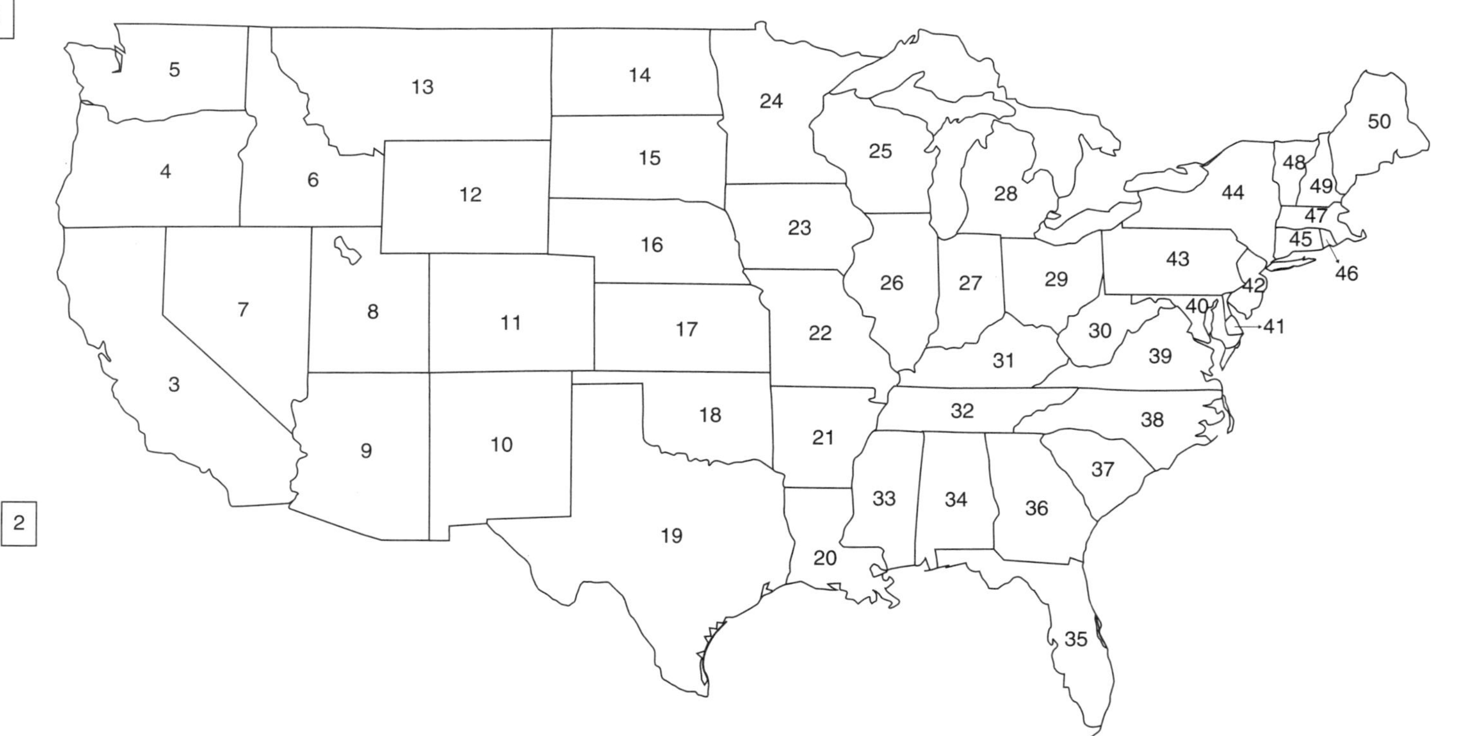

Figure 10.1 The 50 states of the USA in a serpentine ordering.

Table 10.5 Approximate structure of ABS master sample of private dwellings in 2000

	In total	In LFS[1] sample
Numbers of persons aged $\geq$15 in private dwellings	14 m	63 000
Numbers of private dwellings	7.2 m	31 000[2]
Number of strata	312	312
Number of PSUs	856	124[3]
Number of CDs	34 000	5200
Number of Blocks	n.a	5200
Number of dwelling clusters	1.1 m	5200[4]
Number of private dwellings per stratum	23 000	100[2]
Number of PSUs per stratum	7 or 8	1–3[5]
Number of CDs per PSU	6 or 7	2–4
Number of Blocks per CD	About 8	1
Numbers of clusters per Block		
urban areas	4–8	1
rural areas	1–3	1
Numbers of dwellings per cluster in SRAs[6]		
inner metro city[7]	4	4
inner metro settled[7]	6	6
metro settled[8]	7	7
metro outer growth[8]	5	5
metro rural[8]	8	8
extra-metro large towns[9]	8	8
extra-metro small towns	8	8
extra-metro rural	10	10
Number of dwellings per cluster in sampled areas		
urban	8	8
rural	10	10
Number of dwellings per cluster in sparse areas	10	10
Number of dwellings per cluster in indigenous areas	9	9
Number of dwellings per cluster in growth areas	5	5

n.a. No estimate available.
[1] LFS: Labour Force Survey.
[2] Average number of household schedules per stratum processed for LFS; 31 000/312 $\cong$ 100.
[3] Selected PSUs in sample sector only; selected from 41 strata containing 3424 CDs in sampled areas (urban and rural) and from 11 strata containing 572 CDs in sparse areas. The remaining 260 strata, containing some 30 000 CDs, are predominantly in SRAs, and provide most of the sample of private dwellings.
[4] ABS practice in 2000 was to select only one cluster from every sample block.
[5] Depended on number of dwellings in stratum divided by state skip interval. If this ratio was up to 50, one was selected; if it was more than 50 and a maximum of 75, two were selected; if it was more than 75, three were selected.
[6] SRAs: self-representing areas.
[7] Australia's two largest cities, Sydney and Melbourne, only.
[8] Includes Canberra, Sydney, Melbourne, Brisbane, Perth and Adelaide. Excludes Hobart and Darwin.
[9] Includes also Hobart and Darwin.
Source: Various ABS sample design and maintenance documents, 1996.

Unfortunately, sampling systematically from a deliberately ordered population biases the customary estimator of variance, and usually upwards. One of our earlier reports (Chapter 9) contains a discussion of this problem and suggests an alternative estimator. A full consideration of such strategies is, however, out of place in a discussion predicated on the use of sampling with replacement. For now, the point to be made is simply that stratification is seldom (if ever) used at stages other than the first.

The following description of the structure of the ABS master sample of dwellings at the turn of the millennium is intended only as a general guide. It has been greatly simplified, and the numbers given are in many cases orders of magnitude only.

It must be remembered that the ABS sample was designed primarily for its Labour Force Survey, which uses a rather short interview questionnaire. In consequence, travel time is more important for that survey than it would be for one that required an in-depth interview. The optimal sample design for such a survey would have fewer sample dwellings per cluster (at every stage) than that described by Table 10.5.

Remark 10.29.1 Finally, before settling for this or any other quick fix, the number of times that the sample design will be used must be taken into consideration. If it is a one-off survey, the effort saved by not having to find a really close approximation to the optimum is relatively important, and a quick fix is likely to be a sensible choice. If, however, the design is to be used again and again, considerable resources might be profitably channelled into finding such an approximation. As a compromise, a quick fix could be used for the first few survey rounds, and the data gathered so far then used to calculate a better design.

Acknowledgement from Supervisor

10.30 Thank you for your report on multistage sampling with replacement. It seems to cover the ground I was asking for, but it is longer than I expected and I shall need time to absorb it. Please continue with the companion report on multistage sampling without replacement. I intend to comment on both of them together in due course.

Exercises

10.1 Derive formulae for an unbiased estimator of total, its design-variance, and design-unbiased estimators for the variances of each stage, for a three-stage sample of m PSUs, mn CDs and $mn\bar{t}$ dwellings drawn in accordance with the principles set out in this chapter.

10.2 Using the cost equation $C = C_0 m^{1/2} + C_1 m + C_2 mn + C_3 mn^{1/2} + C_4 mn\bar{t}$, derive an optimum allocation of the sample of Exercise 10.1 (see Hansen *et al.*, 1953, Vol. 1, pp. 404–407).

11

Multistage Area Sampling for Household Surveys: Sampling without Replacement

Report for Supervisor: Introduction 209
Selecting a Multistage Equal Probability Sample of Dwellings without Replacement 209
Estimation Formulae for Multistage Samples Selected without Replacement 212
Variance Estimation Formulae for Multistage Samples Selected without Replacement 214
Estimating $Y^*_{\bullet\bullet}$ Using Combined Design-Based and Prediction-Based Inference 219
Estimating the Prediction-Based, Design-Based and Anticipated Variances of $\hat{Y}^*_{\bullet\bullet}$ (Totals and Components) 223
Estimation of Variance Using Jackknife, Bootstrap and Other Resampling Methods 228
Response from Supervisor 229
Exercises 229

Report for Supervisor: Introduction

11.1 This report is a sequel to the one we wrote for you on multistage sampling with replacement. Sampling without replacement is not very different operationally and, being more efficient, is used more widely. We have, as far as possible, kept to the same format for this report as for its predecessor (Chapter 10) so that the differences can easily be discovered by comparing corresponding passages. We do not, however, repeat material which would simply be identical for the two procedures.

The selection process for sampling without replacement is actually somewhat the simpler of the two, and it is certainly simpler to describe. The only drawback of selection without replacement is that the variance formulae and the expressions for the estimators of variance are appreciably more complicated.

Selecting a Multistage Equal Probability Sample of Dwellings without Replacement

11.2 Since the Australian Bureau of Statistics now uses selection without replacement exclusively, the description which follows will resemble quite closely what is currently done in that Bureau. The principal difference is that the ABS uses

Table 11.1 Example of PSU selection

Sample fraction 1/147		Number of sample PSUs 2		Cluster size 32.8	
PSU no.	No. of dwellings	No. of clusters	Cumulated clusters	Selection number	Within-PSU sample fraction
1	1550	47	47		
10	639	20	67		
7	728	22	89		
5	1055	32	121	103	1/32
9	732	22	143		
2	911	28	171		
6	553	17	188		
3	1153	35	223		
4	1457	44	267	250	1/44
8	873	27	294		
Total	9651	294			

systematic selection from deliberately ordered populations, in fact from populations arranged in serpentine orderings, whereas we will assume systematic selection from randomly ordered populations.

The reason why we are assuming random systematic selection, as opposed to systematic selection from a meaningfully ordered list, is that the random ordering permits the variances to be estimated almost without bias. It is a moot point whether it is better to aim for a lower MSE when the attainment of that lower MSE prevents you from knowing how much lower it is. What is certain is this: if we describe what can be done with random ordering, it will be easy for you to make the transition to non-random ordering; but if we describe only what can be done with non-random ordering, the transition in the other direction would be next to impossible. So we will present the random approach, and allow you to decide whether or not you want to use it.

Table 11.1 shows how we selected two PSUs (from the same stratum as figured in Table 10.1) using systematic selection from a randomly ordered population with inclusion probabilities proportional to size (*random systematic πpswor*). In the ABS, the ordering would be serpentine, but in all other respects the selection procedure would be identical with theirs.

The random ordering of the PSUs and the systematic selection of the sample from them are the only differences between this table and Table 10.1. For the definitions of the columns, the determination of the cluster size and the forcing of the numbers of clusters to add to 294, see our comments in **10.5**. However, instead of selecting two random numbers in the range 1–294 independently, a single selection number in the range 1–147 was chosen randomly, and the other selection number was obtained by adding 147. The randomly selected number, 103, selected PSU 3 and the other number, 250, selected PSU 4.

We said just now that 103 was a random number in the range 1–147, and indeed we would have picked a random number in that range had we been starting from scratch. In this instance, however, we wanted to maximize comparability with

Table 11.2 Example of SSU selection from PSU 4

Sample fraction 1/44		Number of sample SSUs 4		Cluster size 8.28	
CD no.	No. of dwellings	No. of clusters	Cumulated clusters	Selection numbers	Within-CD sample fraction
5	282	34	34		
1	220	27	61	37	1/26
4	280	34	95	81	1/34
2	198	24	119		
6, 7, 8	260	31	150	125	1/32
3	217	26	176	169	1/26
Total	1457	176			

what we did in Chapter 10, so we invoked the Keyfitz (1951) technique to *ensure* that we picked PSU 4 again. The 'lottery tickets' held by PSU 4 were numbered 224–267. That meant that we had to restrict the choice of random number to the range from 224 *minus* 147 to 267 *minus* 147, or 77 to 120, but in doing so we still kept in all essentials to the rules set by design-based inference. (A purist might query the comparability of the inclusion probability we are using now to the 'probability of selection' as defined in that last report, but following our experience with the elephants we know that there is little point in being completely pure about the probabilities used to select a small sample, and in any case we were only constructing an example here. If we had been selecting a large sample for use in a real investigation, we might have decided to be more circumspect!) The within-PSU sampling fractions are as shown in column 6.

11.3 The selection of SSUs (CDs) within the selected PSUs follows a similar pattern. Table 11.2 illustrates the manner in which the two CDs were selected within the second of these sample PSUs (PSU 4), again using random systematic *πpswor*.

To select our four sample CDs, we first chose a single selection number. This was notionally in the range 1–44, but because we were using the Keyfitz technique to retain CD 4 it had to be either in the range 18–44 or else in the range 1–7. (We are sure you will be able to work out why we used those particular ranges!) The random number that came up was 37. The other three selection numbers were obtained by adding 44 to it three times, yielding 81, 125 and 169. The corresponding selected CDs were 1, 4, 6–8 combined and 3, respectively. The within-CD sampling fractions are as shown in column 6.

11.4 The same pattern was again followed for the selection of third-stage or tertiary sample units (TSUs or blocks). Table 11.3 illustrates the manner in which the three blocks were selected within CD 4, again using random systematic *πpswor*.

This time we only had to select a single sample of three blocks from CD 4. We selected a random start notionally in the interval 1–34 but, because we wished to retain block 2, our random start was in fact in the interval 4–12. The random start

Table 11.3 Example of block selection from CD 4

Sample fraction 1/34		Number of sample blocks 3		Anticipated cluster size 2.76	
Block no.	No. of dwellings	No. of clusters	Cumulated clusters	Selection numbers	Within-block sample fraction
5	90	30	30	4	1/30
1	34	12	42	38	1/12
4	87	29	71		
2	27	9	80	72	1/9
3	65	22	102		
Total	303	102			

was 4 and the subsequent selection numbers were 38 and 72. The selected blocks were therefore 5, 1 and 2, respectively. The within-block sampling fractions are as shown in column 6.

11.5 The fourth and last stage of selection is that of dwellings within a selected block. For that purpose it was once again necessary to have a list of the dwellings in that block and identify them unambiguously for the survey interviewer. On this occasion we used the same list as previously compiled for block 2 (Table 10.4).

At this fourth stage the selection becomes a little tricky. Ideally we would like the sample to be a high-entropy one with each of the joint inclusion probabilities taking the *srswor* value, which in the more familiar single-stage notation we would write as $n(n-1)/\{N(N-1)\}$.

If the block were to remain completely unchanged in its composition until the next complete redesign of the sample, we could in fact use *srswor*. Not all sample blocks are that stable but, if the changes were moderate in extent, the Keyfitz technique described in Chapter 4 could be used to update the sample in a minimally disruptive fashion. The problem then would be how well interviewers could be trained in how to use it.

But even if that turns out not to be practicable, the *srswor* theory would probably still be usable if initially the sample were to be selected using random systematic selection without replacement, and new dwellings were simply added onto the end of the list and selected systematically using the same skip interval. Whatever practical compromise might be adopted, however, it would be necessary to keep an eye on it to make sure that the ideal was not being departed from in too abandoned a fashion.

At this point in our report we will avoid repetition of the issues raised in **10.9–10.12** and skip straight to the question of estimation.

Estimation Formulae for Multistage Samples Selected without Replacement

11.6 Estimators of total are even simpler for *πpswor* than for *ppswr*. The notation is simpler, because we no longer have any possibility of multiple selections and therefore have no need to make any distinctions among them. Hence no hybrid notation is needed and we can use such expressions as $\delta_i Y_{i\bullet\bullet\bullet}$, $\delta_{ij} Y_{ij\bullet\bullet}$, and $\delta_{ijk} Y_{ijk\bullet}$ without ambiguity. Note, however, the difference between the meaning of δ_{ijkl} under such a convention, and the meaning that it had in Chapter 10, where the *ijk*, though not the *l*, referred to units in the sample rather than to units in the population.

We can then write the total for the *ijk*th block as $Y_{ijk\bullet}$, and a design-unbiased estimator of it, if that block is in sample, as $\hat{Y}_{ijk\bullet} = g_{ijk} \sum_{l=1}^{T^*_{ijk}} \delta_{ijkl} Y_{ijkl}$, where (as in Chapter 10) T^*_{ijk} denotes the number of dwellings found in the *ijk*th block at the time the survey interviewer is sent into the field, as opposed to T_{ijk}, the number listed as being in the *ijk*th block at the time 'clusters' of dwellings were initially defined.

We can similarly write the total for the *ij*th sample CD as $Y_{ij\bullet\bullet}$ and the corresponding unbiased estimator of it as $\hat{Y}_{ij\bullet\bullet} = \sum_{k=1}^{Q_{ij}} \delta_{ijk}(g_{ij}/g_{ijk})\hat{Y}_{ijk\bullet}$. Again correspondingly, we may write the PSU total as $Y_{i\bullet\bullet\bullet}$ and estimate it by $\hat{Y}_{i\bullet\bullet\bullet} = \sum_{j=1}^{N_i} \delta_{ij}(g_i/g_{ij})\hat{Y}_{ij\bullet\bullet}$, where δ_{ij} is 1 when the *j*th CD within the *i*th PSU is in sample and 0 otherwise, and where δ_{ijk} is 1 when the *k*th block within the *j*th CD within the *i*th PSU is in sample and 0 otherwise. The grand total, $Y_{\bullet\bullet\bullet\bullet}$, is similarly estimated by

$$
\begin{aligned}
\hat{Y}_{\bullet\bullet\bullet\bullet} &= \sum_{i=1}^{M} \delta_i (g/g_i)\hat{Y}_{i\bullet\bullet\bullet} \\
&= \sum_{i=1}^{M} \delta_i (g/g_i) \sum_{j=1}^{N_i} \delta_{ij}(g_i/g_{ij}) \sum_{k=1}^{Q_{ij}} \delta_{ijk}(g_{ij}/g_{ijk}) g_{ijk} \sum_{l=1}^{T_{ijk}} \delta_{ijkl} Y_{ijkl} \\
&= g \sum_{i=1}^{M} \sum_{j=1}^{N_i} \sum_{k=1}^{Q_{ij}} \sum_{l=1}^{T^*_{ijk}} \delta_{ijkl} Y_{ijkl}. \qquad (11.1)
\end{aligned}
$$

Since each final-stage unit has the same unconditional probability of inclusion in sample, g^{-1}, (11.1) is the HTE of total. An attractive alternative to (11.1) is, however,

$$
\begin{aligned}
\hat{Y}^*_{\bullet\bullet\bullet\bullet} &= \sum_{i=1}^{M} \delta_i (g/g_i) \sum_{j=1}^{N_i} \delta_{ij}(g_i/g_{ij}) \sum_{k=1}^{Q_{ij}} \delta_{ijk}(T^*_{ijk}/t_{ijk}) \sum_{l=1}^{T^*_{ijk}} \delta_{ijkl} Y_{ijkl} \\
&\vdots \\
&= g \sum_{i=1}^{M} \sum_{j=1}^{N_i} \sum_{k=1}^{Q_{ij}} g_{ijk}^{-1}(T^*_{ijk}/t_{ijk}) \sum_{l=1}^{T^*_{ijk}} \delta_{ijkl} Y_{ijkl}. \qquad (11.2)
\end{aligned}
$$

This has the same advantages over (11.1) as (10.4) had over (10.3).

Variance Estimation Formulae for Multistage Samples Selected without Replacement

11.7 At this point we again switch to the discussion of a two-stage design, since that covers all the concepts needed for writing down the formulae for a three- or four-stage sample design in a more lengthy but still straightforward fashion. This time we will go straight to the consideration of a design that is not necessarily self-weighting. We may then choose our estimator of total to be

$$\hat{Y}^*_{\bullet\bullet} = \sum_{i=1}^{M} \delta_i (g/g_i)(T^*_i/t_i) \sum_{l=1}^{T^*_i} \delta_{il} Y_{il}$$

$$= \sum_{i=1}^{M} \delta_i (g/g_i) \hat{Y}^*_{i\bullet} \tag{11.3}$$

$$= \sum_{i=1}^{M} \delta_i w_i \sum_{l=1}^{T^*_i} \delta_{il} Y_{il}, \tag{11.4}$$

where $\hat{Y}^*_{i\bullet} = (T^*_i/t_i) \sum_{l=1}^{T^*_i} \delta_{il} Y_{il}$ and $w_i = (g/g_i)(T^*_i/t_i)$. As noted earlier in relation to (10.22)–(10.24), (11.4) with this definition of w_i is not quite a design-unbiased estimator, but it is close enough to being unbiased for most practical purposes. However, from this point on, we will work in terms of a yet more general version of (11.4) where w_i is not necessarily equal even to $(g/g_i)(T^*_i/t_i)$ but is nevertheless still close enough to $(g/g_i)(T_i/t_i)$ for the departure from design unbiasedness to be negligible.

11.8 We shall now, therefore, develop formulae relating to the design variance of the $\hat{Y}^*_{\bullet\bullet}$ of (11.4), using the more general definition of w_i introduced at the end of Section **11.7**. For this purpose we shall use the notation π_i in preference to g_i/g. It is more general and more compact than g_i/g, and it is now permissible to use π_i, since the sampling is $\pi pswor$.

The total design variance of $\hat{Y}^*_{\bullet\bullet}$ is, by definition, $\mathrm{V}\hat{Y}^*_{\bullet\bullet} \equiv \mathrm{E}(\hat{Y}^*_{\bullet\bullet} - \mathrm{E}_p\hat{Y}^*_{\bullet\bullet})^2$. Since we are making the assumption here that $\hat{Y}^*_{\bullet\bullet}$ is almost design-unbiased, that is, that $\mathrm{E}\hat{Y}^*_{\bullet\bullet} \cong Y_{\bullet\bullet}$, we may write

$$\mathrm{V}\hat{Y}^*_{\bullet\bullet} \cong \mathrm{E}(\hat{Y}^*_{\bullet\bullet} - Y_{\bullet\bullet})^2$$

$$= \mathrm{E}_{[1]}\mathrm{E}_{[2]}\left[\sum_{i=1}^{M} \delta_i \left\{(g/g_i)\hat{Y}^*_{i\bullet} - m^{-1}Y_{\bullet\bullet}\right\}\right]^2, \tag{11.5}$$

$$= \mathrm{E}_{[1]}\mathrm{E}_{[2]}\left[\sum_{i=1}^{M} \delta_i \left\{\hat{Y}^*_{i\bullet}\pi_i^{-1} - m^{-1}Y_{\bullet\bullet}\right\}\right]^2, \tag{11.6}$$

where $E_{[1]}$ denotes the expectation over all possible first-stage samples and $E_{[2]}$ denotes the expectation over all possible final-stage samples, holding the first-stage sample fixed.

As noted in our previous report (Remark 10.17.2), Theorem 10.17.1 is valid regardless of whether sampling is with replacement (*ppswr*, as in Chapter 10) or without replacement (π*pswor*, as in the present chapter). The proof is nevertheless similar. It only needs to take explicit account of the cross product terms from the first stage that were zero in (10.10) but are no longer zero when sampling is without replacement.

Hence we know that the (design) variance of $\hat{Y}^*_{..}$ – being very nearly an HTE – can be well approximated by the sum of two components, one from sampling at the first stage and the other from sampling at the second stage. More specifically, applying Theorem 10.17.1 to (11.6),

$$\begin{aligned} V\hat{Y}^*_{..} &\cong E_{[1]}E_{[2]}\left\{\sum_{i=1}^{M}\delta_i\left(\hat{Y}^*_{i.}\pi_i^{-1} - m^{-1}Y_{..}\right)\right\}^2 \\ &= E_{[1]}\left[\sum_{i=1}^{M}\delta_i\left\{Y_{i.}\pi_i^{-1} - m^{-1}Y_{..}\right\}\right]^2 \\ &\quad + E_{[1]}\sum_{i=1}^{M}\delta_i\pi_i^{-2}E_{[2]}(\hat{Y}^*_{i.} - Y_{i.})^2, \end{aligned} \tag{11.7}$$

the first term in (11.7) being the first-stage component of variance, $V_{[1]}\hat{Y}^*_{..}$, and the second term the second or final stage of variance, $V_{[2]}\hat{Y}^*_{..}$.

11.9 When the π*pswor* selection procedure is of high entropy, as for instance when selection is systematic from a randomly ordered population, expression (11.7) is capable of further development. The crucial result is (9.9), an approximate expression for the high-entropy variance of the HTE. In this context, (9.9) indicates that the first-stage component of the variance in expression (11.7) is closely approximated by

$$V_{p[1]}(\hat{Y}^*_{..}) \cong \sum_{i=1}^{M}\pi_i(1 - c_i\pi_i)\left(Y_{i.}\pi_i^{-1} - Y_{..}m^{-1}\right)^2, \tag{11.8}$$

where c_i is a quantity that can be defined (depending on the situation) by (9.11), (9.12), (9.13) or (9.26), the sample size n in those equations being replaced here, of course, by the first-stage sample size m.

The second- or final-stage component of variance is also straightforward, with the dwellings (not clusters of dwellings as in Chapter 10) as the final-stage units. We then have, from (11.4) and from the *srswor* formulae of Chapter 1, that

$$V_{[2]}\hat{Y}^*_{i.} = T_i^*(T_i^* - t_i^*)t_i^{*-1}(T_i^* - 1)^{-1}\sum_{l=1}^{T_i^*}(Y_{il} - \bar{Y}_{i.})^2, \tag{11.9}$$

where $\bar{Y}_{i\bullet}$ is the arithmetic mean of the values $\bar{Y}_{ij}, j = 1, 2, \ldots, t_i^*$. It then follows from (11.3) and (11.7) that the second- or final-stage component of the design variance of $\hat{Y}_{\bullet\bullet}^*$ is

$$\mathrm{V}_{[2]}\hat{Y}_{\bullet\bullet}^* \cong \sum_{i=1}^{M} \pi_i.\pi_i^{-2}\mathrm{V}_{[2]}(\hat{Y}_{i\bullet}^*). \tag{11.10}$$

In (11.10) the first π_i is the expectation of the δ_i in (11.3) and the π_i^{-2} is the square of the g/g_i in the same equation. Substituting the expression in (11.9) for $V_{[2]}^2\hat{Y}_{i\bullet}^*$,

$$\mathrm{V}_{[2]}\hat{Y}_{\bullet\bullet}^* \cong \sum_{i=1}^{M} \pi_i^{-1}T_i^*(T_i^* - t_i^*)t_i^{*-1}(T_i^* - 1)^{-1}\sum_{l=1}^{T_i^*}(Y_{il} - \bar{Y}_{i\bullet})^2. \tag{11.11}$$

There is something of an interpretation problem with (11.11), in that strictly speaking t_i^* is not defined unless the ith first-stage unit has been selected and a final-stage sample has been selected within it, but this is a problem that pervades all estimation procedures that are conditioned on particular outcomes. In practice, we only use sample estimates of such variances, and since the corresponding estimators are defined in terms of known sample outcomes, there is no problem either in specifying those estimators or in using those estimators to evaluate the variance estimates using our knowledge of those sample outcomes.

11.10 The straightforward sample estimator corresponding to (11.8) is, from (9.22),

$$\hat{\hat{\mathrm{V}}}_{[1]}\hat{Y}_{\bullet\bullet}^* = \sum_{i=1}^{M} \delta_i\left(c_i^{-1} - \pi_i\right)\left(\hat{Y}_{i\bullet}^*\pi_i^{-1} - \hat{Y}_{\bullet\bullet}^*m^{-1}\right)^2, \tag{11.12}$$

but this is not an unbiased estimator of the first-stage variance nor even an unbiased estimator of the total variance, although the corresponding expression in Theorem **10.21.1** was an unbiased estimator of the total variance for *ppswr*. Approximately unbiased estimators will be derived below for *πpswor*, but the derivation is not quite as simple as for *ppswr*.

If we sidestep the problem of interpretation raised in Section **11.9**, regarding the definition of the second-stage variance when estimation is conditioned on the achieved sample size, it is also possible to write down an unbiased estimator for the second-stage variance of (11.11), conditioned on the achieved sample size, namely

$$\hat{\mathrm{V}}_{[2]}\hat{Y}_{\bullet\bullet}^* = \sum_{i=1}^{M} \delta_i\pi_i^{-2}T_i^*(T_i^* - t_i^*)t_i^{*-1}(t_i^* - 1)^{-1}\sum_{l=1}^{T_i^*}\delta_{il}(Y_{il} - \hat{\bar{Y}}_{i\bullet})^2. \tag{11.13}$$

It will be seen that (11.13) is a (design-)unbiased estimator of (11.11), conditional on the T_i^* and the t_i^* being specified for all the first-stage units. This clarifies the sense in which (11.11) can be regarded as an unbiased estimator of second-stage variance. It is satisfactory for estimating variances but, should the t_i^* vary greatly from PSU to PSU, the estimator of the total itself becomes inefficient. That is why we indicated in Chapter 10 that, should the block counts be found so inaccurate that the number of actual sample units in a particular block differed sharply from the target number, the possibility of field-counting all the blocks in the vicinity should be considered.

11.11 We are now in a position to derive approximately unbiased estimators of first stage and total variance. The expectation of (11.12) over all possible samples is

$$
\begin{aligned}
\mathrm{E}\hat{\hat{\mathrm{V}}}_{[1]}\hat{Y}^*_{\bullet\bullet} &= \mathrm{E}_{[1]}\mathrm{E}_{[2]}\sum_{i=1}^{M}\delta_i\big(c_i^{-1}-\pi_i\big)\big(\hat{Y}^*_{i\bullet}\pi_i^{-1}-\hat{Y}^*_{\bullet\bullet}m^{-1}\big)^2 \\
&= \mathrm{E}_{[1]}\mathrm{E}_{[2]}\sum_{i=1}^{M}\delta_i\big(c_i^{-1}-\pi_i\big)\big[\big\{Y_{i\bullet}\pi_i^{-1}+\big(\hat{Y}^*_{i\bullet}\pi_i^{-1}-Y_{i\bullet}\pi_i^{-1}\big)\big\} \\
&\quad -m^{-1}\big\{\hat{Y}_{\bullet\bullet[1]}+\big(\hat{Y}^*_{\bullet\bullet}-\hat{Y}_{\bullet\bullet[1]}\big)\big\}\big]^2 \\
&= \mathrm{E}_{[1]}\mathrm{E}_{[2]}\sum_{i=1}^{M}\delta_i\big(c_i^{-1}-\pi_i\big)\big[\big\{Y_{i\bullet}\pi_i^{-1}-\hat{Y}_{\bullet\bullet[1]}m^{-1}\big\} \\
&\quad +\{(\hat{Y}^*_{i\bullet}-Y_{i\bullet})\pi_i^{-1}-(\hat{Y}^*_{\bullet\bullet}-\hat{Y}_{\bullet\bullet[1]})m^{-1}\}\big]^2 \\
&= \mathrm{E}_{[1]}\sum_{i=1}^{M}\delta_i\big(c_i^{-1}-\pi_i\big)\big\{Y_{i\bullet}\pi_i^{-1}-\hat{Y}_{\bullet\bullet[1]}m^{-1}\big\}^2 \\
&\quad +2\mathrm{E}_{[1]}\sum_{i=1}^{M}\big[\delta_i\big(c_i^{-1}-\pi_i\big)\big(Y_{i\bullet}\pi_i^{-1}-\hat{Y}_{\bullet\bullet[1]}m^{-1}\big) \\
&\quad \times \mathrm{E}_{[2]}\big\{(\hat{Y}^*_{i\bullet}-Y_{i\bullet})\pi_i^{-1}-(\hat{Y}^*_{\bullet\bullet}-\hat{Y}_{\bullet\bullet[1]})m^{-1}\big\}\big] \\
&\quad +\mathrm{E}_{[1]}\sum_{i=1}^{M}\delta_i\big(c_i^{-1}-\pi_i\big)\mathrm{F}_{[2]} \\
&\quad \times\big\{(\hat{Y}^*_{i\bullet}-Y_{i\bullet})\pi_i^{-1}-(\hat{Y}^*_{\bullet\bullet}-\hat{Y}_{\bullet\bullet[1]})m^{-1}\big\}^2. \qquad (11.14)
\end{aligned}
$$

The first term in (11.14) is known from (9.22) to be a close approximation to the first-stage variance $\mathrm{V}_{[1]}\hat{Y}^*_{\bullet\bullet}$ of $\hat{Y}^*_{\bullet\bullet}$ set out in (11.8). The second term is zero because, conditionally on the T_i^* and the t_i^*, $\mathrm{E}_{[2]}(\hat{Y}^*_{i\bullet}-Y_{i\bullet})=0$ and $\mathrm{E}_{[2]}(\hat{Y}^*_{\bullet\bullet}-\hat{Y}_{\bullet\bullet[1]})=0$. The third term is $\sum_{i=1}^{M}\pi_i(c_i^{-1}-\pi_i)\{(\mathrm{V}_{[2]}\hat{Y}^*_{i\bullet})\pi_i^{-2}-(\mathrm{V}_{[2]}\hat{Y}^*_{\bullet\bullet})m^{-2}\}$, which we can see from (11.10) to be of the same order as (though still somewhat different from) $\mathrm{V}_{[2]}\hat{Y}^*_{\bullet\bullet}$, the second-stage variance of $\hat{Y}^*_{\bullet\bullet}$. We therefore have, from (11.14),

$$
\begin{aligned}
\mathrm{E}\hat{\hat{\mathrm{V}}}_{[1]}\hat{Y}^*_{\bullet\bullet} &\cong \mathrm{V}_{[1]}(\hat{Y}_{\bullet\bullet})+\sum_{i=1}^{M}\pi_i\big(c_i^{-1}-\pi_i\big) \\
&\quad \times\Big\{(\mathrm{V}_{[2]}\hat{Y}^*_{i\bullet})\pi_i^{-2}-(\mathrm{V}_{[2]}\hat{Y}^*_{\bullet\bullet})m^{-2}\Big\}. \qquad (11.15)
\end{aligned}
$$

[Check: $\mathrm{V}_{[1]}\hat{Y}_{\bullet\bullet}$ is $O(M^2m^{-1})$ by definition, $\sum_{i=1}^{M}\pi_i(c_i^{-1}-\pi_i)(\mathrm{V}_{[2]}\hat{Y}_{i\bullet}^*)\pi_i^{-2}$ is $O\{M.(m/M).1.(\bar{T}^{*2}/\bar{t}^*)(M^2/m^2)\}$ or $O(M^2\bar{T}^{*2}/m\bar{t}^*)$ (where $\bar{T}^*$ is the mean of the T_i^* and $\bar{t}^*$ is the mean of the t_i^*), correct for a second-stage variance, and $\sum_{i=1}^{M}\times\pi_i(c_i^{-1}-\pi_i)(\mathrm{V}_{[2]}\hat{Y}_{\bullet\bullet}^*)m^{-2}$ is $O\{M(m/M).1.(M^2\bar{T}^{*2}/m\bar{t}^*)(1/m^2)\}$ or $O(M^2\bar{T}^{*2}/m^2\bar{t}^*)$, which looks at first sight like a small adjustment term to that second-stage variance. Since usually $m=2$, however, this term is seldom small in fact.]

It follows that nearly unbiased estimators of the first-stage variance, $\mathrm{V}_{[1]}\hat{Y}_{\bullet\bullet}^*$, of the second-stage variance, $\mathrm{V}_{[2]}\hat{Y}_{\bullet\bullet}^*$, and of the total variance $\mathrm{V}\hat{Y}_{\bullet\bullet}^*$ of $\hat{Y}_{\bullet\bullet}^*$ are, respectively,

$$\hat{\mathrm{V}}_{[1]}\hat{Y}_{\bullet\bullet}^* = \hat{\hat{\mathrm{V}}}_{[1]}\hat{Y}_{\bullet\bullet}^* - \sum_{i=1}^{M}\delta_i\left(c_i^{-1}-\pi_i\right)\left\{(\hat{\mathrm{V}}_{[2]}\hat{Y}_{i\bullet}^*)\pi_i^{-2} - (\hat{\mathrm{V}}_{[2]}\hat{Y}_{\bullet\bullet}^*)m^{-2}\right\}, \quad (11.16)$$

$$\begin{aligned}\hat{\mathrm{V}}_{[2]}\hat{Y}_{\bullet\bullet}^* &= \sum_{i=1}^{M}\delta_i\pi_i^{-2}\hat{\mathrm{V}}_{[2]}\hat{Y}_{i\bullet}^* \\ &= \sum_{i=1}^{M}\delta_i\pi_i^{-2}T_i^*(T_i^*-t_i^*)t_i^{*-1}(t_i^*-1)^{-1}\sum_{l=1}^{T_i^*}\delta_{il}(Y_{il}-\bar{Y}_{i\bullet})^2 \qquad (11.13)\end{aligned}$$

and

$$\begin{aligned}\hat{\mathrm{V}}\hat{Y}_{\bullet\bullet}^* &= \hat{\hat{\mathrm{V}}}_{[1]}(\hat{Y}_{\bullet\bullet}^*) - \sum_{i=1}^{M}\delta_i\left(c_i^{-1}-\pi_i\right)\{(\hat{\mathrm{V}}_{[2]}\hat{Y}_{i\bullet}^*)\pi_i^{-2} \\ &\quad - (\hat{\mathrm{V}}_{[2]}\hat{Y}_{\bullet\bullet}^*)m^{-2}\} + \hat{\mathrm{V}}_{[2]}\hat{Y}_{\bullet\bullet}^* \qquad (11.17) \\ &= \hat{\hat{\mathrm{V}}}_{[1]}\hat{Y}_{\bullet\bullet}^* - \sum_{i=1}^{M}\delta_i\left(c_i^{-1}-\pi_i\right)(\hat{\mathrm{V}}_{[2]}\hat{Y}_{i\bullet}^*)\pi_i^{-2} \\ &\quad + m^{-2}\left\{\sum_{j=1}^{M}\delta_j\left(c_j^{-1}-\pi_j\right)\right\}\sum_{i=1}^{M}\delta_i\pi_i^{-2}\hat{\mathrm{V}}_{[2]}\hat{Y}_{i\bullet}^* \\ &\quad + \sum_{i=1}^{M}\delta_i\pi_i^{-2}\hat{\mathrm{V}}_{[2]}\hat{Y}_{i\bullet}^* \\ &= \hat{\hat{\mathrm{V}}}_{[1]}\hat{Y}_{\bullet\bullet}^* - \sum_{i=1}^{M}\delta_i(\hat{\mathrm{V}}_{[2]}\hat{Y}_{i\bullet}^*)\pi_i^{-2} \\ &\quad \times\left[c_i^{-1}-\pi_i-1-m^{-2}\left\{\sum_{j=1}^{M}\delta_j\left(c_j^{-1}-\pi_j\right)\right\}\right]. \qquad (11.18)\end{aligned}$$

It is tempting to think about what happens if m is large, because then the terms in the square brackets in (11.18) nearly cancel, as you can see for yourself if you use (9.12) to define c_i, which makes the workings simple. But since m is rarely large, and most often $m=2$, that second term in (11.18) looks dangerous to ignore. Nevertheless it does seem to be substantially smaller than the second-stage variance. For earlier work on this topic, see Durbin (1967) and Brewer and Hanif (1970).

Remark 11.11.1 When $m = 2$, the two half-stratum estimates are $\hat{Y}_{1\bullet}\pi_1^{-1}$ and $\hat{Y}_{2\bullet}\pi_2^{-1}$, and their sum is the stratum estimate, as was the case under *ppswr*. If c_i is defined by (9.13), which appears to be more accurate than (9.11) and (9.12) and is certainly simpler than (9.26), the estimator $\hat{\hat{\mathrm{V}}}_{[1]}\hat{Y}^*_{\bullet\bullet}$ of (11.12) becomes $\left(1 - \pi_1 - \pi_2 + 0.5\sum_{k=1}^{M}\pi_k^2\right)\left(\hat{Y}_{1\bullet}\pi_1^{-1} - \hat{Y}_{2\bullet}\pi_1^{-1}\right)^2$, implying a finite-sample correction factor of $1 - \pi_1 - \pi_2 + 0.5\sum_{k=1}^{M}\pi_k^2$. When sampling is *srswor*, $1 - \pi_1 - \pi_2 + 0.5\sum_{k=1}^{M}\pi_k^2$ becomes $(M - 2)/M$, in accordance with the *srswor* formula for the variance estimator when $m = 2$. (The same is also true for the other three definitions offered for c_i.)

11.12 The underlying principles behind the expression (11.17) may be summarized in prose as follows. For a general multistage design in which the estimators of total used at every stage are design-unbiased, an estimator of total variance can be calculated using the convenient fiction that the totals of the first-stage units have been measured without error. That estimator, the $\hat{\hat{\mathrm{V}}}_{[1]}\hat{Y}^*_{\bullet\bullet}$ of (11.12), incorporates an almost design-unbiased estimator of the first-stage variance, but a biased estimator of the components of variance from the lower stages. This bias may be removed by subtracting the contribution that those lower stages make to $\hat{\hat{\mathrm{V}}}_{[1]}\hat{Y}^*_{\bullet\bullet}$ and adding an unbiased estimator of the lower-stage components of variance – for example, the $\hat{\mathrm{V}}_{[2]}\hat{Y}^*_{\bullet\bullet}$ of (11.13).

Should we instead wish to estimate the first-stage variance only, it would only be necessary to omit that unbiased estimator of the variance arising from the remaining stages of sampling (the $\hat{\mathrm{V}}_{[2]}\hat{Y}^*_{\bullet\bullet}$).

As was the case with *ppswr* in Chapter 10, in deriving the variance component formulae for a two-stage design, we have had to cover all the concepts needed for a more general multistage design, so we will not consider three- or four-stage designs explicitly here. Similarly, there is nothing specifically new that need be said regarding optimal levels of clustering. The general principles are identical with those set out in Chapter 10 and, however complex the resulting equations might turn out to be, the necessary adjustments to allow for *πpswor* are straightforward in principle.

Estimating $Y^*_{\bullet\bullet}$ Using Combined Design-Based and Prediction-Based Inference

11.13 In Chapter 10 we employed design-based inference exclusively because we were sampling with replacement. That selection procedure does not lend itself to prediction-based inference. Although it did not prevent us from using a prediction model when imputing variance components to help us design an efficient sample, we would not have used one when estimating totals for a client or for the public!

Now, however, we are sampling without replacement, so it is feasible to use both inferences simultaneously to estimate $Y^*_{\bullet\bullet}$. As noted in Remark 8.8.2, the HTE is itself a cosmetically calibrated estimator provided either that the sample size is fixed in advance or else that the 'inclusion probabilities' used in the HTE are adjusted by conditioning on the achieved sample size (Furnival *et al.*, 1987). Although in this case the sample size is not, strictly speaking, fixed beforehand, the population size and the sample skip interval are fixed, so, if we can ignore the end-effect, the sample size can also be regarded as fixed. The end-effect introduces a small variability in the achieved sample size, but this is compensated for when the sample weight is defined as the ratio of the actual number of dwellings in the selected first-stage unit to the number of sample dwellings selected from that unit. Inverting the sample weight, we arrive at the 'adjusted inclusion probability' (i.e. the one conditioned on the achieved sample size).

$\hat{Y}^*_{i\bullet}$ is thus both a GREG estimator *and* a predictor of $Y^*_{i\bullet}$. It has in fact sounder claims to both these descriptions than it has to being an HTE! It is only a modified HTE, the modification being its conditioning on the achieved sample size. Despite this modification, we can analyse it as though it were the HTE obtained from a sample of fixed size, that size being the achieved size of the actual sample. Using this approach, its (randomization- or) design-based variance is that displayed in (11.9), and a design-unbiased estimator of it is given in (11.13).

The analysis at the end of Chapter 1 indicated that the prediction-based variance of the expansion estimator was identical in form to its design-based variance under *srswor*, and in consequence its anticipated variance under *srswor* was also exactly the same expression. These results were, however, dependent on using the extremely simple model

$$\xi: \quad Y_i = \mu + U_i; \quad \mathrm{E}_\xi U_i = 0; \quad \mathrm{E}_\xi U_i^2 = \sigma^2; \quad \mathrm{E}_\xi U_i U_j = 0, \quad j \neq i; \quad i = 1, 2, \ldots, N$$

of Section **1.11**. Our mentor used this model in Chapter 1, partly because we had no knowledge about the variability of the individual elephant weights (so it seemed sensible to assume that they all had the same population variance) but also partly because then we were complete newcomers to prediction-based estimation and she wanted to keep things as simple as possible. Now we know a little more, we can profitably choose a somewhat more general form for the variance function and expand the whole model to accommodate two stages. Our basic parameter is still μ, the model mean value per household over the entire superpopulation. The first-stage parameters, μ_i, are the model mean values per household over the individual first stage units. Our complete model specification is

$$\begin{aligned} \xi^*: \quad & \mu_i = \mu + U_{1i}; \quad \mathrm{E}_{\xi^*} U_{1i} = 0; \quad \mathrm{E}_{\xi^*} U_{1i}^2 = \sigma_{1i}^2; \\ & i = 1, 2, \ldots, M, \quad \mathrm{E}_{\xi^*}(U_{i_1} U_{i_2}) = 0, \ i_2 \neq i_1. \\ & Y_{ij} = \mu_i + U_{2ij}; \quad \mathrm{E}_{\xi^*} U_{2ij} = 0; \quad \mathrm{E}_{\xi^*} U_{2ij}^2 = \sigma_{2ij}^2; \\ & i = 1, 2, \ldots, M; \quad j = 1, 2, \ldots, T_i^*. \end{aligned} \tag{11.19}$$

$$\mathrm{E}_{\xi^*}(U_{2ij_1} U_{2ij_2}) = 0, \; j_2 \neq j_1.$$

$$Y_{i\bullet} = \sum_{j=1}^{T_i^*} Y_{ij} = \sum_{j=1}^{T_i^*} (\mu_i + U_{2ij}) = T_i^* \mu_i + \sum_{j=1}^{T_i^*} U_{2ij}$$
$$= T_i^* \mu + T_i^* U_{1i} + U_{2i\bullet}$$

We are aiming for design-based and model-based estimators of total that coincide numerically, so we have, for every first-stage unit included in sample, from design-based inference:

$$\hat{Y}^*_{i\bullet} = \sum_{l=1}^{T_i^*} \delta_{il} Y_{il} / \pi^*_{l|i}$$
$$= (T_i^* / t_i^*) \sum_{l=1}^{T_i^*} \delta_{il} Y_{il}$$
$$= \sum_{l=1}^{T_i^*} \delta_{il} Y_{il} + \{(T_i^* - t_i^*)/t_i^*\} \sum_{l=1}^{T_i^*} \delta_{il} Y_{il} \tag{11.20}$$

where $\pi^*_{l|i} = t_i^* / T_i^*$ is the inclusion probability of each of the T_i^* dwellings in the ith block, adjusted for the achieved sample size t_i^*. We also have, from inference based on the model ξ^*,

$$\hat{Y}^*_{i\bullet} = \sum_{l=1}^{T_i^*} \delta_{il} Y_{il} + (T_i^* - t_i^*)\hat{\mu}_i. \tag{11.21}$$

Equating (11.20) and (11.21), we obtain as our estimator for each sample μ_i,

$$\hat{\mu}_i = \sum_{l=1}^{T_i^*} \delta_{il} Y_{il} / t_i^* = \hat{Y}^*_{i\bullet} / T_i^*, \tag{11.22}$$

which is the sample mean for the ith PSU (block).

For the population total $Y_{\bullet\bullet}$ we then have the design-based estimator

$$\hat{Y}^*_{\bullet\bullet} = \sum_{i=1}^{M} \delta_i \hat{Y}^*_{i\bullet} (g/g_i) = \sum_{i=1}^{M} \delta_i \hat{Y}^*_{i\bullet} \pi_i^{-1}, \tag{11.23}$$

but when it comes to model-based estimation we have

$$\hat{Y}^*_{\bullet\bullet} = \sum_{i=1}^{M} \delta_i t_i^* \hat{\mu}_i + \sum_{i=1}^{M} \delta_i (T_i^* - t_i^*)\hat{\mu}_i + \sum_{i=1}^{M} (1 - \delta_i) T_i^* \hat{\mu}_i$$
$$= \sum_{i=1}^{M} \delta_i \hat{Y}^*_{i\bullet} + \sum_{i=1}^{M} (1 - \delta_i) T_i^* \hat{\mu}_i, \tag{11.24}$$

the second term of which involves both unspecified estimators, $\hat{\mu}_i$, of the non-sample μ_i and unknown non-sample values of T_i^*. If these T_i^* were known, the $\hat{\mu}_i$ would be no problem, for we could then replace each of them with an estimator of μ, which we could denote by $\hat{\mu}$, obtaining

$$\hat{Y}_{\bullet\bullet}^* = \sum_{i=1}^{M} \delta_i \hat{Y}_{i\bullet}^* + \hat{\mu} \sum_{i=1}^{M} (1 - \delta_i) T_i^*. \tag{11.25}$$

Equating (11.25) with (11.23), we would obtain the following expression for $\hat{\mu}$:

$$\hat{\mu} = \left\{ \sum_{i=1}^{M} (1 - \delta_i) T_i^* \right\}^{-1} \sum_{i=1}^{M} \delta_i (\pi_i^{-1} - 1) \hat{Y}_i^* \tag{11.26}$$

Clearly we must in fact replace the unknown T_i^* in (11.26) with $\hat{T}_i^*$, an as yet unspecified estimator of the dwelling count that would have been made in the field if the ith block in this summation had been selected at the first stage. Unfortunately, all the non-zero values of $1 - \delta_i$ relate to blocks that have *not* been selected at the first stage!

What can be done? There are basically three possibilities.

(i) Conduct field counts for each of the non-selected blocks and obtain exact values for their T_i^*.
(ii) Use all the available information short of conducting field counts of the non-selected blocks to form partly subjective estimates of their T_i^*.
(iii) Replace $\sum_{i=1}^{M} T_i^*$ by its design-based estimate $\sum_{i=1}^{M} \delta_i T_i^* \pi_i^{-1}$, obtaining

$$\hat{\mu} = \left\{ \sum_{i=1}^{M} \delta_i (\pi_i^{-1} - 1) T_i^* \right\}^{-1} \sum_{i=1}^{M} \delta_i (\pi_i^{-1} - 1) \hat{Y}_i^*. \tag{11.27}$$

Option (i) is obviously expensive. Option (ii) is a tempting possibility when the information required is known to be both cheap and plausibly reliable, but this combination is a rare one. Option (iii) is always open, and can make good sense even to those who are exclusively modellers when (as in the case now) the design-based estimator of μ is also a plausible ratio estimator.

Adopting option (iii), (11.24) becomes

$$\begin{aligned}
\hat{Y}_{\bullet\bullet}^* &= \sum_{i=1}^{M} \delta_i \hat{Y}_{i\bullet}^* + \hat{\mu} \sum_{i=1}^{M} (1 - \delta_i) T_i^* \\
&= \sum_{i=1}^{M} \delta_i \hat{Y}_{i\bullet}^* + \sum_{i=1}^{M} \delta_i \left(\pi_i^{-1} - 1\right) \hat{Y}_i^* \\
&= \sum_{i=1}^{M} \delta_i \pi_i^{-1} \hat{Y}_i^*,
\end{aligned} \tag{11.28}$$

confirming the status of $\hat{Y}^*_{..}$ as a cosmetically calibrated estimator. This is not to suggest that option (iii) is superior to either of its alternatives; only that even if a model-oriented sampling statistician has to fall back on option (iii), the resulting estimator is supported by design assisted prediction inference.

Estimating the Prediction-Based, Design-Based and Anticipated Variances of $\hat{Y}^*_{..}$ (Totals and Components)

11.14 The variance function in our model ξ^* differs substantially from that in model ξ of Chapter 1. In ξ the U_i were *homoscedastic* (i.e. they all shared the same population variance, σ^2). In ξ^* both the U_i and the U_{ij} are heteroscedastic, each having its own population variance, σ^2_{1i} and σ^2_{2ij} respectively. This complicates the estimation of variance, but (since PSUs and households are not all of the same size) it is more realistic.

When selecting the sample it makes sense to consider the 'first stage' first, but when estimating the variance the reverse is true. We will consider the second-stage variance first. The relevant model is the second stage part of (11.19), and the model-based estimator of the second-stage population variance is quite straightforward to derive.

Theorem 11.14.1 The model ξ^*-based variance of $\hat{Y}^*_{i.}$ is

$$g^*_i(g^*_i - 2)g^*_i \sum_{l=1}^{T^*_i} \delta_{il}\sigma^2_{2il} + \sum_{l=1}^{T^*_i} \sigma^2_{2il},$$

where $g^*_i = T^*_i/t^*_i$.

Proof. From (11.20), $\hat{Y}^*_{i.} = (T^*_i/t^*_i)\sum_{l=1}^{T^*_i} \delta_{il}Y_{il}$ and

$$\begin{aligned}
V_{\xi^*}\hat{Y}^*_{i.} &= E_{\xi^*}(\hat{Y}^*_{i.} - Y^*_{i.})^2 \\
&= E_{\xi^*}\left\{(T^*_i/t^*_i)\sum_{l=1}^{T^*_i}\delta_{il}Y_{il} - \sum_{l=1}^{T^*_i}Y_{il}\right\}^2 \\
&= E_{\xi^*}\left\{g^*_i\sum_{l=1}^{T^*_i}\delta_{il}U_{2il} - \sum_{l=1}^{T^*_i}U_{2il}\right\}^2 \\
&= E_{\xi^*}\left\{(g^*_i - 1)\sum_{l=1}^{T^*_i}\delta_{il}U_{2il} - \sum_{l=1}^{T^*_i}(1-\delta_{il})U_{2il}\right\}^2 \\
&= (g^*_i - 1)^2\sum_{l=1}^{T^*_i}\delta_{il}\sigma^2_{2il} + \sum_{l=1}^{T^*_i}(1-\delta_{il})\sigma^2_{2il}
\end{aligned}$$

$$= \{g_i^{*2} - 2g_i^* + 1\} \sum_{l=1}^{T_i^*} \delta_{il}\sigma_{2il}^2 + \sum_{l=1}^{T_i^*} (1 - \delta_{il})\sigma_{2il}^2$$

$$= g_i^*(g_i^* - 2) \sum_{l=1}^{T_i^*} \delta_{il}\sigma_{2il}^2 + \sum_{l=1}^{T_i^*} \sigma_{2il}^2. \tag{11.29}$$

◇

This formula is satisfactory for the variance, but inappropriate for the estimation of variance if the σ_{2il}^2 are to be estimated individually, since this can only be attempted for the sample dwellings. Noting that $g_i^* \sum_{l=1}^{T_i^*} \delta_{il}\sigma_{2il}^2$ is the HTE of $\sum_{l=1}^{T_i^*} \sigma_{2il}^2$, it is convenient to approximate (11.29) by

$$\tilde{\mathrm{V}}_{\xi^*} \hat{Y}_{i\bullet}^* = g_i^*(g_i^* - 1) \sum_{l=1}^{T_i^*} \delta_{il}\sigma_{2il}^2 \tag{11.30}$$

and to estimate this approximation by

$$\hat{\tilde{\mathrm{V}}}_{\xi^*} \hat{Y}_{i\bullet}^* = g_i^*(g_i^* - 1) \sum_{l=1}^{T_i^*} \delta_{il}\hat{\sigma}_{2il}^2. \tag{11.31}$$

All that then remains to complete the second-stage variance estimation process is to find a suitable formula for the sample $\hat{\sigma}_{2il}^2$.

Theorem 11.14.2 A model ξ^*-unbiased estimator of σ_{2ij}^2 is

$$\hat{\sigma}_{ij}^2 = (t_i^* - 2)^{-1} \left\{ t_i^*(Y_{ij} - \hat{Y}_{i\bullet}^*)^2 - (t_i^* - 1)^{-1} \sum_{k=1}^{T_i^*} \delta_{ik}(Y_{ij} - \hat{Y}_{i\bullet}^*)^2 \right\}.$$

Proof. We will be estimating σ_{2il}^2 using some function of $(Y_{ij} - \hat{Y}_{i\bullet}^*)^2$. The expectation of that expression is

$$\mathrm{E}_{\xi^*}(Y_{ij} - \hat{Y}_{i\bullet}^*)^2 = \mathrm{E}_{\xi^*} \left(U_{2ij} - t_i^{*-1} \sum_{k=1}^{T_i^*} \delta_{ik} U_{2ik} \right)^2$$

$$= \mathrm{E}_{\xi^*} \left\{ U_{2ij}(1 - t_i^{*-1}) - t_i^{*-1} \sum_{\substack{k=1 \\ k \neq j}}^{T_i^*} \delta_{ik} U_{2ik} \right\}^2$$

$$= \sigma_{2ij}^2 \left(1 - t_i^{*-1}\right)^2 + t_i^{*-2} \sum_{\substack{k=1 \\ k \neq j}}^{T_i^*} \delta_{ik}\sigma_{2ik}^2$$

$$= \sigma_{2ij}^2 \left(1 - 2t_i^{*-1}\right) + t_i^{*-2} \sum_{k=1}^{T_i^*} \delta_{ik}\sigma_{2ik}^2. \tag{11.32}$$

Hence an unbiased estimator of σ^2_{2il} can be obtained by solving

$$\hat{\sigma}^2_{2ij} = \left(1 - 2t_i^{*-1}\right)^{-1} \left\{ \left(Y_{ij} - \hat{Y}^*_{i\bullet}\right)^2 + t_i^{*-2} \sum_{k=1}^{T_i^*} \delta_{ik} \hat{\sigma}^2_{2ik} \right\}. \tag{11.33}$$

Cross-multiplying and summing over the sample units,

$$\begin{aligned}
\left(1 - 2t_i^{*-1}\right) \sum_{k=1}^{T_i^*} \delta_{ik} \hat{\sigma}^2_{2ij} &= \sum_{k=1}^{T_i^*} \delta_{ik} \left\{ (Y_{ij} - \hat{Y}^*_{i\bullet})^2 - t_i^{*-2} \sum_{k=1}^{T_i^*} \delta_{ik} \hat{\sigma}^2_{2ik} \right\} \\
&= \sum_{k=1}^{T_i^*} \delta_{ik} (Y_{ij} - \hat{Y}^*_{i\bullet})^2 - t_i^{*-1} \sum_{k=1}^{T_i^*} \delta_{ik} \hat{\sigma}^2_{2ik}.
\end{aligned} \tag{11.34}$$

Hence

$$\left(1 - t_i^{*-1}\right) \sum_{k=1}^{T_i^*} \delta_{ik} \hat{\sigma}^2_{2ij} = \sum_{k=1}^{T_i^*} \delta_{ik} (Y_{ij} - \hat{Y}^*_{i\bullet})^2$$

so

$$\sum_{k=1}^{T_i^*} \delta_{ik} \hat{\sigma}^2_{2ij} = \left(1 - t_i^{*-1}\right)^{-1} \sum_{k=1}^{T_i^*} \delta_{ik} (Y_{ij} - \hat{Y}^*_{i\bullet})^2. \tag{11.35}$$

Substituting (11.35) into (11.33),

$$\begin{aligned}
\hat{\sigma}^2_{2ij} &= \left(1 - 2t_i^{*-1}\right)^{-1} \left\{ (Y_{ij} - \hat{Y}^*_{i\bullet})^2 - t_i^{*-2} \left(1 - t_i^{*-1}\right)^{-1} \sum_{k=1}^{T_i^*} \delta_{ik} (Y_{ij} - \hat{Y}^*_{i\bullet})^2 \right\} \\
&= (t_i^* - 2)^{-1} \left\{ t_i^* (Y_{ij} - \hat{Y}^*_{i\bullet})^2 - (t_i^* - 1)^{-1} \sum_{k=1}^{T_i^*} \delta_{ik} (Y_{ij} - \hat{Y}^*_{i\bullet})^2 \right\}.
\end{aligned} \tag{11.36}$$

◇

Substituting the $\hat{\sigma}^2_{2ij}$ of (11.36), with the dummy suffix changed from j to l, for the σ^2_{2il} in (11.30) completes the definition of the unbiased estimator of the approximate second-stage variance given in (11.31).

Remark 11.14.1 When $t_i^* < 3$, (11.34) is indeterminate. An estimator can be found for $t_i^* = 2$, but only by making an additional assumption as to the relative sizes of the two $\hat{\sigma}^2_{2il}$. A similar situation has already been considered in **5.5**.

11.15 As with design-based inference, we cannot deal directly with the estimation of first-stage variance. What we have to do is estimate the total variance, and subtract from that an estimate of the variance from the second stage (and lower stages if any).

Most of the task of estimating the total variance is comparatively straightforward. The rounded dwelling counts provide not only the inclusion probabilities for the first stage of sampling but also the auxiliary variable in the two-stage prediction model of (11.19). The first-stage sample size is fixed in advance and there is no end-effect. However, the prediction-based variance, which follows the pattern set by (8.29), is logically distinct from the design-based variance, which was approximated by (11.8) and estimated, almost without bias, by (11.18).

As pointed out in Chapter 8 – and as paralleled by the developments in **11.14** – the prediction-based variance may be approximated by the first term in (8.29), namely $\sum_{i=1}^{M} \delta_i w_i(w_i - 1)\sigma_i^2$, where the w_i are the general first-stage sample weights. (Remember that these w_i were described at the end of **11.7** as 'not necessarily equal even to $(g/g_i)(T_i^*/t_i)$ but ... nevertheless still close enough to $(g/g_i)(T_i/t_i)$ for the departure from design unbiasedness to be negligible'. For the design variance and the hybrid anticipated variance the w_i may be replaced by the π_i^{-1}.)

It therefore only remains to show how the approximate sample variances $\sum_{i=1}^{M} \delta_i w_i(w_i - 1)\sigma_i^2$ for the prediction variance and $\sum_{i=1}^{M} \delta_i \pi_i^{-1}(\pi_i^{-1} - 1)\sigma_i^2$ for both the design and anticipated variance (all of them first- and second-stage variances combined) can be estimated from the sample data. For that we need an unbiased estimator of the σ_i^2.

Theorem 11.15.1 A model ξ^*-unbiased estimator of σ_i^2 is

$$\hat{\sigma}_i^2 = \pi_i^2(1 - 2m^{-1})^{-1}\{(\hat{Y}_{i\bullet}^*\pi_i^{-1} - m^{-1}\hat{Y}_{\bullet\bullet}^*)^2 - \hat{S}^2\}$$

where

$$\hat{S}^2 = m^{-1}(m-1)^{-1}\sum_{k=1}^{M} \delta_k \left(\hat{Y}_{k\bullet}^*\pi_k^{-1} - m^{-1}\hat{Y}_{\bullet\bullet}^*\right)^2.$$

Proof. Consider the model expectation of $(\hat{Y}_{i\bullet}^*\pi_i^{-1} - m^{-1}\hat{Y}_{\bullet\bullet}^*)^2$:

$$\begin{aligned}
\mathrm{E}_{\xi^*}(\hat{Y}_{i\bullet}^*\pi_i^{-1} - m^{-1}\hat{Y}_{\bullet\bullet}^*)^2 &= \mathrm{E}_{\xi^*}\left(U_i\pi_i^{-1} - m^{-1}\sum_{k=1}^{M}\delta_k U_k \pi_k^{-1}\right)^2 \\
&= \mathrm{E}_{\xi^*}\left\{U_i\pi_i^{-1}(1 - m^{-1}) - m^{-1}\sum_{\substack{k=1\\k\neq i}}^{M}\delta_k U_k\pi_k^{-1}\right\}^2 \\
&= \sigma_i^2\pi_i^{-2}(1 - m^{-1})^2 + m^{-2}\sum_{\substack{k=1\\k\neq i}}^{M}\delta_k\sigma_k^2\pi_k^{-2} \\
&= \sigma_i^2\pi_i^{-2}(1 - 2m^{-1}) + m^{-2}\sum_{k=1}^{M}\delta_k\sigma_k^2\pi_k^{-2}. \qquad (11.37)
\end{aligned}$$

Writing $S^2 = m^{-2}\sum_{k=1}^{M}\delta_k\sigma_k^2\pi_k^{-2}$, we then have

$$\mathrm{E}_{\xi^*}\left(\hat{Y}^*_{i\bullet}\pi_i^{-1} - m^{-1}\hat{Y}^*_{\bullet\bullet}\right)^2 = \sigma_i^2\pi_i^{-2}(1-2m^{-1}) + S^2$$

so that

$$\sigma_i^2 = \pi_i^2(1-2m^{-1})^{-1}\left\{\mathrm{E}_{\xi^*}\left(\hat{Y}^*_{i\bullet}\pi_i^{-1} - m^{-1}\hat{Y}^*_{\bullet\bullet}\right)^2 - S^2\right\} \tag{11.38}$$

and

$$\hat{\sigma}_i^2 = \pi_i^2(1-2m^{-1})^{-1}\left\{\left(\hat{Y}^*_{i\bullet}\pi_i^{-1} - m^{-1}\hat{Y}^*_{\bullet\bullet}\right)^2 - \hat{S}^2\right\}, \tag{11.39}$$

where $\hat{S}^2 = m^{-2}\sum_{k=1}^{M}\delta_k\hat{\sigma}_k^2\pi_k^{-2}$.

To obtain an explicit formula for $\hat{\sigma}_i^2$, however, we need one for $\hat{S}^2$ that does not depend on $\hat{\sigma}_i^2$. We obtain that as follows. From (11.38),

$$\sigma_i^2\pi_i^{-2} = (1-2m^{-1})^{-1}\left\{\mathrm{E}_{\xi^*}\left(\hat{Y}^*_{i\bullet}\pi_i^{-1} - m^{-1}\hat{Y}^*_{\bullet\bullet}\right)^2 - S^2\right\}.$$

Multiplying both sides by m^{-2} and summing over the sample first-stage units,

$$S^2 = m^{-2}\sum_{k=1}^{M}\delta_k(1-2m^{-1})^{-1}\left\{\mathrm{E}_{\xi^*}\left(\hat{Y}^*_{k\bullet}\pi_k^{-1} - m^{-1}\hat{Y}^*_{\bullet\bullet}\right)^2 - S^2\right\},$$

which simplifies to

$$S^2 = m^{-1}(m-1)^{-1}\sum_{k=1}^{M}\delta_k\mathrm{E}_{\xi^*}\left(\hat{Y}^*_{k\bullet}\pi_k^{-1} - m^{-1}\hat{Y}^*_{\bullet\bullet}\right)^2. \tag{11.40}$$

The explicit formula required for $\hat{S}^2$ is therefore

$$\hat{S}^2 = m^{-1}(m-1)^{-1}\sum_{k=1}^{M}\delta_k\left(\hat{Y}^*_{k\bullet}\pi_k^{-1} - m^{-1}\hat{Y}^*_{\bullet\bullet}\right)^2 \tag{11.41}$$

as required. ◇

As mentioned above, the first-stage components of variance may be obtained by subtracting the second-stage components from the total. This can be done for the individual first-stage sample units as follows.

The total population variance of the ith first-stage sample unit is estimated without bias by the $\hat{\sigma}_i^2$ of (11.39). The second-stage component of that is the estimated second-stage variance of $\hat{Y}_i^*\pi_i^{-1}$. The first-stage population variance of the ith first-stage sample unit is therefore estimated without bias by $\hat{\sigma}_i^2 - \sum_{j=1}^{T_i^*}\hat{\sigma}_{ij}^2\pi_i^{-2}$. (Like $\hat{\sigma}_i^2$ itself, this estimator can yield negative estimates, but since they are unbiased, the errors will tend to cancel on aggregation.) The σ_{ij}^2 themselves may be estimated in exactly the same way as the σ_i^2, or, bearing in mind that households are reasonably similar in size (at least as compared with businesses), the σ_{ij}^2 may be modelled as sharing a common value, either within a block or over the entire population. If one of these modelling options is chosen, the relevant σ_{ij}^2 would share a common estimator, and that could be arrived at routinely by least squares.

When $m = 2$, Theorem 11.15.1 does not yield meaningful estimates of variance, and it is necessary to make an additional assumption of some kind regarding the relative sizes of the two sample population variances.

Estimation of Variance Using Jackknife, Bootstrap and Other Resampling Methods

11.16 It is quite common (at the time we write this report) to avoid the complications involved with estimating variances under multistage *πpswor* by resorting to non-parametric resampling methods such as the jackknife and the bootstrap. Such resampling methods involve estimating the desired statistic (in our case here, a variance of an estimated mean or total) using various portions of the sample, and comparing these part-sample estimates in order to arrive at an estimate of the variance of the whole-sample estimate.

Without going into detail at this point, we may say that non-parametric resampling methods can be very useful when the primary statistic being estimated (in our case a mean or total) is a complicated one and it is difficult to derive a simple analytical expression for its variance. In our case, the primary statistics are usually very simple: means and totals. Until recently, however, it had been difficult to estimate directly the variance of the HTE (and consequently also the variance of the GREG estimators that incorporate the HTE in their structure). This was because the only exact analytical expressions for the HT variance required reasonably accurate knowledge of the sample π_{ij} (the probabilities of inclusion of the ith and jth units together in the same sample).

Certain approximate expressions for this variance are now known to be of usable accuracy, including (9.9) with the c_i defined by (9.11), (9.12), (9.13) or (9.26), all of which return much the same values. Other things being equal, it is preferable to use direct estimates of one of these approximate variances, such estimates being based on the whole sample, rather than use non-parametric resampling methods. Reasons for this preference include the following:

1. The formulae used for direct estimation of variance contain information regarding the nature of the variance that is ignored if such resampling methods are used instead.
2. If there is already an estimator of variance that uses efficiently all the relevant information provided by the sample, it is logically impossible to obtain any more accurate estimate of variance using comparisons between part-sample estimates. (The very name 'bootstrap' sends an implicit warning to this effect.)
3. Non-parametric methods ignore certain kinds of information that might be available about the population being sampled. The information that the sample has been selected without replacement is one such piece of information,

though the jackknife (but not the bootstrap) can be modified by the inclusion of a finite-population correction factor. The fact that the population has been stratified is another such piece of information. To use resampling methods efficiently, it is necessary to use them within each stratum separately. But when the number of units selected within a stratum is small, resampling methods cannot provide accurate estimates of variance, and the repeated subsampling employed by the bootstrap in particular may give a false impression of accuracy.

4. Resampling methods in principle require much larger amounts of computer (CPU) time, memory and storage than are required for direct estimation. Although this objection may eventually be overcome by the use of short-cut formulae such as 5.4.6 in Valliant *et al.* (2000, p. 143) – which in its present form applies only to the delete-one jackknife – it is generally the case at present that the choice of a resampling method has required the use of this additional CPU time, memory and storage.

In view of these considerations, it does not seem necessary to go into any further detail, at least in this report, on the use of resampling methods.

Response from Supervisor

11.17 I have now managed to absorb reasonably well both the reports you have written for me on multistage sampling. They cover a lot of ground in a short space, and, apart from certain topics you refer to as being reasonably tractable but unreasonably tedious to include, I cannot think of any others in multistage sampling that I might need briefing on in the foreseeable future.

My big surprise was with what you had to say about resampling methods. Everyone else seems to use these as a matter of course, and your views on them must be at least as controversial as the stand you took on the relationship between randomization- or design-based and prediction- or model-based sampling inference. If I may read between the lines, you are not yet finished with that topic, and I am looking forward with some curiosity as to what you might have to say about it later on!

In the meantime, however, I am more immediately concerned about methods for dealing with non-response, a problem which seems to be growing more and more serious as time goes on. Is it also true, as I have heard rumoured, that methods for coping with it are simultaneously becoming more powerful? Once you have completed your present project, please make that your next priority.

Exercises

11.1 Derive formulae for an unbiased estimator of total, its design variance, and design-unbiased estimators for the variances of each stage, for a three-stage sample of m PSUs, mn CDs and $mn\bar{t}$ dwellings drawn using $\pi pswor$ at all stages except the last and *srswor* at the third or last stage.

11.2 A nationwide and self-weighting four-stage survey sample is being selected. The four stages are the selection of PSUs, of CDs, of blocks and of dwellings, in that order. At the first three stages it is being drawn with unequal probabilities without replacement. At the fourth stage, dwellings are being selected systematically with equal probabilities (and therefore without replacement) from geographically ordered block lists.

At the second stage of selection, a particular selected PSU consists of six CDs. The required sample fraction within this PSU is one in 15, and at the most recent Census there were 1406 dwellings in it, distributed over a serpentine listing of the CDs as follows: 260 dwellings in CD 1, 176 in CD 2, 222 in CD 3, 312 in CD 4, 128 in CD 5 and 308 in CD 6. Two sample CDs are to be selected from this PSU.

(a) Draw up a table showing the numbers of dwellings in each CD, the numbers of clusters that should be assigned to each of them, and the cumulated numbers of clusters going down the list.
(b) Take or derive the selection numbers from the first usable entries to be found in the table of random numbers below. Enter them in the table also, together with the corresponding within-block sample fractions.

38 67	53 70	59 66	86 10	48 63	37 18	49 31	57 38	42 28	02 10
04 49	23 42	40 88	11 54	44 25	20 17	03 04	29 65	94 70	10 33
23 17	51 55	94 49	06 57	94 60	92 52	38 61	48 64	74 49	78 71

12

Multiphase Sampling, Repeated Sampling and Non-response

Introduction 231
Report on Non-response and Related Topics 231
Response from Supervisor 244
Exercises 244

Introduction

12.1 Our supervisor's most recent request was for information on ways to deal with non-response. No sooner had we started to tackle the subject, however, than we found that to deal with it properly, we had to deal with two-phase sampling first. Two-phase sampling, also known as double sampling, is the simplest case of multiphase sampling. In multiphase sampling from a finite population of N units, an initial *first-phase sample* of n_1 units is selected, usually *srswor*, then a *second phase sample* of n_2 from the n_1 first phase units, again usually *srswor*, and so on until selection at the required number of phases has been completed.

Non-response and two-phase sampling are related in this fashion. The simplest way to deal with non-response is to treat the sample of respondents as if those respondents had constituted the whole of the target sample or, equivalently, as though the sample units' choices between response and non-response were all governed by a known random process. The target sample is then a first-phase sample and the set of respondents effectively a second-phase sample.

As soon as we realized this, we asked our supervisor for permission to expand the scope of our report to include multiphase sampling. Further, since a special theory involving multiphase techniques is also used when samples are repeatedly drawn from the same population, we asked permission to cover that theory as well. That permission was granted. We now present the report we prepared on this basis.

Report on Non-response and Related Topics

12.2 This report covers three related topics. The first and simplest is two-phase sampling. We mention also its generalization to multiphase sampling and deal briefly with the theory of repeated sampling. The relevance of these topics to procedures for ameliorating the effects of non-response is considered in some detail.

Two-Phase Sampling with a Single Supplementary Variable

12.3 Often, in addition to the survey variable of interest, y, there is a potential supplementary variable, x, information regarding which is not immediately available but may be obtained with comparatively little effort. Two-phase sampling is then a useful procedure to adopt. A relatively large *first-phase* sample is selected, using *srswor*, to collect data on the supplementary variable only, and a smaller *second-phase* sample is also selected, again using *srswor*, to collect data on the survey variable itself.

Variations on this theme are also possible, such as *srswr* or *πpswor* selection at different phases, stratification and/or multistage selection. In fact, there is almost always the need for one or more such complications in any real survey. The skill of the sampling statistician lies largely in picking out which building blocks are required in what order, and in being able to construct them into a harmonious edifice. Since it is obviously impossible to deal with all the possible combinations that might arise in practice, we limit ourselves here to the simplest possible situation: a population of N units within which the first-phase sample of n_1 units is selected *srswor*, and within which in turn a second-phase subsample of n_2 units is selected, also *srswor*.

This situation may be analysed in one of two ways. The first option treats two-phase sampling as a generalization of ratio estimation, one in which the supplementary variable is known only for a random sample of the population units. Classical ratio estimation is applied to estimate the total of the survey variable for the first-phase sample only, and the expansion estimator's raising factor, N/n_1, is then applied to convert that estimate into one for the entire population. The second option uses the supplementary variable, x, to impute values for those $n_1 - n_2$ units that appear in the first-phase sample but not in the second. It then uses these imputed values, as well as the n_2 known y-values, to form the whole-population estimate. These two options produce identical estimates.

12.4 For the time being, we will use only the first of these options. Classical ratio estimation, using the second-phase sample values of y and the first-phase sample values of x, is initially applied in an unmodified fashion to arrive at an estimate of the first-phase sample total, namely

$$\hat{Y}_{\bullet R2|1} = \frac{\sum_{i=1}^{N} \delta_{2i}\delta_{1i}Y_i}{\sum_{i=1}^{N} \delta_{2i}\delta_{1i}X_i} \sum_{i=1}^{N} \delta_{1i}X_i.$$

Since δ_{2i} can only take the value one if δ_{1i} also has the value one, $\delta_{2i}\delta_{1i} = \delta_{2i}$ and

$$\hat{Y}_{\bullet R2|1} = \frac{\sum_{i=1}^{N} \delta_{2i}Y_i}{\sum_{i=1}^{N} \delta_{2i}X_i} \sum_{i=1}^{N} \delta_{1i}X_i = \bar{R}_2 \sum_{i=1}^{N} \delta_{1i}X_i, \tag{12.1}$$

where $\bar{R}_2 = \sum_{i=1}^{N} \delta_{2i}Y_i / \sum_{i=1}^{N} \delta_{2i}X_i$.

We next multiply $\hat{Y}_{\bullet R2|1}$ by the ratio of the number of units in the population to the number in the first-phase sample to obtain the two-phase estimator $\hat{Y}_{\bullet R2P}$ of $Y_{\bullet}$:

$$\begin{aligned}
\hat{Y}_{\bullet R2P} &= \frac{N}{n_1}\bar{R}_2 \sum_{i=1}^{N} \delta_{1i} X_i \\
&= N \frac{\sum_{i=1}^{N} \delta_{2i} Y_i}{\sum_{i=1}^{N} \delta_{2i} X_i} \frac{\sum_{i=1}^{N} \delta_{1i} X_i}{\sum_{i=1}^{N} \delta_{1i}} \qquad (12.2) \\
&= N \frac{\hat{\bar{Y}}_2}{\hat{\bar{X}}_2} \hat{\bar{X}}_1, \qquad (12.3)
\end{aligned}$$

where $\hat{\bar{Y}}_2 = \sum_{i=1}^{N} \delta_{2i} Y_i / n_2$ is the second-phase estimator of the population mean, $\bar{Y} = Y_{\bullet}/N$; $\hat{\bar{X}}_2 = \sum_{i=1}^{N} \delta_{2i} X_i / n_2$ is the second-phase estimator of the population mean, $\bar{X} = X_{\bullet}/N$; and $\hat{\bar{X}}_1 = \sum_{i=1}^{N} \delta_{1i} X_i / n_1$ is the first-phase estimator of that same $\bar{X}$.

12.5 Using the same kind of Taylor expansion analysis as was introduced in **3.7**, and used in **3.8** to arrive at the expressions leading up to (3.7) for the variance of $\hat{Y}_{\bullet R}$, we can similarly arrive at

$$\frac{\mathrm{V}(\hat{\bar{Y}}_2/\hat{\bar{X}}_2)}{\bar{Y}^2/\bar{X}^2} \cong \frac{\mathrm{V}\hat{\bar{Y}}_2}{\bar{Y}^2} - \frac{2\mathrm{C}(\hat{\bar{Y}}_2, \hat{\bar{X}}_2)}{\bar{Y}\bar{X}} + \frac{\mathrm{V}\hat{\bar{X}}_2}{\bar{X}^2}. \qquad (12.4)$$

Writing, for convenience, $\bar{R}, \hat{\bar{R}}$ interchangeably with $\bar{X}, \hat{\bar{X}}$, and using the same logic as for (12.4), we can similarly arrive at

$$\begin{aligned}
&\frac{V(\hat{\bar{R}}_2 \hat{\bar{R}}_1)}{\bar{R}_2^2 \bar{R}_1^2} - \frac{\mathrm{V}\{(\hat{\bar{Y}}_2/\hat{\bar{X}}_2), \hat{\bar{X}}_1\}}{(\bar{Y}^2/\bar{X}^2)\bar{X}_1^2} \\
&\cong \frac{\mathrm{V}\hat{\bar{Y}}_2}{\bar{Y}^2} + \frac{\mathrm{V}\hat{\bar{X}}_2}{\bar{X}^2} + \frac{\mathrm{V}\hat{\bar{X}}_1}{\bar{X}^2} - 2\frac{\mathrm{C}(\hat{\bar{Y}}_2, \hat{\bar{X}}_2)}{\bar{Y}\bar{X}} + 2\frac{\mathrm{C}(\hat{\bar{Y}}_2, \hat{\bar{X}}_1)}{\bar{Y}\bar{X}} - 2\frac{\mathrm{C}(\hat{\bar{X}}_2, \hat{\bar{X}}_1)}{\bar{X}^2}
\end{aligned} \qquad (12.5)$$

The first four of these six terms may be written, by reference to (3.7), as

$$\begin{aligned}
&\frac{\mathrm{V}\hat{\bar{Y}}_2}{\bar{Y}^2} = N^{-1}(N - n_2)n_2^{-1} S_Y^2 \bar{Y}^{-2}, \quad \frac{\mathrm{V}\hat{\bar{X}}_2}{\bar{X}^2} = N^{-1}(N - n_2)n_2^{-1} S_X^2 \bar{X}^{-2}, \\
&\frac{\mathrm{V}\hat{\bar{X}}_1}{\bar{X}^2} = N^{-1}(N - n_1)n_1^{-1} S_X^2 \bar{X}^{-2} \quad \text{and} \quad -2\frac{\mathrm{C}(\hat{\bar{Y}}_2, \hat{\bar{X}}_2)}{\bar{Y}\bar{X}} \\
&= -2N^{-1}(N - n_2)n_2^{-1} S_{Y,X} \bar{Y}^{-1} \bar{X}^{-1}
\end{aligned} \qquad (12.6)$$

where $S_{Y,X} = (N-1)^{-1} \sum_i (Y_i - \bar{Y})(X_i - \bar{X})$.

The last two, however, being covariances between expressions based on samples of different sizes, require some further analysis. We start this with

$$\begin{aligned}\mathrm{C}(\hat{\bar{Y}}_2, \hat{\bar{X}}_1) &= n_2^{-1} n_1^{-1} \mathrm{C}\left(\sum_i \delta_{2i} Y_{2i}, \sum_i \delta_{1i} X_{1i}\right) \\ &= n_2^{-1} n_1^{-1} (N-1) S_{Y,X} \mathrm{C}(\delta_{2i}, \delta_{1i}) \qquad (12.7)\end{aligned}$$

where δ_{1i} and δ_{2i} are the inclusion indicators for the first and second phase samples respectively.

Now

$$\begin{aligned}\mathrm{C}(\delta_{2i}, \delta_{1i}) &\equiv \mathrm{E}(\delta_{2i}\delta_{1i}) - \mathrm{E}\delta_{1i}\mathrm{E}\delta_{2i} = n_2 N^{-1} - n_1 n_2 N^{-2} \\ &= n_2 N^{-1}\left(1 - n_1 N^{-1}\right). \qquad (12.8)\end{aligned}$$

Hence

$$\begin{aligned}\mathrm{C}(\hat{\bar{Y}}_2, \hat{\bar{X}}_1) &= n_2^{-1} n_1^{-1} (N-1) S_{Y,X} n_2 N^{-1}\left(1 - n_1 N^{-1}\right) \\ &= (N-1) S_{Y,X} n_1^{-1} N^{-1}\left(1 - n_1 N^{-1}\right) \\ &= \mathrm{C}(\hat{\bar{Y}}_1, \hat{\bar{X}}_1), \qquad (12.9)\end{aligned}$$

and, similarly,

$$-\mathrm{C}(\hat{\bar{X}}_2, \hat{\bar{X}}_1) = -\mathrm{V}\hat{\bar{X}}_1 \qquad (12.10)$$

It follows that the last two terms in (12.5) are

$$2\frac{\mathrm{C}(\hat{\bar{Y}}_2, \hat{\bar{X}}_1)}{\bar{Y}\bar{X}} = 2\frac{\mathrm{C}(\hat{\bar{Y}}_1, \hat{\bar{X}}_1)}{\bar{Y}\bar{X}} = -2N^{-1}(N - n_1) n_1^{-1} S_{Y,X} \bar{Y}^{-1} \bar{X}^{-1} \qquad (12.11)$$

and

$$-2\frac{\mathrm{C}(\hat{\bar{X}}_2, \hat{\bar{X}}_1)}{\bar{Y}\bar{X}} = -2\frac{\mathrm{V}\hat{\bar{X}}_1}{\bar{X}^2} = -2N^{-1}(N - n_1) n_1^{-1} S_X^2 \bar{X}^{-2}. \qquad (12.12)$$

The sum of the six terms in (12.5) may now be written as

$$\begin{aligned}\frac{\mathrm{V}(\hat{\bar{R}}_2 \hat{\bar{R}}_1)}{\bar{R}_2^2 \bar{R}_1^2} &= \frac{\mathrm{V}\hat{\bar{Y}}_2}{\bar{Y}^2} + \frac{\mathrm{V}\hat{\bar{X}}_2}{\bar{X}^2} + \frac{\mathrm{V}\hat{\bar{X}}_1}{\bar{X}^2} - 2\frac{\mathrm{C}(\hat{\bar{Y}}_2, \hat{\bar{X}}_2)}{\bar{Y}\bar{X}} + 2\frac{\mathrm{C}(\hat{\bar{Y}}_1, \hat{\bar{X}}_1)}{\bar{Y}\bar{X}} - 2\frac{\mathrm{V}\hat{\bar{X}}_1}{\bar{X}^2} \\ &= \frac{\mathrm{V}\hat{\bar{Y}}_2}{\bar{Y}^2} + \frac{\mathrm{V}\hat{\bar{X}}_2}{\bar{X}^2} - 2\frac{\mathrm{C}(\hat{\bar{Y}}_2, \hat{\bar{X}}_2)}{\bar{Y}\bar{X}} - \frac{\mathrm{V}\hat{\bar{Y}}_1}{\bar{Y}^2} - \frac{\mathrm{V}\hat{\bar{X}}_1}{\bar{X}^2} + 2\frac{\mathrm{C}(\hat{\bar{Y}}_1, \hat{\bar{X}}_1)}{\bar{Y}\bar{X}} + \frac{\mathrm{V}\hat{\bar{Y}}_1}{\bar{Y}^2} \\ &= \bar{Y}^{-2}\left\{\mathrm{V}\hat{\bar{Y}}_{R2} - \mathrm{V}\hat{\bar{Y}}_{R1} + \mathrm{V}\hat{\bar{Y}}_1\right\}. \qquad (12.13)\end{aligned}$$

Hence also

$$\begin{aligned}\mathrm{V}\hat{Y}_{\bullet R2P} &= \mathrm{V}\hat{Y}_{\bullet R2} - \mathrm{V}\hat{Y}_{\bullet R1} + \mathrm{V}\hat{Y}_{\bullet 1} \\ &= N(N - n_2) n_2^{-1} S_{(Y-RX)}^2 - N(N - n_1) n_1^{-1} S_{(Y-RX)}^2 + N(N - n_1) n_1^{-1} S_Y^2 \\ &= N^2\left\{\left(n_2^{-1} - n_1^{-1}\right) S_{(Y-RX)}^2 + \left(n_1 - N^{-1}\right) S_Y^2\right\} \qquad (12.14)\end{aligned}$$

This may be compared with $\mathrm{V}\hat{Y}_{\bullet 2}$, the reduction being due to the extra information supplied by the X_i values in the first stage sample. That reduction is

$$\mathrm{V}\hat{Y}_{\bullet 1} - \mathrm{V}\hat{Y}_{\bullet R2P} = N^2\left(n_2^{-1} - n_1^{-1}\right)\left(S_Y^2 - S_{(Y-RX)}^2\right), \qquad (12.15)$$

an expression which is both simple and intuitively appealing.

There is nothing unfamiliar regarding the estimation of the variance expression in (12.14), so that topic is omitted here and throughout the rest of this report.

Two-Phase Sampling with Two Supplementary Variables

12.6 The sampling strategy described in **12.2** is a sensible one to adopt if there is only a single supplementary variable and its value is not immediately available for all population units. A situation somewhat more frequently met, however, is the one where there are two supplementary variables, one whose value is known for all population units, and one for which it is known (or can be discovered at small cost) only for a sample of units (size n_1) that includes all those in the current survey sample (size n_2). Let the supplementary variable known for all population units be denoted by x, and the other supplementary variable by z. Then the question of interest is to what extent two-phase sampling could improve on the classical ratio estimator, $\left(\sum_i \delta_{2i} Y_i / \sum_i \delta_{2i} X_i\right) \sum_i X_i$, that relates the survey variable to x, but ignores z. The two-phase estimator in question may be written

$$\begin{aligned}\hat{Y}_{R\bullet 2} &= \left(\sum_i \delta_{2i} Y_i \Big/ \sum_i \delta_{2i} Z_i\right)\left(\sum_i \delta_{1i} Z_i \Big/ \sum_i \delta_{1i} X_i\right) X_{\bullet} \\ &= \hat{\bar{R}}_2 \hat{\bar{R}}_1 X_{\bullet}, \end{aligned} \qquad (12.16)$$

where $\hat{\bar{R}}_1 = \hat{\bar{Z}}_1 / \hat{\bar{X}}_1$ and $\hat{\bar{R}}_2 = \hat{\bar{Y}}_2 / \hat{\bar{Z}}_2$.

An expression for the variance of this estimator may be obtained using the same style of derivation as in **12.5**. It takes the form

$$\begin{aligned}\mathrm{V}\hat{Y}_{\bullet R2} &= \mathrm{V}\{(\hat{\bar{Y}}_2/\hat{\bar{Z}}_2)(\hat{\bar{Z}}_1/\hat{\bar{X}}_1)X_{\bullet}\} \\ &\cong N^2\left[(n_2^{-1} - n_1^{-1})S_{(Y-\bar{R}_2 Z)}^2 + (n_1^{-1} - N^{-1})S_{(Y-\bar{R}_2\bar{R}_1 X)}^2\right]\end{aligned} \qquad (12.17)$$

where $S_{(Y-\bar{R}_2\bar{R}_1X)}^2 = (N-1)^{-1}\sum_{i=1}^N (Y_i - \hat{\bar{R}}_2\hat{\bar{R}}_1 X_i)^2$ and $S_{(Y-\bar{R}_2 Z)}^2 = (N-1)^{-1} \times \sum_{i=1}^N (Y_i - \hat{\bar{R}}_2 Z_i)^2$.

The variance of the classical ratio estimator is approximately $N^2(n_2^{-1} - N^{-1})S_{(Y-\bar{R}_1\bar{R}_2X)}^2$, so the approximate reduction in variance brought about by two-phase sampling is $N^2\left(n_2^{-1} - n_1^{-1}\right)\left\{S_{(Y-\bar{R}_2\bar{R}_1X)}^2 - S_{(Y-\bar{R}_2Z)}^2\right\}$, an expression entirely analogous to that of (12.15).

The sample estimation of the variance in (12.17) is omitted, as foreshadowed at the end of the previous section.

Sampling on Repeated Occasions: Sample Rotation

12.7 An obvious example of the situation described in **12.6** is that where a census has been conducted, supplying complete information on the variable x, and a survey has since been conducted using sample size n_1 to supply information on the supplementary variable y_1, but where the sample size for the initial survey has randomly been reduced to the size n_2 before being used to obtain information on variable y_2.

This does not sound a very likely scenario, but a scenario quite close to it is very common indeed. This is one where the sample of n_1 units has been partially rotated. In this process, n_{21} of the old units have been retained, the remaining $n_1 - n_{21}$ have been rotated out, and n_{22} replacement units have been selected from the remaining $N - n_1$ (where n_{22} is close to but not necessarily the same as $n_1 - n_{21}$) to restore the sample to something like its original size.

Now we have a situation where we have two *srswor* samples on which the survey variable y_2 is to be measured. One of these consists of the n_{21} retained units, and for this sample the available supplementary variables are y_1 (on a larger sample of n_1 units) and x (on every unit in the population). This makes it possible to estimate the population total $Y_{\bullet}$ using the two-phase sampling strategy of **12.4**. The other consists of the n_{22} newly selected units, for which the only supplementary variable is x, and for that the appropriate estimator is usually the classical ratio estimator of Chapter 3.

The estimates of $Y_{\bullet}$ obtained from these two samples are not quite independent, because the samples themselves were not drawn independently. (They were drawn one after the other using *srswor* throughout.) The estimates are in fact slightly negatively correlated. If we denote them by $\hat{Y}_{2\bullet1}$ and $\hat{Y}_{2\bullet2}$ respectively, and their variances and covariance by $\mathrm{V}\hat{Y}_{2\bullet1}$, $\mathrm{V}\hat{Y}_{2\bullet2}$ and $\mathrm{C}(\hat{Y}_{2\bullet1}, \hat{Y}_{2\bullet2})$ respectively, the *composite estimator* supplied by the weighted average $\hat{Y}_{2\bullet w} = w_1\hat{Y}_{2\bullet1} + (1 - w_1)\hat{Y}_{2\bullet2}$ will have the variance

$$\mathrm{V}\hat{Y}_{2\bullet w} = w_1^2\mathrm{V}\hat{Y}_{2\bullet1} + (1 - w_1)^2\mathrm{V}\hat{Y}_{2\bullet2} + 2w_1(1 - w_1)\mathrm{C}(\hat{Y}_{2\bullet1}, \hat{Y}_{2\bullet2}). \tag{12.18}$$

This is a minimum with respect to w_1 when its differential coefficient with respect to w_1 is zero, that is, when

$$2w_1\mathrm{V}\hat{Y}_{2\bullet1} - 2(1 - w_1)\mathrm{V}\hat{Y}_{2\bullet2} + 2(1 - 2w_1)\mathrm{C}(\hat{Y}_{2\bullet1}, \hat{Y}_{2\bullet2}) = 0, \tag{12.19}$$

and the corresponding optimal value of w_1 is

$$w_{1opt} = \frac{\mathrm{V}\hat{Y}_{2\bullet2} - \mathrm{C}(\hat{Y}_{2\bullet1}, \hat{Y}_{2\bullet2})}{\{\mathrm{V}\hat{Y}_{2\bullet1} - \mathrm{C}(\hat{Y}_{2\bullet1}, \hat{Y}_{2\bullet2})\} + \{\mathrm{V}\hat{Y}_{2\bullet2} - \mathrm{C}(\hat{Y}_{2\bullet1}, \hat{Y}_{2\bullet2})\}}. \tag{12.20}$$

For most practical purposes, however, it is sufficient to use the simpler formula,

$$w_{1opt} \cong \frac{\mathrm{V}\hat{Y}_{2\bullet2}}{\mathrm{V}\hat{Y}_{2\bullet1} + \mathrm{V}\hat{Y}_{2\bullet2}}, \tag{12.21}$$

particularly since, as with most optimum choices in sampling, the loss function is nearly flat over a considerable range. The approximate expression in (12.21) corresponds to the usual rule of thumb, 'weight inversely to the variance', which holds exactly when the estimates are independent.

Note, in addition, that since it is usual to rotate the sample fairly slowly, seldom more than 20% between successive surveys, and further since two-phase estimation is more accurate than classical ratio estimation, $V\hat{Y}_{2\bullet 2}$ typically exceeds $V\hat{Y}_{2\bullet 1}$ by a considerable factor. In consequence, the value of w_{1opt} is likely to be substantially closer to unity than to zero, so that the optimal estimator is typically rather closer to $\hat{Y}_{2\bullet 1}$ than to $\hat{Y}_{2\bullet 2}$.

The relationship between the samples used for second and third survey rounds can usefully be chosen to be closely analogous to that which has just been described between the samples used for the first and second rounds. Some extra accuracy is theoretically obtainable by breaking the current sample down into even smaller subsets and using three or more supplementary variables, such as y_2, y_1 and x, to estimate the survey variable y_3 at the third sample survey round; however, the complications rapidly become more cumbersome to handle and the potential reductions in variance are progressively less worthwhile. The use of two-phase sampling at the mth survey round, with y_{m-1} and x as the supplementary variables, appropriates most of the improvements in accuracy possible from the use of successive sampling, and it is also reasonably easy to handle. An idea of what can be achieved by introducing a time series model of dependence between the y_m from one survey period to the next may be found in Patterson (1950).

12.8 We have already explicitly assumed that the rate of sample rotation from survey to survey will be substantial but less than 50%, but we have not yet justified that assumption, nor is it straightforward to do so. It would be nice if we could set up some obvious criterion of optimality and show how to achieve it, but in fact there are competing advantages achievable with faster and slower rotation rates, and the choice between them is necessarily subjective.

If the rate of rotation is zero, serious problems with respondent burden and sample fatigue are almost inevitable. Respondents retained in surveys for the entire period between successive census-based redesigns, which may be up to ten years, will eventually feel that they are being called on to shoulder more than their fair share in the work of producing statistical data (response burden), and even if they nominally remain as respondents, their responses will usually be produced with diminishing care and accuracy (sample fatigue). Conventional wisdom is that most businesses will perform reasonably cheerfully and accurately for about five successive surveys, and households a little longer. One pattern for household response used by the US Bureau of the Census is 'four months in, eight months out, four months in again and then out permanently'. Such practical considerations set a lower bound to the extent of sample rotation between surveys.

Given that some rotation is necessary, why should it be chosen to be relatively slow? One advantage of slow rotation is that new respondents typically need a period of 'breaking in' before they perform optimally. (This fact is something that should be borne in mind when conducting 'one-off' surveys. Attempting to collect a great deal of information from respondents in a one-off survey is asking for trouble, unless a certain amount of softening up can be done beforehand.) The other principal advantage of slow rotation is that a sample that remains relatively constant over time provides relatively good measures of change between one survey period and another.

Conversely, the principal advantage of fast rotation is that the effective sample size for measuring the average level of activity over a lengthy period can be several times the size of the sample used in any given survey round. Changes in level are measured relatively poorly, but the average level over a number of surveys is measured with considerably greater accuracy than would be the case if the rotation were slow. It is also particularly difficult, when redesigning a slowly rotating sample following a census, to keep the overlap between the old and the new sample as high as it has been over the period between censuses. There is likely to be an easily detectable change in the levels between the old and new sample designs in consequence. Such breaks in the series are awkward for analysts to handle and may be embarrassing if they have to be explained to the public.

Obviously the choice of the rotation speed calls for compromise, and the existence of theoretical optima (slow for measures of change, fast for measures of level) is seldom particularly relevant. The psychological and practical management considerations are likely to be paramount. The theory of successive sampling on several occasions is more relevant to the question of how best to operate with a given rate of rotation than it is to the choice of an optimal rate.

Coping with Non-response

12.9 One of the most important uses of multiphase sampling is in reducing the impact of non-response. Non-response is arguably the most serious practical problem encountered in survey sampling. Not only does it reduce the intended number of responses – that is handled easily enough by increasing the size of the target sample – but also, more seriously, it tends to distort the nature of the contact sample. This can happen both in subtle and in not so subtle ways. As a rule of thumb, one can say that a high non-response rate tends to cut out the extremes of potential respondents, such as the very rich, the very poor, those who are seldom home, those who have no home at all, and very small businesses. (Large businesses are usually well enough organized and prepared to respond, at least to compulsory surveys and prestigiously sponsored ones.)

Non-response has its least impact in those official government surveys where response is a legal requirement and can be backed up by the threat of a fine if it is refused. In such circumstances, even where the fine is purely nominal, refusal rates are usually quite low, although non-response caused by failure to contact can still be a serious problem. Where such compulsion cannot be exercised, refusal to respond can be quite serious, often of the order of 50% or worse. As a rule of thumb that might be used in such circumstances, a combined non-response rate (failure to contact plus refusal to co-operate) can often be defended as respectable if it can be limited to 35% or less, but a lower rate than that should always be aimed for. A useful reference on methods for reducing non-response in non-compulsory business surveys is Paxson *et al.* (1995).

Even where the principal source of non-response is failure to contact, the differential rates of response between those whom it is easy to contact and those who are hard to trace can serve to distort the sample estimates quite appreciably. Consequently, the simplest way of dealing with non-response – treating the respondents as though they constitute a random sample of that fixed size – can be quite seriously biased. This is especially the case where there is no supplementary variable available and the only feasible estimator is the expansion estimator of Chapter 1. If a suitable supplementary variable is available for the whole population, the ratio estimator of Chapter 3 can be used, but the randomization-based theory presented in that chapter is not really valid because the selection is not random, therefore not *srswor*. In fact the sample is not a probability sample of any kind, as there are no knowable probabilities of inclusion in sample. The prediction-based theory of Chapter 5 is, however, valid to the extent that the corresponding prediction model, along the lines of the ξ_R of **5.2**, is valid. The decision as to whether that is the case or not has to be taken on the basis of subject-matter knowledge regarding the population.

The next simplest way to cope with non-response at the estimation stage is to use some item known for the entire target sample, but not for the non-sampled units, as an additional supplementary variable for two-phase sampling. Such an additional supplementary variable might well be the 'current survey variable' from the previous survey round. (This is what was used in **12.7**.) But whether a previous survey round is the source of the additional supplementary variable or not, the fact that we have such a variable takes us back to the situation described in **12.6**. Formally, the two cases are almost identical. There is one supplementary variable, x, whose values are known for all population units, and another one, z, which is known for all units in the target sample. Moreover, (by definition) that sample includes all the responding units. The only difference is that the respondent sample is not a probability sample.

12.10 Once again, however, to the extent that the relevant prediction models represent useful assumptions, prediction-based inference can still be useful. In this case the appropriate model is

$$\begin{aligned}\xi_2:\quad & Z_i = \beta_{zx}X_i + U_{zxi};\quad \mathrm{E}_{\xi_2}U_{zxi} = 0;\quad \mathrm{E}_{\xi_2}U_{zxi}^2 = \sigma_{zxi}^2;\quad \mathrm{E}_{\xi_2}(U_{zxi}U_{zxj}) = 0;\\ & Y_i = \beta_{yz}Z_i + U_{yzi};\quad \mathrm{E}_{\xi_2}U_{yzi} = 0;\quad \mathrm{E}_{\xi_2}U_{yzi}^2 = \sigma_{yzi}^2;\quad \mathrm{E}_{\xi_2}(U_{yzi}U_{yzj}) = 0;\\ & \mathrm{E}_{\xi_2}(U_{zxi}U_{yzi}) = \rho\sigma_{zxi}\sigma_{yzi};\quad j \neq i \text{ throughout};\quad i,j = 1,2,\ldots,N.\end{aligned} \tag{12.22}$$

If we choose our estimators of β_{yz}, β_{zx} and β_{yx} to be

$$\hat{\beta}_{yz} = \frac{\sum_{i=1}^{N}\delta_{2i}Y_i}{\sum_{i=1}^{N}\delta_{2i}Z_i}, \tag{12.23}$$

$$\hat{\beta}_{zx} = \frac{\sum_{i=1}^{N} \delta_{1i} Z_i}{\sum_{i=1}^{N} \delta_{1i} X_i}, \tag{12.24}$$

$$\hat{\beta}_{yx} = \hat{\beta}_{yz}\hat{\beta}_{zx} = \frac{\sum_{i=1}^{N} \delta_{2i} Y_i \sum_{i=1}^{N} \delta_{1i} Z_i}{\sum_{i=1}^{N} \delta_{2i} Z_i \sum_{i=1}^{N} \delta_{1i} X_i}, \tag{12.25}$$

a plausible prediction estimator for $Y_{\bullet}$ is

$$\hat{Y}_{\bullet} = \sum_{i=1}^{N} \delta_{2i} Y_i + \hat{\beta}_{yz} \sum_{i=1}^{N} (\delta_{1i} - \delta_{2i}) Z_i + \hat{\beta}_{yx} \sum_{i=1}^{N} (1 - \delta_{1i}) X_i. \tag{12.26}$$

The first term is the respondents' sample take, and appears without modification in (12.26) because the respondents' values of Y_i are known – and notionally known exactly, although of course respondents do make 'response errors'! Only the balance of the population needs to be 'prediction-estimated'.

In the second and third terms these prediction estimates appear as imputed values for the individual units; in the second term for the non-responding sample units and in the third term for the non-sampled units. (We are now using the second option for two-phase estimation described at the close of **12.3**.) The expression for non-responding sample units in the second term takes the form it does because the imputed values for Y_i are $\hat{\beta}_{yz} Z_i$ and because the non-response set consists, by definition, of those units for which $\delta_{1i} - \delta_{2i} = 1 - 0 = 1$. The expression for the non-sample units in the third term, for which (somewhat similarly) $1 - \delta_{1i} = 1 - 0 = 1$, nevertheless takes a slightly different form, because the imputed values for Y_i are then $\hat{\beta}_{yz}\hat{\beta}_{zx} X_i$.

The estimators of β_{yz} and $\beta_{yz}\beta_{zx}$ used for the prediction-based analysis are the same as those used for $\bar{R}_2$ and $\bar{R}_2\bar{R}_1$ in the randomization-based analysis, namely $\sum_i \delta_{2i} Y_i / \sum_i \delta_{2i} Z_i$ and $\left(\sum_i \delta_{2i} Y_i / \sum_i \delta_{2i} Z_i\right)\left(\sum_i \delta_{1i} Z_i / \sum_i \delta_{1i} X_i\right)$, respectively.

It is not immediately obvious that the prediction-based $\hat{Y}_{\bullet}$ of (12.26) is identical to the randomization-based $\hat{Y}_{R\bullet}$ of (12.16), but in fact it is. This may be seen as follows:

$$\hat{Y}_{\bullet} = \sum_{i=1}^{N} \delta_{2i} Y_i + \hat{\beta}_{yz} \sum_{i=1}^{N} (\delta_{1i} - \delta_{2i}) Z_i + \hat{\beta}_{yz}\hat{\beta}_{zx} \sum_{i=1}^{N} (1 - \delta_{1i}) X_i \tag{12.26}$$

$$= \sum_{i=1}^{N} \delta_{2i} Y_i + \hat{\beta}_{yz} \sum_{i=1}^{N} \delta_{1i} Z_i - \hat{\beta}_{yz} \sum_{i=1}^{N} \delta_{2i} Z_i + \hat{\beta}_{yz}\hat{\beta}_{zx} \sum_{i=1}^{N} X_i - \hat{\beta}_{yz}\hat{\beta}_{zx} \sum_{i=1}^{N} \delta_{1i} X_i$$

$$= \sum_{i=1}^{N} \delta_{2i} Y_i + \left(\sum_i \delta_{2i} Y_i \Big/ \sum_i \delta_{2i} Z_i\right) \sum_{i=1}^{N} \delta_{1i} Z_i - \left(\sum_i \delta_{2i} Y_i \Big/ \sum_i \delta_{2i} Z_i\right)$$

$$\times \sum_{i=1}^{N} \delta_{2i} Z_i + \left(\sum_i \delta_{2i} Y_i \Big/ \sum_i \delta_{2i} Z_i\right)\left(\sum_i \delta_{1i} Z_i \Big/ \sum_i \delta_{1i} X_i\right) X_{\bullet}$$

$$- \left(\sum_i \delta_{2i} Y_i \Big/ \sum_i \delta_{2i} Z_i\right)\left(\sum_i \delta_{1i} Z_i \Big/ \sum_i \delta_{1i} X_i\right) \sum_{i=1}^{N} \delta_{1i} X_i$$

$$= \sum_{i=1}^{N} \delta_{2i} Y_i + \left(\sum_i \delta_{2i} Y_i \Big/ \sum_i \delta_{2i} Z_i\right) \sum_{i=1}^{N} \delta_{1i} Z_i - \sum_i \delta_{2i} Y_i$$

$$+ \left(\sum_i \delta_{2i} Y_i \Big/ \sum_i \delta_{2i} Z_i\right)\left(\sum_i \delta_{1i} Z_i \Big/ \sum_i \delta_{1i} X_i\right) X_{\bullet}$$

$$- \left(\sum_i \delta_{2i} Y_i \Big/ \sum_i \delta_{2i} Z_i\right) \sum_i \delta_{1i} Z_i$$

$$= \left(\sum_i \delta_{2i} Y_i \Big/ \sum_i \delta_{2i} Z_i\right)\left(\sum_i \delta_{1i} Z_i \Big/ \sum_i \delta_{1i} X_i\right) X_{\bullet}$$

$$= \hat{R}_2 \hat{R}_1 X_{\bullet}. \qquad (12.16)$$

The identity of these two differently supported estimators means that (12.16) is the randomization-based and (12.26) is the prediction-based form of the same cosmetically calibrated estimator. Despite their identity, however, their randomization variance (12.17) and their prediction-based variance, being differently defined, assume different forms.

Paradoxically, however, their prediction-based variance can be a little more directly estimated from (12.16) than from (12.26):

Theorem 12.10.1 For large samples, the prediction variance of the two-phase estimator denoted by $\hat{Y}_{R\bullet}$ in (12.16) and by $\hat{Y}_{\bullet}$ in (12.26) is approximately given by

$$\mathrm{V}_{\xi_2} \hat{Y}_{\bullet} = \mathrm{E}_{\xi_2} (\hat{Y}_{\bullet} - Y_{\bullet})^2 \cong w(w-1) \sum_{i=1}^{N} \delta_i \sigma_i^2, \qquad (12.27)$$

where $w = \left(\sum_i \delta_{1i} Z_i / \sum_i \delta_{2i} Z_i\right)\left(X_{\bullet} / \sum_i \delta_{1i} X_i\right)$.

Proof. From **8.12** we have that if $\hat{Y}_{\bullet P}$ is any prediction-unbiased estimator of the form $\hat{Y}_{\bullet PRED} = \sum_{i=1}^{N} \delta_i w_i Y_i$, the prediction variance of $\hat{Y}_{\bullet PRED}$ – defined there, to avoid ambiguity, as the variance of $\hat{Y}_{\bullet PRED} - Y_{\bullet}$ – is given by

$$\mathrm{V}_{\xi}(\hat{Y}_{\bullet PRED} - Y_{\bullet}) = \sum_{i=1}^{N} \delta_i w_i (w_i - 1) \sigma_i^2 + \sum_{i=1}^{N} \sigma_i^2 - \sum_{i=1}^{N} \delta_i w_i \sigma_i^2, \qquad (8.28)$$

or equivalently by

$$\mathrm{V}_{\xi}(\hat{Y}_{\bullet PRED} - Y_{\bullet}) = \sum_{i=1}^{N} \delta_i w_i (w_i - 1)\sigma_i^2 + \left(\sum_{i=1}^{N} \sigma_i^2 - \sum_{i=1}^{N} \delta_i \pi_i^{-1} \sigma_i^2\right) - \left(\sum_{i=1}^{N} \delta_i w_i \sigma_i^2 - \sum_{i=1}^{N} \delta_i \pi_i^{-1} \sigma_i^2\right). \quad (8.29)$$

For the reasons given in that section, both the bracketed terms in (8.29) can be ignored for large samples, leaving only the single term $\sum_{i=1}^{N} \delta_i w_i (w_i - 1)\sigma_i^2$.

In (12.16), the weight applied to each of the Y_i is identical at $w = \left(1/\sum_k \delta_{2k} Z_k\right)\left(\sum_k \delta_{1k} Z_k / \sum_k \delta_{1k} X_k\right) X_{\bullet}$, so the prediction variance of $\hat{Y}_{\bullet}$ is

$$\mathrm{V}_{\xi_2}(\hat{Y}_{\bullet}) = \mathrm{E}_{\xi_2}(\hat{Y}_{\bullet} - Y_{\bullet})^2 \cong w(w-1) \sum_{i=1}^{N} \delta_i \sigma_i^2. \qquad \diamond$$

Corollary 12.10.1 The approximate expression given in (12.27) for the prediction variance of the $\hat{Y}_{\bullet}$ of (12.26) may be estimated without bias by

$$\hat{\mathrm{V}}_{\xi_2} \hat{Y}_{\bullet} = w(w-1) \sum_{i=1}^{N} \delta_i \tilde{\sigma}_i^2,$$

where the $\tilde{\sigma}_i^2$ are the unbiased estimators of the σ_i^2 obtained in the same way as the $\tilde{\sigma}_{hi}^2$ were in Theorem 5.3.1.

12.11 It is time to take stock of the relevance of the results in **12.10** to straightforward two-phase ratio estimation with *srswor* on the one hand, and to the non-response situation on the other hand.

For straightforward two-phase sampling with *srswor*, a randomization-based estimator will always be valid by definition (though not necessarily useful, for instance when the sample and/or population are very small). If the sample and/or population are too small for the randomization-based inference to be helpful, a good model can come to the rescue. A prediction-based estimator based on model ξ_2 is useful only to the extent that ξ_2 is itself a useful approximation, but if is, the prediction-based estimator will often be preferable. Conversely, if the model is unrealistic, a large enough sample and population can obviate the need for a better model.

The estimator defined by either (12.16) or (12.26), or both together, is cosmetically calibrated and combines the merits of both the randomization-based and prediction-based estimators. The case is, however, still desperate if both support bases are deficient – that is, if sample and/or population are small *and* ξ_2 is not a useful model. Wearing both belt and braces (suspenders) will not stop your pants from falling down if both are broken!

Isaki and Fuller (1982) showed that if an estimator was doubly unbiased – that is to say, both over all possible samples and under a prediction model – the randomization expectation of the model variance and the model expectation of the randomization variance would be equal. Any substantial difference between the estimates of these two quantities is therefore a signal that something is awry with at least one of these analyses. Random samples with any given degree of imbalance will occur in a potentially calculable proportion of selections, and poor balance is quite a likely explanation if the sample (or the part of the sample within the relevant domain) is small. For large samples, the more likely explanation would be model breakdown, so in that case it would be appropriate to inspect the data for unexpected features.

In any case, the prediction-based variance is the more appropriate one to measure the precision of estimates based on the particular sample selected. The randomization variance is more relevant to the design of the next sample, than to the reliability of the current one.

12.12 In cases where the second-phase sample is a self-selected set of respondents, the randomization-based variance is considerably less likely to provide a reliable guide to the accuracy of the sample estimate than it is in the case of two-phase *srswor*. The accuracy of prediction-based variance, however, is not affected by the manner in which the sample is selected, so relatively more attention might legitimately be paid to it, provided the model is believed valid for the whole population.

A problem of particular importance can arise when ratio estimation is used to allow for non-response in a completely enumerated or 'take-all' stratum. Sometimes there is an unwritten rule in the survey organization that the ratio adjustment will not be applied unless and until one or two very large and well-known businesses have responded. If that is what is done in practice, that is the way in which the analysis should be conducted. There should be a separation into two strata, the genuinely completely enumerated stratum of large or unusual units where non-response simply cannot be tolerated, and another stratum consisting of the smaller and less unusual (but still nominally 'take-all') units which are always in the target sample but whose response is not regarded as essential. Unless this distinction is made, the randomization variance (which treats units in these two quite different classes as equally likely to be found in the response set) can and usually will greatly overestimate the actual sample error in the undivided 'take-all' stratum.

12.13 The simple two-phase sampling procedures described in this report are not the only ways in which non-response can be allowed for. For instance, it is possible to select a random (or even a balanced) sample of non-respondents for more intensive follow-up, and to treat any later responses so obtained as being typical of all those who initially failed to respond. This involves a poststratification of the target sample into initial respondents and initial non-respondents.

Another alternative is to keep track of the times at which the responses come in, and to attempt to model the way in which these responses change with 'time required to respond'. The assumption then used is that the extent of this delay in responding can provide clues as to the potential responses of those who delay so long that they never respond at all (or at least miss the cut-off for inclusion in the estimation process). This assumption is rather dangerous though, since the hard core of those who steadfastly refuse to respond under all circumstances can be quite different from those who eventually succumb to repeated requests.

Yet another device used by some organizations is *network sampling*, in which information regarding the target sample is sought from relatives and neighbours. This has been used successfully by Nathan (1976) and Johnson (1995), but it requires very careful organization and analysis.

Research into ways of dealing with non-response will almost certainly continue for a long time, but the two-phase sampling that we have described is a simple and effective tool. We recommend that this be used unless there is a clearly demonstrable need for something more elaborate.

Response from Supervisor

12.14 This latest report of yours contains much useful information, but as usual opens up as many new questions as it answers.

One topic I clearly need to know about is the methods that can be used to select these repeated samples that you refer to. How do you prevent them getting in each other's way and selecting some respondents too many times?

Another is the way to go about 'inspecting the data for unusual features'. This, I imagine, would cover how to detect and cope with unusually large or otherwise atypical observations.

But that topic can wait for the moment. Please tell me first how to go about selecting lots of different samples, both one-off and repeated, from the same sample frame.

Exercises

12.1 Use the Taylor expansion to verify equations (12.6) and (12.7).

12.2 Use the type of analysis set out in **12.5** to derive equation (12.17) for the variance of the estimator $\hat{Y}_{\bullet R2}$, as defined in equation (12.16) of **12.6**.

12.3 For the third survey round using a sample with 20% rotation between rounds, there are five samples with different survey histories: (i) one with size n_1 that was surveyed only in round 1; (ii) one with size n_{12} that was surveyed only in rounds 1 and 2; (iii) one with size n_{123} that was surveyed in all three rounds; (iv) one with size n_{23} that was surveyed only in rounds 2 and 3; and (v) one with size n_3 that was surveyed only in round 3.

(a) Draw a diagram illustrating the rotation of the sample through the three survey rounds, and the relative sizes of the five samples.

(b) Write down two formulae for the estimation of the total $Y_{3\bullet}$ of the survey variable y_3, the first using y_2, y_1 and x as supplementary variables, and the other using y_2 and x only.

(c) Without deriving a variance formula for either of these estimators, indicate in which of these samples, and why, the variance of the first estimator will be smaller than the variance of the second.

13

Tracking and Rotating Samples

Introduction 246
Permanent Random Number Sampling 247
Bernoulli Sampling 247
Poisson Sampling 248
Rotation and Control of a Poisson Sample 248
The Problem with Having a Random Sample Size 251
Estimation and Variance Estimation for a Poisson Sample 252
Two Ways of Viewing the Horvitz–Thompson Ratio Estimator 254
Alternatives to Poisson Sampling 256
Response from Supervisor 266
Exercises 266

Introduction

13.1 When a single survey is repeated a number of times and the sample is rotated between survey rounds, the requirement of fairness in spreading the response burden is potentially in conflict with keeping the selection process simple. The best compromise involves keeping track of which population units have been in sample on what occasions, in order to ensure, for instance, that no unit is dropped from sample in one round only to be reselected again in the next.

The need for such information is heightened when more than just one survey is being rotated through the same population. Usually it is the aim of the survey organization to minimize the overlap between any given survey's sample and every other survey's sample, but occasionally it is preferable for one survey's sample to be identical with another survey's sample.

The situation is further complicated by the need to allow for 'births' of new units, 'deaths' of those that exit the population for whatever reason, and important events such as a 'change of description' for a retail establishment – where, for example, a chemist's shop might be sold to a new owner and reopened as a butcher's at the same address. The movement from one size stratum to another is another such event, and quite a common one.

Yet another feature that needs to be taken into account is that while many population units have no legal or operational link with any other, many others do have such links. A retail establishment might be part of a chain (local, national or multinational), a business in one industry might be a subsidiary of a business in the same or another industry, and so on. It is generally considered convenient to define groups of related *establishments* as *enterprises*, and sometimes intermediate levels of structural integration also need to be recognized. This grouping can affect a survey's sample design quite appreciably. For instance, surveys of financial activities are more easily conducted using samples of enterprises, but surveys of employment, personnel, leave etc. typically require samples of establishments.

Permanent Random Number Sampling

13.2 One way of facilitating sample rotation and control is to allocate a unique *permanent random number* (PRN), in the range between zero and one, to every population unit. If the sample is to be selected with equal probabilities without replacement within any given stratum, the decision whether a given unit is to be in sample or not can be made solely on the value of its PRN. If the sample is defined as consisting of all those units having PRNs in the interval $[0.4, 0.6)$, the probability of inclusion in sample for every population unit will be 0.2.

Remark 13.2.1 'The interval $[0.4, 0.6)$' is another way of describing the range of PRN values for which $0.4 \leq \text{PRN} < 0.6$. Intervals such as $(0.4, 0.6)$ are called *open* intervals. Those such as $[0.4, 0.6]$ are called *closed* intervals. PRNs are defined over the half-open interval $[0, 1)$ for convenience only. If, for instance, they are in fact 12-digit numbers generated by computers, their range is from 000 000 000 000 to 999 999 999 999. The smallest number in that range is interpreted as exactly zero, and the greatest as 0.999 999 999 999, completely filling the range $[0, 1)$ to 12 decimal places. ◇

Note, however, that although the selection is with equal probabilities and without replacement, it is not *srswor*. With *srswor*, the number of units to be selected is fixed in advance. Using the procedure described above, each unit in the population has a probability of inclusion in sample that is very nearly independent of that of every other population unit. (It is not quite independent, because there is not an infinity of numbers that the computer can recognize between, say, 000 000 000 000 and 999 999 999 999. However, the number of potential PRNs it is able to recognize should always be large compared with the size of any finite population for which it is likely to be generating them.)

Bernoulli Sampling

13.3 Imagine for a moment that each population unit has the same inclusion probability as every other, and that these inclusion probabilities are strictly independent of each other. The most straightforward way of selecting a sample of this nature is to conduct a random trial for each population unit in turn. If a unit's PRN is smaller than its inclusion probability, it is included in sample; otherwise it is not. Trials of this kind are known as *Bernoulli trials*, and the entire sampling procedure is known as *Bernoulli sampling*. It is obviously incompatible with the setting of a fixed sample size in advance.

Poisson Sampling

13.4 Bernoulli sampling is a special case of the more general sampling scheme in which, once again, each unit in the population has a probability of inclusion in sample that is independent of that of every other population unit, but for which the inclusion probabilities need not be equal. This more general sampling scheme is called *Poisson sampling*. It is, in its turn, a special case of sampling with unequal probabilities without replacement, or $\pi pswor$ (Chapter 4).

The optimal inclusion probabilities are, as indicated in Chapter 8, proportional to the square root of the variance function, which can usually be modelled as a power function of a measure of overall size, say $Z_i^{2\gamma}$, where Z_i is the overall size measure and γ is the coefficient of heteroscedasticity defined in **5.2**. In that case the optimal inclusion probabilities, π_{iO}, satisfy $\pi_{iO} \propto Z_i^{\gamma}$, where typically $0.5 \leq \gamma \leq 1$.

Poisson sampling was first described by Hájek (1964). Because the samples selected using Poisson sampling did not have a sample size that could be fixed in advance, Hájek did not envisage any practical application for this procedure. He used it only as a tool for investigating the properties of other estimators.

The first practical application of Poisson sampling came in forestry (Grosenbaugh, 1964, 1965). Poisson sampling was used in this context because it was not practicable to select a probability sample of trees in any other way, without first undertaking the awkward and expensive tasks of identifying each tree individually and making a list of them. The first practical use of Poisson sampling outside forestry was in the United States Bureau of the Census's Annual Survey of Manufacturers (Ogus and Clark, 1971). The idea was quickly picked up in Sweden (see Atmer *et al.*, 1975; and Thulin, 1976). It was also developed conceptually in Australia by Brewer *et al.* (1972). (Despite the later publication dates, the Swedish application predated the Australian.)

Kröger *et al.* (1999) introduced a version of Poisson sampling called *Pomix sampling* in which the inclusion probabilities have a minimum value $\pi_i = B$ at $Z_i = 0$, and increase linearly with z_i to take some maximum value less than or equal to unity for the largest unit in the sampled portion of the population. (The units for which Z_i exceeds that maximum value are placed in a take-all stratum.) This represents a simple approximation to Poisson sampling with optimal inclusion probabilities, and has the further advantage that no unit has an inclusion probability smaller than B. Unequal probability samples in which the smallest units have only tiny inclusion probabilities are notoriously unstable and should always be avoided.

Rotation and Control of a Poisson Sample

13.5 Brewer *et al.* (1972) produced a chart very similar to Figure 13.1 showing how Poisson sampling could be used for a population that is stratified by size into three sampled strata and a completely enumerated sector. The units of the

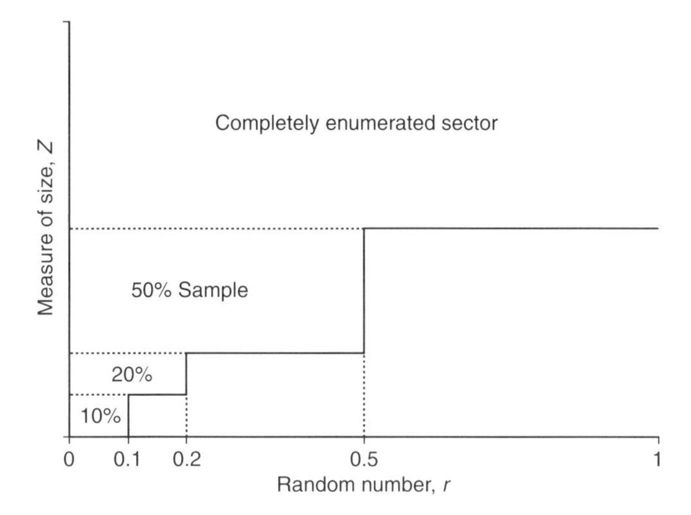

Figure 13.1 Stratified random Poisson sample.

population correspond to points on the chart specified by the PRN (r on the horizontal axis) and its measure of size (z on the vertical axis). The sample initially selected consists of all points to the left of the stepped unbroken line.

Rotation of the sample can be effected by shifting the sampled area to the right. If the rightward shift in r is 0.02, all units for which $r < 0.02$ are rotated out of sample, and are replaced by units for which $0.10 \leq r < 0.12$ for the lowest sampled stratum, $0.20 \leq r < 0.22$ for the middle sampled stratum and $0.50 \leq r < 0.52$ for the highest sampled stratum. This implies rotation rates of 20% for the lowest stratum, 10% for the middle one and 4% for the highest. The consequence is that the larger the business, the longer it remains in sample. For the completely enumerated or 'take-all' sector, the chart must be imagined to be cylindrical, so that the units with $r < 0.02$, which are notionally 'rotated out', are in fact rotated back in again immediately with values of r notionally in the range $1.00 \leq r < 1.02$, but actually in the range $0.00 \leq r < 0.02$.

Figure 13.1 illustrates only the special case of Bernoulli sampling within each of the sampled strata individually. The next chart produced by Brewer *et al.* (Figure 13.2) does, however, relate to Poisson sampling more generally, with all the points in the triangular region AOB constituting the initial sample. In its original form, the vertical axis still indicated the measure of size, Z_i, for the ith unit, but since Brewer *et al.* were assuming the inclusion probabilities to be proportional to that measure of size, the vertical axis was effectively indicating inclusion probability also, and it is that inclusion probability, π_i, that is shown in our version of their diagram.

Figure 13.2 also indicates two ways in which a PRN sample can be rotated. The original sample consists of all units contained in the triangular region AOB. One method of rotation, similar to that used in Figure 13.1, shifts the sample region bodily to the right as far as A′O′B′. As in Figure 13.1, however, the percentage

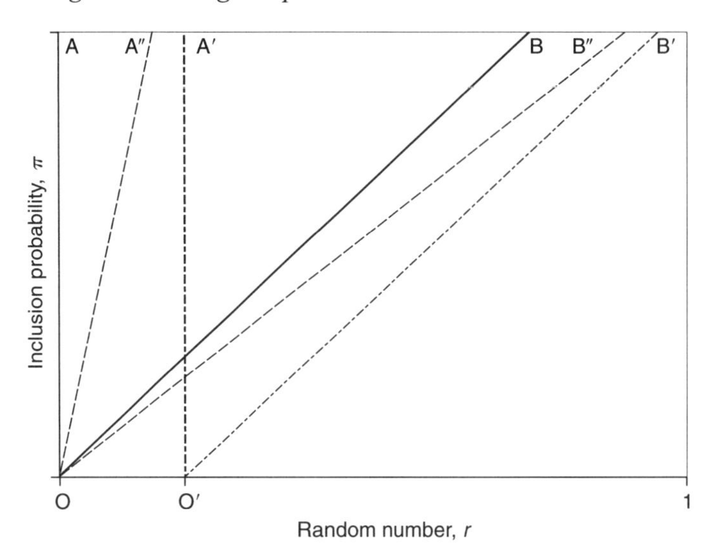

Figure 13.2 Two ways of rotating a πps Poisson sample.

rotation rate is not uniform over all sizes. It is faster for points in the vicinity of O (which represent small units) than for those higher up (that represent units with larger measures of size). There is no completely enumerated sector in this diagram but, if there were, it would consist of a single horizontal line (as opposed to a region with depth, as in Figure 13.1), and along that line the inclusion probabilities would all be unity.

An alternative method of rotation is represented by the sample region being moved from AOB to A″OB″. The percentage rotation rate is now constant over the entire sample. There are two reasons, however, why this alternative is less convenient than moving the sample region to A′O′B′. The first is that small units are less heavily sampled than larger ones, for good reasons, and it is not appropriate to allow just a few of them to be saddled with the response burden over a long time period while others escape it entirely. The second reason has to do with keeping track of the sample when decisions are being made as to who is to be in sample and who is not. It is obvious to the eye that A″OB″ is a thinner triangular region than A′O′B′. If the rotation were continued for six or eight survey rounds, the sample region would not be a compact triangle any longer, but a thin strip, narrow at the bottom and wide at the top, wrapped several times around the 'cylinder'. Not only would such a region be awkward to keep track of, but small changes in the size of the unit, moving it small distances vertically up and down the 'cylinder', would cause it to move in and out of the sample region unnecessarily rapidly. The uniform rightward shift is preferable on both counts.

Similar considerations arise when there is more than one sample to be selected from the same population. Minimum overlap between samples is usually regarded as advantageous, as it spreads the response burdens equably, but occasions arise where a survey sample should be obtained by subsampling from another. The virtue of diagrams such as Figures 13.1 and 13.2 is that they enable the relations between the various samples to be seen at a glance. It becomes obvious, for instance, that if two survey samples are to have minimum overlap, this will be easier to organize if both rotate by the same horizontal amount at any given time.

For Pomix sampling, Kröger *et al.* (1999) prefer to use a modified version of Figures 13.1 and 13.2 in which the vertical axis is not π but Z. The triangular regions AOB and A′O′B′ then translate into trapezia, each sample region extending over a rectangular area of width B, together with a downward-pointing triangular area immediately to the right of it.

The Problem with Having a Random Sample Size

13.6 Bernoulli sampling is subject to the problem that the sample size cannot be fixed beforehand, as is Poisson sampling more generally. In the extreme case, no population unit at all might be selected in sample. (Such a sample may be referred to as *null* or *empty*.) Empty samples can be selected with non-negligible probability if the target sample size is small, and this can happen if the extent of stratification is particularly demanding (say, by type of business, size, and small geographical area). If and when the sample selected is empty, the Horvitz–Thompson estimate of the population total is zero, and nothing can be done to remedy the situation other than to make a guess at that total or to select another sample. If another sample is selected, the probabilities of inclusion in sample differ from the values originally chosen. This fact can be accommodated using certain variants on Poisson sampling (see **13.11**ff.), but the elegant simplicity of Poisson sampling itself and the ease with which it can be rotated and controlled are to various extents compromised.

A second aspect of the same problem is that random variations in sample size can interfere with forward planning. If the optimal sample size is 100 units, and the sample selected is 120, extra work and expense are involved in collection, and in a manner that cannot be forecast beforehand. Although sample design optima are almost always very flat (so that little if any additional effort is actually wasted) survey managers are usually expected to plan beforehand exactly what levels of work and expenditure will be required, and shortfalls in them are almost as unwelcome as the opposite. Nothing can be done about this, short of reversion to a selection method that can guarantee a given sample size.

The problem's third aspect is that the HTE in particular has a much greater design variance for Poisson sampling than it does for any selection method that guarantees a fixed sample size. This is because the HTE of total is the sum of n terms, one from each sample unit, and usually these terms are all much the same in size. The contribution to variance coming from variation in the number of sample units then exceeds, and typically exceeds by an order of magnitude, the contribution coming from the variability between the terms in the HT sum.

This third drawback can be overcome fairly satisfactorily, as will be seen in the next section, but to deal with the first two, a more radical solution will be needed (see **13.11**ff.).

Estimation and Variance Estimation for a Poisson Sample

13.7 Poisson sampling assigns the ith unit in the population ($i = 1, 2, \ldots, N$) an individual inclusion probability π_i. To select a Poisson sample, a sequence of N trials is carried out to determine whether each unit in turn is to be selected in the sample or not. Using PRN sampling, the same goal is achieved by random allocation to an area in a diagram, and that allocation will determine whether and when the unit is included in sample.

As indicated in **13.4**, the inclusion probabilities, π_i, used to draw a Poisson sample are usually better chosen to be proportional to Z_i^{γ} rather than to Z_i itself. The special features of Poisson sampling are, however, more easily understood if we consider first the simple case where the Y_i are roughly proportional to the Z_i and also the π_i are chosen to be exactly proportional to the Z_i. In these circumstances the ordinary HTE is an obvious estimator to use (though as we shall soon see, not really a good one).

Under Poisson sampling, the HTE of the population total, $Y_{\bullet} = \Sigma_i Y_i$, is

$$\hat{Y}_{\bullet HT} = \sum_i \delta_i Y_i \pi_i^{-1}. \tag{13.1}$$

The variance of $\hat{Y}_{\bullet HT}$ given in Chapter 4 as (4.6) may also be written as

$$\mathrm{V}\hat{Y}_{\bullet HT} = \sum_{i=1}^{N} Y_i^2 \pi_i^{-1} + \sum_{i=1}^{N} \sum_{j \notin i}^{N} \pi_{ij} Y_i \pi_i^{-1} Y_j \pi_j^{-1} - Y_{\bullet}^2.$$

Since in Poisson sampling the binomial draws are conducted independently of each other, we have $\pi_{ij} = \pi_i \pi_j$ and the HTE's variance simplifies to

$$\mathrm{V}\hat{Y}_{\bullet HT} = \sum_i \pi_i^{-1}(1 - \pi_i) Y_i^2 \tag{4.12}$$

$$= \sum_i \left(\pi_i^{-1} - 1\right) Y_i^2, \tag{13.2}$$

which is estimated without bias by

$$\hat{\mathrm{V}}_1 \hat{Y}_{\bullet HT} = \sum_i \delta_i \pi_i^{-1} \left(\pi_i^{-1} - 1\right) Y_i^2, \tag{13.3}$$

or more efficiently (though not quite without bias) by

$$\hat{\mathrm{V}}_2 \hat{Y}_{\bullet HT} = n^{-1}(\mathrm{E}n) \sum_i \delta_i \pi_i^{-1} \left(\pi_i^{-1} - 1\right) Y_i^2, \tag{13.4}$$

where En is the expected number of units included in sample, or *target sample size*, and therefore also the population sum of the inclusion probabilities, that is, $\mathrm{E}n = \sum_i \pi_i$.

As already indicated, however, most of the variance of $\hat{Y}_{\bullet HT}$ under Poisson sampling is due to the variability in the sample size, n. It is therefore misleading to use the design variance (13.2) of $\hat{Y}_{\bullet HT}$ as a measure of its imprecision. That variance is a measure of the estimate's variability over all possible samples, so cannot vary from sample to sample. By contrast, the imprecision of any particular $\hat{Y}_{\bullet HT}$ is a function of n, the number of units in the particular sample upon which it is based.

This is not to say, however, that the imprecision of $\hat{Y}_{\bullet HT}$ diminishes monotonically as the achieved sample size increases. A sample with $n > \mathrm{E}n$ will tend to overestimate the population total, and one with $n < \mathrm{E}n$ will tend to underestimate it. And not even when $n = \mathrm{E}n$ will the imprecision of $\hat{Y}_{\bullet HT}$ be reflected by its design variance.

When it comes to estimating $\mathrm{V}\hat{Y}_{\bullet HT}$ using the $\hat{\mathrm{V}}_1 \hat{Y}_{\bullet HT}$ of (13.3), the situation is still worse. A sample with $n > \mathrm{E}n$ will tend to overestimate that variance and one with $n < \mathrm{E}n$ will tend to underestimate it. If we are rash enough to treat (13.3) as an indication of the imprecision in any particular HT estimate, the situation becomes more paradoxical still. Despite the fact that when $n < \mathrm{E}n$, the imprecision in $\hat{Y}_{\bullet HT}$ is relatively large, there are fewer than En terms in the summation of $\hat{\mathrm{V}}_1 \hat{Y}_{\bullet HT}$, so the latter is relatively small. Conversely, when $n > \mathrm{E}n$, the imprecision in $\hat{Y}_{\bullet HT}$ is relatively small, but there are more than En terms in the summation of $\hat{\mathrm{V}}_1 \hat{Y}_{\bullet HT}$, so the latter is relatively large.

13.8 A better estimator of the population total is the *HT ratio estimator* (HTRE),

$$\hat{Y}_{\bullet HTR} = n^{-1}(\mathrm{E}n)\hat{Y}_{\bullet HT} = n^{-1}(\mathrm{E}n)\sum_i \delta_i Y_i \pi_i^{-1}. \tag{13.5}$$

The use of this estimator greatly reduces the third aspect of the problem described in **13.6**, eliminating the component of variance due to the unequal numbers of contributions to the HTE, one from each 'successful' trial (meaning each trial that results in the inclusion of the relevant population unit in the sample).

It does nothing to ameliorate either of the other two aspects of the problem, however. The second aspect, the deviations from the planned workload and expenditure, is unchanged in its impact. The first, the non-zero probability of selecting an empty sample, is arguably made even more problematical. For the HTE itself, the estimate of total for an empty sample is unequivocally zero. It needs to be zero in order to preserve the design unbiasedness. For the HTRE, by contrast, there is no zero design unbiasedness to preserve, and a zero estimate for an empty sample is likely to provide a major contribution to both the design variance and the design MSE. In practice, it is highly unlikely that a zero estimate would ever be tolerated. Some of the more respectable alternatives will be mentioned in **13.11**ff., but even an informed guess would be better than zero!

Two Ways of Viewing the Horvitz–Thompson Ratio Estimator

13.9 The HTRE may be looked at in two ways. The first, obviously, is as a classical ratio estimator, the relevant supplementary variable being π_i, of which the population total or benchmark value is En, the target or expected number of units to be included in the sample. Using the Taylor series expansions of Chapter 3, we then obtain the following formulae for the variance and estimated variance of $\hat{Y}_{\bullet HTR}$:

$$\mathrm{V}\hat{Y}_{\bullet HTR} \cong \mathrm{V}\hat{Y}_{\bullet HT} + \left(\frac{Y_{\bullet}}{\mathrm{E}n}\right)^2 \mathrm{V}n - 2\left(\frac{Y_{\bullet}}{\mathrm{E}n}\right) \mathrm{C}(\hat{Y}_{\bullet HT}, n) \qquad (13.6)$$

and

$$\hat{\mathrm{V}}\hat{Y}_{\bullet HTR} \cong \hat{\mathrm{V}}\hat{Y}_{\bullet HT} + \left(\frac{\hat{Y}_{\bullet HT}}{n}\right)^2 \hat{\mathrm{V}}n - 2\left(\frac{\hat{Y}_{\bullet HT}}{n}\right) \hat{\mathrm{C}}(\hat{Y}_{\bullet HT}, n). \qquad (13.7)$$

(The expression in (13.7) is the variance estimator used by Brewer *et al*. (1972), and denoted by Brewer and Gregoire (2001) in their Table 3 simply as 'BEJ'.) Here, of course,

$$\mathrm{V}n = \sum_i (\pi_i^{-1} - 1)\pi_i^2 = \sum_i \pi_i(1 - \pi_i) = \mathrm{E}n - \sum_i \pi_i^2, \qquad (13.8)$$

$$\hat{\mathrm{V}}n = \sum_i \delta_i \pi_i^{-1}(\pi_i^{-1} - 1)\pi_i^2 = \sum_i \delta_i(1 - \pi_i) = n - \sum_i \delta_i \pi_i, \qquad (13.9)$$

$$\mathrm{C}(\hat{Y}_{\bullet HT}, n) = \sum_i (\pi_i^{-1} - 1)Y_i\pi_i = Y_{\bullet} - \sum_i Y_i\pi_i \qquad (13.10)$$

and

$$\mathrm{C}(\hat{Y}_{\bullet HT}, n) = \sum_i \delta_i \pi_i^{-1}(\pi_i^{-1} - 1)Y_i\pi_i = \sum_i \delta_i(\pi_i^{-1} - 1)Y_i$$
$$= \hat{Y}_{\bullet HT} - \sum_i \delta_i Y_i. \qquad (13.11)$$

There is, however, a residual problem with treating $\hat{Y}_{\bullet HTR}$ as a classical ratio estimator, in that its variance and MSE are defined over all possible samples, which are of different sizes, while the precision of the estimated total based on the actual or realized sample is in fact a function of the size of that particular sample.

This is, we believe, the principal reason why Brewer and Gregoire (2001) found that 'BEJ' (13.7) performed less well as an estimator of MSE (even over all possible samples) than their alternative estimator, '$\hat{\hat{\mathrm{V}}}\hat{Y}_{\bullet 3P7}$', did. This alternative estimator was constructed using the second way of looking at the HTRE, namely as the HTE conditioned on the achieved sample size, n.

In other words, Brewer and Gregoire (2001) estimated the variance of $\hat{Y}_{\bullet HTR}$ as though their actual Poisson sample had instead been selected with *srswor*, that *srswor* sample size being fixed at the size, n, of their Poisson sample. Note that their Poisson sampling estimator, $\hat{Y}_{\bullet HTR}$, was numerically identical to the one that would have been the HTE, $\hat{Y}_{\bullet HT}$, had their sample actually been selected in the way that they were pretending it was. (For simple estimation of a close approximation to the variance of the HTE, together with a generalization to the variances of regression estimators based on the HTE, see Chapter 9.)

13.10 Up to this point, we have been working only in terms of the HTE itself and of the particular HTRE for which the auxiliary variable is the sample size. But, as indicated in **13.4**, optimal inclusion probabilities are seldom proportional to the auxiliary variable that is best for ratio estimation, which we will denote here by x. In more normal circumstances the inclusion probabilities, π_i, would be proportional either to a power of the x_i or to some completely different auxiliary variable. It is then tempting to opt for the ratio estimator $\left(\sum_i \delta_i Y_i / \sum_i \delta_i X_i\right) X_{\bullet}$ and ignore the π_i entirely. Under the purely prediction-based paradigm, that would be the only sensible course of action. But we are now strongly of the opinion that it is better to use estimators that are supported by the design-based inference as well. Under this mixed paradigm the appropriate two-step ratio estimator is

$$\hat{\hat{Y}}_{\bullet HTR} = \frac{\hat{Y}_{\bullet HTR}}{\hat{X}_{\bullet HTR}} X_{\bullet} = \frac{\sum_i \delta_i Y_i \pi_i^{-1}}{\sum_i \delta_i X_i \pi_i^{-1}} X_{\bullet}.$$

We have already recommended that $\hat{Y}_{\bullet HTR}$ (and by implication also $\hat{X}_{\bullet HTR}$) be treated as HTEs conditioned on their achieved sample size. Hence, to find and estimate the variance or MSE of the two-step ratio estimator, all that is needed is to incorporate the ratio estimation theory of Chapter 3 into the unequal probability sampling theory of Chapter 9. This is just one more instance where the 'special skill of the sampling statistician' that we mentioned in our most recent report (**12.3**), is required to 'construct ... a harmonious edifice', so we will leave this to you and any other reader (Exercise 13.1).

Much the same may be said regarding the problem of estimation in the context of a rotating sample. This matter has already been touched on in **12.7**. We recommended there that the sample be split into two or more portions, depending on the inclusion history of their component units. Each portion would provide its own estimate of the population total, and these estimates could then be combined in a close to optimal fashion by weighting them inversely to their variances. (It was not worthwhile, we suggested, taking account of the small negative covariances that arose from sampling without replacement, but that can still be done if the aim is set at perfection.) Thus rotation adds one or even two more levels of complexity to the problem of constructing the relevant 'harmonious edifice'. Taking account of non-response could add yet another (Exercise 13.3).

Alternatives to Poisson Sampling

13.11 All the sampling procedures described in the remainder of this chapter are derivative from Poisson sampling. The only difference of substance is that in all but two of these derivative procedures (modified Poisson sampling and collocated sampling) the sample size is a fixed number. The estimators we therefore recommend are either the HTE conditioned on the achieved sample size, the two-step ratio estimator, $\hat{\hat{Y}}_{\bullet HTR}$, of **13.10**, or, best of all, the regression estimators described in Chapter 9.

Some Early Variations on Poisson Sampling

13.12 While use of the HTRE circumvents one of the three aspects of the problem described in **13.6**, it does little or nothing for the other two. These can only be addressed by eliminating, or at least reducing, the randomness in the sample size.

The earliest suggestion along these lines was *modified Poisson sampling* (Ogus and Clark, 1971; see also Brewer *et al*., 1972, 1984). This was specifically aimed at eliminating the non-zero probability of selecting an empty sample. If an empty sample was selected, another Poisson sample was selected, and this process was repeated if necessary until a non-empty sample eventuated. This idea did not catch on. The essential randomness of the sample size was barely dented, the estimation became more complicated and the elegance of the rotation procedures described in **13.5** was put at risk.

Another early suggestion was collocated sampling. This was described in Brewer *et al*. (1972), elaborated in Brewer *et al*. (1984) and investigated by Brewer and Gregoire (2001). The underlying idea was to spread the PRNs uniformly over the interval [0, 1) instead of randomly. This substantially reduced the variability in the sample size, and eliminated the possibility of selecting an empty sample for almost all but the smallest samples while retaining the essential elegance of the rotation procedures. Brewer and Gregoire's investigation, however, revealed certain problems that arose with the variance estimation of the HTE and related estimators when collocated sampling was used, and these problems seemed to outweigh any advantages.

Synchronized Sampling

13.13 A more successful and practicable variant on Poisson sampling was synchronized sampling (Hinde and Young, 1984). It replaced the use of collocated sampling in the Australian Bureau of Statistics in the early 1980s. At that time, collocated sampling had been used there only in the context of stratified random sampling with equal inclusion probabilities within size strata, and the fact that stratification had to be identical from one survey to another severely reduced the usefulness of collocated sampling. Synchronized sampling was introduced (in the same limited context) largely to overcome that shortcoming, but even so, a certain amount of improvization and compromise was necessary (Hinde and Young, 1984, Section 3.3).

Synchronized sampling within any given stratum may be described as follows. As with Poisson sampling, every unit listed in the sample frame is given a PRN in the range [0, 1). If (as is usual) more than one rotating survey sample is to be selected from that frame, the line [0, 1) is partitioned into smaller non-intersecting half-open intervals called *overlap ranges*, one for each survey.

The initial sample for each survey occupies a specific segment within its overlap range known as the *selection interval*, and the *startpoint* and *endpoint* of that interval are defined so that it holds precisely the target sample number of units. Specifically, one unit is chosen randomly from all the units in the stratum, and its PRN is used to define the startpoint or closed end of the selection interval. At its open end, the selection interval extends right up to (but does not include) the first unit *not* required for the initial sample.

Rotation is effected by shifting a survey's selection interval bodily to the right, but not (as with Poisson or collocated sampling) by a predetermined interval. Instead, the startpoint is shifted through as many PRNs as are to be rotated out, and the endpoint is shifted through as many as are to be rotated in. At each rotation, the PRN of the first unit retained in sample defines the new (closed) startpoint, while its open endpoint extends right up to (but does not include) the first unit *not* required for the newly rotated sample.

Importantly, the entire overlap range for each survey must be regarded as wrapped around in a cylindrical fashion, so that the end of it and the start of it are effectively the same point. For instance, if a particular survey range is [0.3, 0.6), the next number after 0.6 is 0.3 again. (In practice, this would mean that the computer had to treat the next number after 599 999 999 999 as 300 000 000 000.) If the open end of the overlap range is reached during a rotation, the process must 'wrap around', meaning that it must continue again from its closed end (that is to say, from its beginning). This prevents the survey samples from trespassing in each others' territories.

Despite its conceptual simplicity, synchronized sampling is not that easy to operate in practice, and we believe no one should seriously try to use it without first becoming familiar with Hinde and Young (1984). Substantial complications occur when dealing with 'deaths' (businesses taken over or ceasing operations) and 'births' (new businesses starting up). These complications are collectively described as *birth biases* (Hinde and Young, 1984, Sections 3.3.2ff.).

13.14 The birth bias introduced by a single new birth (and no deaths) is the first and simplest of the birth bias problems dealt with by Hinde and Young's (1984) manual, but all of them spring from the same counter-intuitive fact regarding order statistics, namely that if n points are randomly selected on the interval [0, 1), the expected lengths of the $n+1$ intervals $[0, x_1)$, $[x_1, x_2), \ldots, [x_n, 1)$ are all equal at $1/(n+1)$. This result may be obtained from considerations of symmetry: if $n+1$ points are randomly drawn on the circumference of a circle and one of these is then selected randomly to represent the point zero, or for that matter any preselected value in the interval [0, 1), the expected lengths of the $(n+1)$ intervals between the pairs are obviously equal.

To take the simplest possible case, consider a population containing only two units. Each is allocated a PRN randomly in the interval [0, 1). Denote the smaller of them by x_1 and the larger by x_2. A 50% sample is selected by dividing the interval into two selection intervals. The first is $[x_1, x_2)$, which contains only the smaller unit (the larger being just beyond its endpoint), and the second is the union of $[x_2, 1)$ and $[0, x_1)$, which contains only the larger unit, the smaller being just beyond the endpoint of $[0, x_1)$.

Now imagine we have a 'birth', and we want to divide the interval [0, 1) into three in such a way as to give the 'newly born' unit one chance in three of being the sample unit at the next rotation. We will first attempt to achieve that result in the following straightforward but inadequate fashion.

Denote the PRN of the newborn unit by x_b. There are three possible intervals in which x_b can fall. These are $[x_1, x_2)$, $[x_2, 1)$ and $[0, x_1)$, and because the ordered pair $\{x_1, x_2\}$ was chosen randomly in [0, 1), each of these three intervals has the same expected length. So the *a priori* probability of x_b turning up in each of those intervals is one-third.

If x_b falls in the interval $[x_1, x_2)$, the selection interval for the unit at x_1 shortens to $[x_1, x_b)$ and that for the new unit is $[x_b, x_2)$, while that for x_2 remains at the union of $[x_2, 1)$ and $[0, x_1)$. If x_1 is rotated out, wraparound does not occur and the unit rotated in is x_b. If x_2 is rotated out, wraparound does occur and the unit rotated in is x_1.

If, instead, x_b is in the interval $[x_2, 1)$, the selection interval for the unit at x_1 remains at $[x_1, x_2)$, that for the unit at x_2 shortens to $[x_2, x_b)$ and that for the new unit is the union of $[x_b, 1)$ and $[0, x_1)$. If x_1 is rotated out, wraparound does not occur and the unit rotated in is x_2. If x_2 is rotated out, wraparound does occur and the unit rotated in is x_b.

Finally, if x_b is in the interval $[0, x_1)$, the selection interval for the unit at x_1 remains at $[x_1, x_2)$, that for the unit at x_2 shortens to the union of $[x_2, 1)$ and $[0, x_b)$, and that for the new unit is $[x_b, x_1)$. If x_1 is rotated out, wraparound does not occur and the unit rotated in is x_2. If x_2 is rotated out, wraparound does occur and the unit rotated in is x_b.

All six situations are equally probable, and three of them result in the rotation of x_b, so its inclusion probability at that rotation is not one-third, but one-half – a bias in favour of the newly born unit.

One way of dealing with the birth bias problem would be to ensure that the zero PRN was always (or at least nearly always) occupied by a sample unit. At the start of the PRN selection process, one unit could be selected at random to occupy that position and, if and whenever that selected unit 'died', the next available 'newly born' unit could fill the vacancy. That solution breaks down, however, if there is more than one level of stratification – for instance, if one coarse or aggregated stratum were composed of half a dozen fine ones. If each of the fine strata had a unit at zero, the aggregate stratum would have six units at zero, rather defeating the purpose of allocating a separate PRN to each unit!

Hinde and Young's solution is to suggest that wherever the rotation involves a wraparound, the last *fully* open interval in $[0,\ 1)$ is to be omitted from the selection interval. In the example we are examining, this last fully open interval is $(x_2, 1)$. In addition, there is one chance in two of wraparound occurring. There is also one change in the selection result, namely that when x_b is in the interval $[x_2,\ 1)$ and x_2 is rotated out, the new unit rotated in is not x_b but x_1. This change reduces the inclusion probability of x_b from one-half to one-third and the birth bias is eliminated.

In general, when there are originally N units in the population and n in the sample, and a single birth occurs, the probability of wraparound is n/N. To see this, denote the unit with the largest PRN by x_n. Then Hinde and Young's rule requires that when a wraparound occurs, the fully open interval $(x_n,\ 1)$ is to be omitted from the selection interval. This results in the probability of selecting the newly born unit at the next rotation falling from $(n+1)/(N+1)$ to $n/(N+1)$ if wraparound occurs, while remaining at $n/(N+1)$ if there is no wraparound. So the inclusion probability for the newly born unit falls from $(n/N)\{(n+1)/(N+1)\} + \{(N-n)/N\}\{n/(N+1)\} = n/N$ to $(n/N)\{n/(N+1)\} + \{(N-n)/N\}\{n/(N+1)\} = n/(N+1)$, eliminating the birth bias.

Hinde and Young proceed to demonstrate that the same rule can be used to eliminate the birth bias even when there are any number of births and any number of deaths. On that score alone, their solution to the problem is distinctly elegant.

13.15 Among the many other topics dealt with by Hinde and Young are the determination of respondent burden (including, among others, allowances for different rotation rates, different frequencies of collection, different size stratifications, different stratification variables and different selection units), the allocation of PRNs within highly structured businesses, changes to overlap ranges and determining overlap ranges and sample startpoints within them. As mentioned above, synchronized sampling is conceptually very simple, but it can nevertheless be surprisingly complex to operate in practice.

One possible improvement to Hinde and Young's proposals would be to allocate as many births as possible randomly into the positions made vacant by deaths. It seems likely that its adoption would substantially slow the rate of unintended rotation (a phenomenon caused on the one hand by deaths and births, and on the other hand by the requirement that the sample must never be shifted to the left).

Conditional Poisson Sampling

13.16 *Conditional Poisson sampling* is Poisson sampling conditioned on the sample size being set at a predetermined number, n. We shall use Aires's (2000) acronym for it, CPS. A conditional Poisson sample of size n is achieved by selecting successive experimental Poisson samples of expected size n, and choosing the first sample of that exact size. (Naturally, one would immediately abort any attempt that reached a progressive sample size of $n+1$ prior to the completion of the N relevant trials.)

Conditional Poisson sampling appears to have been introduced first by Hájek (1964), under the name *rejective sampling*. In the same paper, Hájek shows that as n approaches infinity, the actual inclusion probabilities for a conditional Poisson sample approach the working inclusion probabilities used in each experiment. In his posthumous book (Hájek, 1981) he further shows that CPS maximizes the entropy of the sample design within the class of those schemes that have the same first-order inclusion probabilities π_i. Entropy, a concept defined by $-\sum_{s \subset U} P(s) \ln P(s)$, where $P(s)$ is the probability of selecting the sample s from the set U of possible samples, is a measure of the randomness of the sample design. Aires (2000) comments that 'this measure informs about how the population is represented in the sample', which suggests that high-entropy samples are likely to be particularly suitable for design-based inference. From the point of view of a design-oriented sampling statistician, that makes CPS the best choice (if only by a whisker) among all possible designs sharing the same set of π_i values.

But what does 'best' imply in this context? If a sample is drawn systematically πps from a randomly ordered population, the HTE is design-unbiased and achieves the minimum possible anticipated variance. The same is true for several other πps sampling schemes. How can this performance be bettered?

The answer seems to lie in the efficiency with which the variance of the HTE can be estimated using purely design-based inference, and in particular using the Sen–Yates–Grundy variance estimator, which requires knowledge of the second-order inclusion probabilities π_{ij}. While it is possible to calculate these π_{ij} exactly if the sample is reasonably small, or to approximate them closely if the sample is large (Hartley and Rao, 1962), the values they assume for small samples do not generally come close to optimizing the efficiency of the Sen–Yates–Grundy variance estimator (Brewer and Hanif, 1983, p. 64). It seems likely that both they and the CPS values of π_{ij} calculated by Aires (2000) would do so, or at least come very close to doing so, for large samples. Whether this is still a matter of practical importance will, however, depend on whether that variance estimator ever comes back into prominence. It has already largely been bypassed by the use of replication methods such as the jackknife and the bootstrap, and the approximations mentioned in Chapter 9 now provide another (and arguably more convenient) bypass route. We would have to say at this stage that any substantial increase in the use of the Sen–Yates–Grundy variance estimator in practical survey sampling seems at best to be a long way off.

Order Sampling Schemes

13.17 There are in any case certain more convenient alternatives to CPS that provide the same or nearly the same values of π_{ij} and therefore almost the same levels of entropy. Aires (2000, p. xii) groups several of the more important of them under the heading of *order sampling*. For an order sample, each unit in the population is assigned an independently but not necessarily identically distributed random variable called a ranking variable. The n distinct units with the smallest ranking variable values constitute an order sample.

The idea of order sampling is most easily picked up by way of examples. We have already described synchronized sampling, which is an important special case of it. For synchronized sampling the ranking variable is simply the PRN itself, a random number picked from the uniform distribution over the interval [0, 1). An initial equal probability (*epsem*) sample of n distinct units is selected by choosing those with the smallest PRNs.

Sequential Poisson Sampling

13.18 It is easy to generalize synchronized sampling to the unequal probability situation by changing the ranking variable. Instead of simply the PRN, r_i, we might choose the PRN divided by the first-order inclusion probability, i.e. r_i/π_i. This kind of order sampling was called *sequential Poisson sampling* by Ohlsson (1990, 1995). Aires (2000, p. xii) mentions that it has been used in the Swedish Consumer Price Index Survey since 1990.

It has a simple graphic representation similar to that used above for Poisson sampling itself. Consider the selection region defined by AOB in Figure 13.2. If the line OB is drawn with a predefined slope, the sample selected is simply a Poisson sample. If, however, it is drawn so as to include in the sample region, AOB, a predetermined number of points representing population units, the sample selected is a sequential Poisson sample.

It would be desirable, when attempting to select a sample in this fashion, to ensure that the region AOB had a horizontal 'ceiling' that stopped well short of stretching over the entire potential range of PRNs from zero to unity, with a take-all stratum of all units above that ceiling. Without that feature, pure chance could cause the number of units in AOB to fall below the required sample size. In theory, the deficiency could be made up by double-counting (or more generally by multiple-counting) some or all of the population units above the ceiling, where notionally the 'inclusion probabilities' would exceed unity. That expedient, however, would be clumsy and inefficient.

Since sequential Poisson sampling is a generalization of synchronized sampling from *epsem* to unequal probability sampling, it is subject to the same problem of birth bias, but some of the problems mentioned in **13.15** would not appear here. For one thing, there would not be any stratification by size (except to separate out the take-all stratum) and hence little or no problem with units changing size stratum, which in synchronized sampling is normally quite a common occurrence. For the same reason, there would be little or no problem with different size stratifications or different stratification variables.

It might, however, be suggested that there would be problems with units having different sizes (and therefore different inclusion probabilities) for surveys having different scopes and hence different survey variables. This need not necessarily be the case, however, for – as indicated in **13.4** – the optimal inclusion probability is proportional to the square root of the variance function, and that function in turn is likely to be more dependent on the overall size of a population unit than on its size as measured within a given sector of its activities. (A business that has a large overall size and many different production items can more easily double its production of a given item than another business that has the same level of production of that item, but whose operations are limited to that item alone.) So it may well be advisable to restrict a population to a given size measure (and hence a given inclusion probability), not merely to keep the selection procedure simple, but from considerations of sampling efficiency as well.

Pareto πps Sampling

13.19 The type of order sampling considered in detail by Aires (2000) is *Pareto πps sampling*. Her acronym for it was PPS, but here we shall use $P\pi ps$ instead. $P\pi ps$ was introduced independently by Saavedra (1995) and Rosén (1997b). It is of particular interest because the second-order inclusion probabilities, π_{ij}, are very close to those of CPS and because they are substantially easier to calculate for $P\pi ps$ than for CPS. Even more important operationally is the fact that $P\pi ps$ samples can be represented graphically in the same way as Poisson and sequential Poisson samples can, while CPS samples cannot.

We saw in **13.18** that whereas synchronized sampling used the PRN, r_i, as its ranking variable, sequential sampling used r_i/π_i. Rosén (2001) uses $\{r_i/(1 - r_i)\}/\{\lambda_i/(1 - \lambda_i)\}$ for $P\pi ps$, where the λ_i are trial values or approximations to the π_i. In fact, the π_i tend asymptotically to the λ_i in this expression. It will be helpful in what follows if we think of the λ_i as virtually the same as the π_i, although they are in fact logically distinct. In Figures 13.4–13.7 we call λ the *measure of size.*

To represent a $P\pi ps$ sample in graphical form, we first calculate our λ_i to be proportional to whatever variable we have chosen or constructed to approximate the square root of the variance function, and thereby we nearly optimize our choice of inclusion probabilities. We also select our PRNs, r_i, as before, from a uniform distribution over the range [0, 1). We then represent each of the N units in the population by a point at $r_i/(1 - r_i)$ to the right of the vertical axis of Figure 13.3 and at $\lambda_i/(1 - \lambda_i)$ above its horizontal axis. To select a $P\pi ps$ sample we rotate the straight line OB clockwise until the required sample number, n, of them lie in the sample zone, above and to the left of OB.

There are, of course, two problems in representing the N population units in this fashion, namely that we would require a very large sheet of paper, and that almost all our points would be crowded in the bottom left-hand corner (close to the origin). More realistically, we might plot r_i to the right of the vertical axis, as in Figure 13.4, and λ_i above its horizontal axis. That reduces the paper size and spreads the points more conveniently, but there remains a problem in defining the sample zone. What we need to plot are contour lines for which $\{r/(1 - r)\}/\{\lambda/(1 - \lambda)\}$ is equal to an arbitrary constant, say k. That condition can be redefined as the contour $\lambda = r/\{r + k - kr\}$. Figure 13.5 shows how this contour varies with k. It always passes through the points $(0, 0)$ and $(1, 1)$ but, as k increases, holding r constant, the value of λ decreases, so that the non-sample zone shrinks downwards and to the right. In other words, smaller units are progressively being included in sample, and the sample size is increasing. The appropriate value of k would be that for which the number of units in the sample zone just became n.

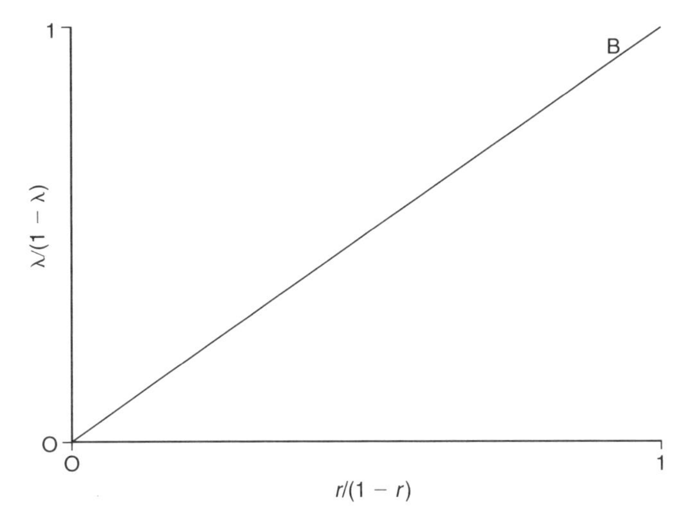

Figure 13.3 Plotting $\lambda/(1-\lambda)$ against $r/(1-r)$ for Pareto πps sampling.

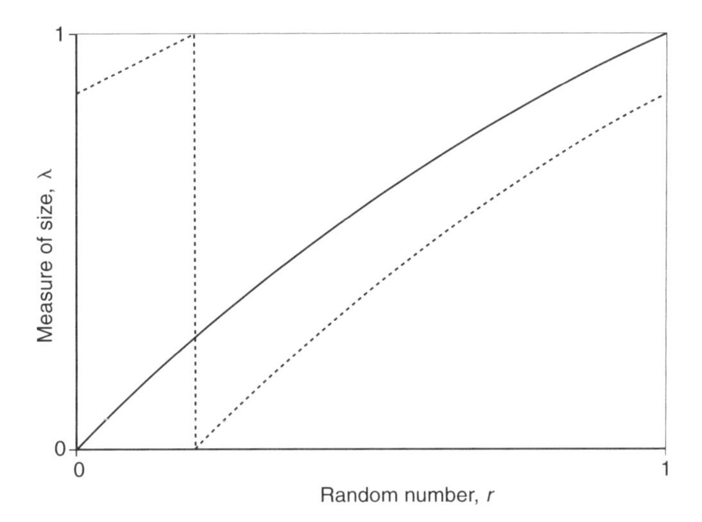

Figure 13.4 Plotting λ against r for Pareto πps sampling for a given value of k.

To rotate this sample with minimum complications, it would be necessary to move the contour lines bodily to the right, and wrap the diagram around cylindrically if necessary. For example, if they were moved a distance d to the right, where $0 \leq d < 1$, the new contour lines would be defined by $\{(r-d)/(1-r+d)\}/\{\lambda/(1-\lambda)\}$ for $r > d$ and $\{(r+1-d)/(d-r)\}/\{\lambda/(1-\lambda)\}$ for $r \leq d$.

A new value of k would need to be determined for each rotation. If the population being sampled is large enough, it should seldom be very different from the old value. Figure 13.6 provides a typical example. There might, however, be the rare occasion where the new *endcurve* (corresponding to the endpoint in synchronized sampling) intersected with the old one.

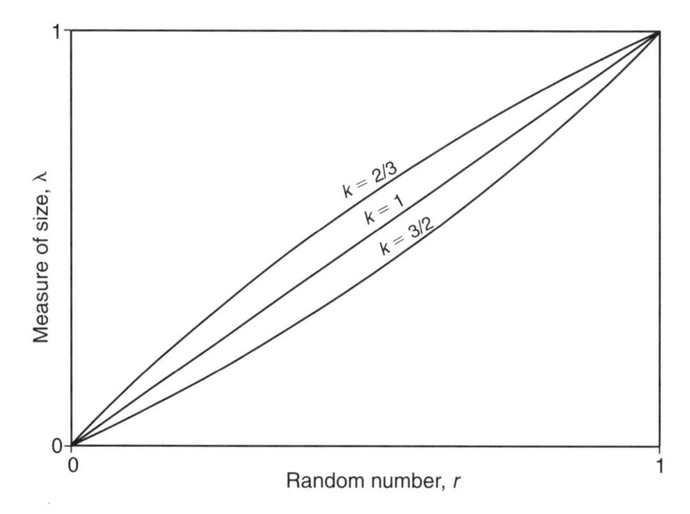

Figure 13.5 Plotting λ against r for Pareto πps sampling for different values of k.

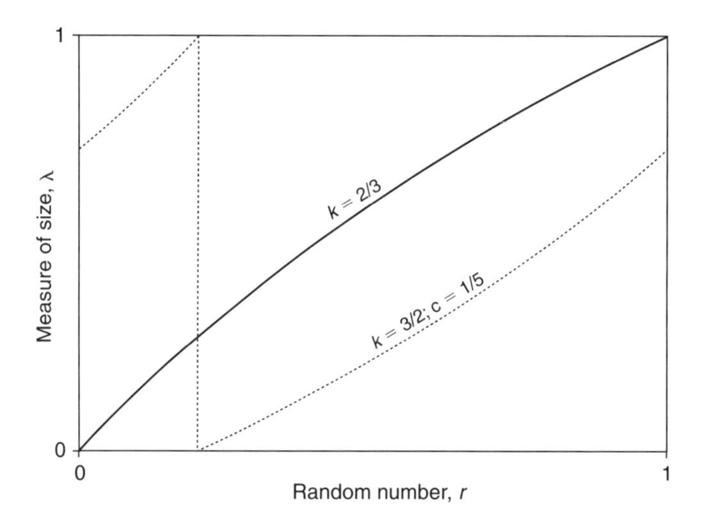

Figure 13.6 A typical rotation for Pareto πps sampling.

To be on the safe side, the program should be written so as to ensure that no part of the new endcurve is allowed to fall behind (that is, to the left of) the old one. Figure 13.7 illustrates how this could happen with the old endcurve OB overlapping with the new one, O′B′. The easiest way of doing this, without changing the sample size, would be to shift the new *startline*, A″O″, which corresponds to the startpoint in synchronized sampling, to the right. It would have to go at least as far as A″O″, and the new endcurve O″B″ with it, until O″B″ and OB barely touched. A little tricky, but not impossible to program.

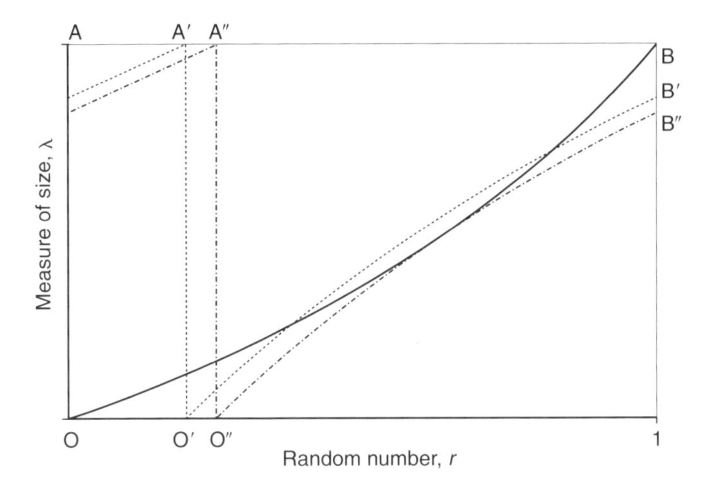

Figure 13.7 An atypical rotation diagram for Pareto πps with new startline and endcurve shifted right to eliminate overlap.

Rotation Groups in Panel Samples

13.20 PRN sampling is not the only method that can be used to control and/or rotate a sample. The most frequently used alternative, one especially useful for the clustered samples of dwellings described in Chapters 10 and 11, is panel sampling with rotation groups (Brewer *et al.*, 1972, pp. 232–233; Sigman and Monsour, 1995, pp. 145–149).

Conceptually, it is not all that different from PRN sampling. To 'pour it into the same mould', we could think of it as the assignment of the same PRN to a number of population units, thereby dividing them into (say) 60 rotation groups. The panel for any given survey round would consist of perhaps five rotation groups, one being rotated out and another being rotated in after each survey round, providing an 80% overlap in the sample between successive survey rounds.

We chose the number 60 because it is exactly divisible by 2, 3, 4, 5, 6, 10, 12, 15, 20 and 30, providing the opportunity to choose among eleven different sample fractions (including 1/60). With 120 rotation groups there are 15 such options. With 360 there are 23. This is less flexible than PRN sampling, which permits samples of any size whatever, but is more convenient particularly where the sample is clustered at various levels and it is convenient to put whole clusters into the same rotation group. For an example, see Brewer *et al.* (1972).

Since single-stage panel sampling is next door to being a special case of PRN sampling, it is not necessary to provide a separate account of estimation or variance estimation. If the sample size is fixed, the relevant theory is that of *srswor* or $\pi pswor$. If it is not fixed, the relevant theory is that of *srswor* or $\pi pswor$ as the case may be, but in any case one conditioned on the achieved sample size. (See also our corresponding comments on the analysis of PRN sampling in **13.11**.)

Multistage sampling is a different matter. It would be difficult, if not impossible, to adapt PRN sampling to the multistage environment. However, each panel is in itself a self-contained multistage sample and the only relevant complication lies in the fact that it is being rotated. The last paragraph of **13.10** is relevant here.

13.21 Sigman and Monsour (1995) discuss, among other relevant topics, the possibility of collecting data from more than one period at each survey round (say, data for period $t-1$ as well as for period t for the round conducted immediately following period t). They call this a *two-level scheme*, or more generally a *multilevel scheme*, of information gathering and point out that, in order to avoid collecting the same data more than once, at least two distinct rotating panels would be needed. If there were two such panels for a monthly survey, one would provide the sample for January, March, ..., November, and the other would provide the sample for February, April, ..., December, but each would supply a complete year's worth of data. This almost halves the work for the collection agency (as compared with having a sample of the same size provide the same data using a one-level scheme), but requires either the preparation of provisional estimates using only half the data that would eventually become available, or a month's delay in the release of the estimate. As so often happens in survey sampling – and indeed in statistics generally – the choice is not amenable to optimization and has to be made subjectively. Fortunately, the optima are almost always flat.

Response from Supervisor

Thanks. I think that meets the first of my queries quite adequately for the moment. Clearly there has been a lot of interest in the topic recently, so don't be surprised if I ask for an update from time to time.

I hardly need to remind you that I also asked for a report on inspecting data for extreme observations and other unusual features, and coping with them once they have been found.

Exercises

13.1 Use the ratio estimation theory of Chapter 3 and the unequal probability sampling theory of Chapter 9 to find an approximate expression for the large-sample variance of the $\hat{\hat{Y}}_{\bullet HTR}$ of **13.10** (that variance being conditioned on the achieved sample size).

13.2 Find a suitable estimator for the approximate variance expression derived in Example 13.1.

13.3 Suggest in principle how the phenomenon of non-response might be taken account of in the estimation of total in the context of **13.10**.

13.4 Suppose synchronized sampling is being used. Verify, diagramatically or otherwise, that when there are originally N units in the population and n in the sample, and a single birth occurs, the probability of wraparound at the next single unit rotation is n/N.

13.5 Suppose once more that there are originally N units in the population and n in the sample, and a single birth occurs. Assume also that the Hinde–Young rule (to omit the last *fully* open interval in $[0, 1)$ from the selection interval wherever the rotation involves a wraparound) has *not* been adopted. Verify, diagramatically or otherwise, that the probability of selecting the newly born unit at the next single unit rotation is n/N.

13.6 Next, assume instead that the Hinde–Young rule *has* been adopted. Verify, diagramatically or otherwise, that the probability of selecting the newly born unit at the next single unit rotation is thereby reduced to $n/(N + 1)$.

14

Coping with Extreme Values and Other Unusual Features

Report for Supervisor: Introduction 268
Relevant and Recognizable Subsets 268
Stratification and Selection of Atypical Units 270
Spurious Extreme Values 271
Genuine Extreme Values 272
Winsorization 274
Spreading the Estimated Bias Back 278
Summary and Concluding Remarks 280
Response from Supervisor 281
Exercises 282

Report for Supervisor: Introduction

14.1 This will be a rather different report from any that we have written for you earlier. In the other reports we were relying largely on written sources, supplementing them where necessary by our own material, but this one will rely principally on Brewer's reminiscences on what we have referred to recently as 'extreme observations and other unusual features'.

To be honest, he had a somewhat idiosyncratic approach to the topic. He avoided wherever possible routine 'cookbook' approaches, emphasizing that each unusual feature was likely to have its own characteristics and merit its own individual treatment. If there were more extreme observations than he could spare the time to investigate, he would refuse to regard them as extreme and insist that they must be treated no differently from the other observations. If there were several of them in the sample, they were most probably representative of others in the population that had not been selected in sample. Whether this attitude is still a practical one to adopt in these days of information overload we are unable to say. For this report, we are supplying you with the best we can conveniently lay our hands on, and for the most part it will be those reminiscences.

Relevant and Recognizable Subsets

14.2 You will no doubt recognize the phrase 'relevant and recognizable subsets' as originating from Sir Ronald Fisher. If a subset can be recognized that is substantially different from the remainder of the set, Fisher insisted on its being treated separately, and Brewer followed his example. Quite early in his statistical career – in the mid-1950s – Brewer was called on to redesign the three business surveys of the Australian Bureau of Statistics: Capital Expenditure, Stocks, and Labour Turnover.

This was the first redesign of those surveys since Ken Foreman returned from the US Bureau of the Census in 1949 with the training he had received there from Morris Hansen and Bill Hurwitz. Consequently, they were being looked at quite differently from the way they had been looked at in the past. Brewer gave them the standard design-based treatment, stratifying the businesses by industry and size and using wages (at the time the only available supplementary variable) for ratio estimation purposes. He also estimated variances from past surveys and used those estimates to allocate the sample units among strata in an optimal fashion (see Chapter 3).

In the course of this work, he came across three industries where a subgroup of sample units had unusually high variability in their ratios of survey variable values to supplementary variable values. In the Capital Expenditure Survey there was an industry category called 'Other', and within that category there was a group of sample businesses that had very high and variable capital expenditures in relation to their wages. Up till then, not much attention had been paid to whether an observation was extreme, so many of them were being ignored, but when one came up that was *obviously* extreme, the standard procedure was to delete it from both the sample and the sample frame, and add it on at the end as an 'extreme observation' – effectively with a sample weight of one.

Brewer felt uncomfortable with either of these options. The subgroup was recognizable and relevant, so it could not be ignored. But its members were not that exceptional, so it would be incurring a large downward bias to give them each a sample weight of unity. He looked at their names in the framework list and found that they were all financial institutions (banks and insurance companies mainly). That made sense; with the amounts of money that they were handling, of course they would be able to undertake substantially larger capital expenditures than businesses that had similar payrolls but were engaged in other activities. He recommended that financial institutions be constituted into a separate industry and completely enumerated – and they were.

In the Stocks Survey there was a similar subgroup in the food and drink industry that had high ratios of stocks to wages. Brewer looked up their names and found that they were all wineries and distilleries, holding large amounts of maturing stocks as 'work in process'. Same problem, same solution.

But again in the Stocks Survey there was a subgroup of wholesalers that also had high ratios of stocks to wages. It looked like the same problem again. They were all wool-selling brokers. All the wool-selling brokers in the sample frame were identified with the intention of constituting them into a separate industry. But then it was discovered that most of the wool-selling brokers in the sample frame did not have high ratios of stocks to wages after all. This anomaly took a little longer to sort out, but it was worth it. The relatively small group of wool-selling brokers with the high ratios of stocks to wages operated their businesses in a different fashion from the remainder. Most wool-selling brokers received and stored wool and sold it on behalf of their clients. Consequently, the stocks they were physically holding did not need to appear in the survey returns – it was not their own wool. Only a small minority actually bought the wool from the growers and resold it. The solution here was therefore to separate out and completely enumerate the group of wool-*buying* brokers.

It may be plausible nowadays to suggest that these were just teething problems, and that most statistical bureau are now well aware of the industry structures they deal with. But similar problems may still arise in new collections, and in countries that are still developing their basic statistical services. The principle remains unchanged: where there are not just one but several extreme-valued sample units, there may be one or more relevant and recognizable subsets. It may be an easy matter to discover what they are, as with the financial institutions and the wineries and distilleries. Or it may be less straightforward, as with the wool-buying brokers. Either way, a knowledge about the population structure is a very useful thing to have, or to acquire!

In fact, right through this chapter, the message will be coming through again and again: know your collection!

Stratification and Selection of Atypical Units

14.3 Not all unusual features give rise to extreme observations, but they still merit recognition and may deserve remedial action. In the late 1950s Brewer was engaged in stratifying the sample frame for the selection of primary sampling units for the ABS Labour Force Survey (see Chapters 10 and 11). One of the local government areas that was potentially a rural PSU in a stratum predominantly given to the raising of sheep for wool was the Shire of Canobolas. This surrounded but did not include the City of Orange. It was not as typical as the surrounding rural LGAs, because there was also a great deal of stone and pome fruit growing in Canobolas, and not elsewhere.

Brewer wanted to avoid putting Canobolas in the same stratum as those other shires. He suggested instead that Orange and Canobolas combined be constituted as a self-representing area. Each normal stratum had two PSUs selected from it, and a multistage 'workload' of 60 dwellings was selected from each of those selected PSUs. Orange–Canobolas, as an SRA with the same population as half a normal stratum, was just the right size to have a single 60-dwelling workload selected from it.

This time, Brewer's suggestion was rejected. The presence of a substantial fruit-growing industry in Canobolas was regarded as insufficiently important to warrant disrupting a certain administrative convenience, namely the distinction between urban and rural workloads. Urban interviewers moved around their workloads on foot or by public transport. They did not need to be able to drive or to have access to a motor vehicle. Rural interviewers needed both, and were paid more in consequence. Orange–Canobolas would have needed an interviewer who was two-thirds urban and one-third rural. The full standard extra payments for driving and using the interviewer's own vehicle would have needed to be paid, even though the workload was two-thirds urban. This was the inconvenience; it was tangible, capable of being costed, and not just a possibility but a certainty. The improvement in precision offered by forming the SRA was difficult to quantify and would only have been relevant if Canobolas was actually going to be selected to represent half its rural stratum. There was only about one chance in five of that happening (and in the event, Canobolas was *not* selected). Many years afterwards, Brewer considered that in all probability the right decision had been made. It is often sensible for considerations of administrative convenience to override the pursuit of variance reduction. The latter may be optimal in terms of a standard cost function, but administrative problems give rise to additional costs that seldom appear in such functions.

14.4 A year or so later, in the course of selecting PSUs from strata already formed, Brewer encountered another atypical situation. In one of the small to medium-sized towns strata, two PSUs (towns) were selected that were the only ones in the stratum to share a certain important feature. Brewer could not remember which towns they were, but was confident that they were important railway junctions, and that in consequence each had a substantial proportion of its labour force employed by the state's railways. He raised the matter with his supervisor, who instructed him to retain one of those towns (effectively by tossing a coin) and to replace the rejected one by one chosen with probability proportional to size from the remaining (non-railway) towns.

At the time, Brewer felt uncomfortable both with the fact that the selection was being tampered with, and with the method of tampering. On reflection, however, he came to see that it was better to have a reasonably well-balanced sample than a pure probability sample that was obviously badly balanced. (In those days, the word 'balanced' would not have been used, but a well-balanced sample would nevertheless have been recognized as 'representative' of the stratum from which it was selected.) He also came to recognize that if one of the two selected towns had to be dropped, it was more logical to decide which one should be dropped by tossing a coin than in any other fashion.

Spurious Extreme Values

14.5 The most important question to consider when dealing with an extreme value is whether the observation is genuine or spurious. The more familiar the sample designer is with the relevant subject matter, the easier it is to spot the difference, but a few general points can still be made.

As evidenced by Brewer's anecdotes about the business surveys in **14.2**, the recognition of relevant subsets can sometimes lead to the clear conclusion that the extreme values are genuine. The presence of a number of extreme values in a file without any obvious pattern is good *prima facie* (first impression) evidence that most of them are spurious, but further acquaintance with a collection will sometimes reveal patterns that were not obvious to begin with. And simple logic indicates that if two collections are of the same quality (contain the same proportion of spurious extremes) but differ substantially in their proportions of *all* extreme values, those extreme values in the collection where they are rarer are necessarily more likely to be spurious.

14.6 One spurious extreme value that Brewer particularly remembered from his later career (after he had left the ABS) was that of a beef cattle station for which the record showed a number of cattle enormously in excess of what was feasible, not merely for the size of the station, but in absolute terms.

At the time, the project on which Brewer was engaged was a purely methodological one, and his chief concern was to compare his methodology with one that had been used by another researcher. That researcher had also been involved in a methodological investigation, and had decided simply to drop the entire record from the file, reducing the sample size by one. For comparability, Brewer did the same, but he knew that if his interests had been substantive rather than methodological, he would have wanted to do something more efficient, and from time to time he used to wonder what he would have done.

Of one thing he was certain: he would have looked at the record on that file and seen whether some simple adjustment, such as moving a decimal point, could make sense of the entire record. If so, it would have been so nearly certain that that was the nature of the error, that the risk involved in making that correction would have been negligible. If, however, it appeared that that field in the record was the only one in error, but the exact nature of the error was not obvious, another way of amending the data would have been to contact the cattle station again and get the correct figure. Failing that, it might still have been possible to estimate the number of cattle on the station using, for instance, an average from other stations of the ratio between the number of cattle and some related item such as income from cattle. (And if the station were in the Northern Territory, another relevant fact would be that, on account of their remoteness, many NT stations only mustered and sold cattle in alternate years.)

If, however, it appeared that more than one field in the record was seriously in error, the conclusion might be arrived at that it was not worth trying to amend the entire record, and that the correct course of action was in fact what the earlier researcher had done – simply discard it from the sample.

Genuine Extreme Values

14.7 As mentioned in **14.2**, when Brewer was a relatively young statistician, the standard method of dealing with an extreme observation known to be real was to delete it both from the sample and the sample frame, and to add it on at the end with a sample weight of unity.

This is still an acceptable procedure to use when common sense suggests that the probability of there being more than one such extreme value in the population is very small. It might be, for instance, that there is one (and only one) unit in the population that is famously or notoriously unlike the rest, but that nobody has yet thought of treating it as genuinely extreme. If such a unit happens to turn up in the sample, straightforward poststratification leads automatically to the old 'delete and add on' procedure described in the paragraph immediately above.

Problems can arise, however, if the well-known unit fails to turn up in the sample, or if there is no single well-known unit. If there is one, and it fails to turn up in sample, there is only a short-term problem. Fairly soon its absence will be noticed, an adjustment will be made, and a revised series will be issued. If, however, no exceptional unit is known, but an extreme value turns up unexpectedly in sample, the question naturally arises, 'Why didn't we know about this?' If it turns out that it should have been known about, we are (at least temporarily) back in the poststratification situation; but we had better make sure that there really are no others like it, because otherwise we will be missing out on a relevant and recognizable subset, and our estimates will be biased (usually downwards) in consequence.

14.8 It is in fact the general rule that the biases induced by ignorance are almost all downwards. If we know that there are classes exhibiting extreme values, we can stratify them out and modify our sampling procedure accordingly. When our knowledge as to their existence is imperfect, so that we sample from a list that contains them but does not identify them, one of two things is bound to happen. Either we fail to select any, in which case our estimate will be below the true value, or else we select one or more of them, in which case our sample estimate will have an unacceptably high estimated variance. Once again, if we pull them out and add them on, the bias will be downwards.

14.9 The prevalence of such downward biases has led to the adoption of methods to mitigate their impact. Most of them fall into one of two classes, weight modification and value modification.

The old 'delete and add on' method is a crude form of weight modification. The affected unit's weight is reduced from the original stratum's sample weight, g (which is generally greater than unity), down to unity. An equally crude value-modification method, in fact one leading to exactly the same numerical results, would be to reduce all the affected unit's variable values by the factor g^{-1}, and then leave it in the sample, so that each value would receive the compensating weight, g. The two methods yield exactly the same (downwards-biased) adjusted sample estimates.

But now compare the unmodified sample estimates with either of these adjusted sample estimates. In the former, an extreme unit receives the ordinary sample weight g. The estimator is unbiased, but has high variance. In the latter, such a unit actually or effectively receives the weight unity instead. The adjusted sample estimate has low variance, but is biased downwards. If the observation is a genuine one, it is not at all clear whether the MSE of the survey's sample estimate will be reduced by deleting the unit and adding it on in this way. How can we work out which is preferable?

The way to answer this apparently intractable question lies in the recognition that in adopting the 'delete and add on' procedure, the analyst is taking a risk on the extreme observation being a genuine rarity. Suppose, for instance, that we are sampling from a population consisting of 995 normal units with mean $\bar{Y}_a$ and 5 very large units with mean $\bar{Y}_b$. The population total is $995\bar{Y}_a + 5\bar{Y}_b$. Suppose, further, that we select a sample of 50, and that it includes one very large value. The mean of the normal units in sample is clearly our best estimator of $\bar{Y}_a$, and the one very large value is our best estimator of $\bar{Y}_b$. Only the weights that we accord to these two estimates are in question.

Our problem is, of course, that we don't know that the actual number of unusual units in sample is five. However, we may be able to guess roughly how many of them there might be, and use that guess to decide between them, for if we use the ordinary expansion estimator, we will effectively have an estimate of $980\bar{Y}_a+20\bar{Y}_b$, but if we use the adjusted estimator we will effectively be estimating $999\bar{Y}_a+\bar{Y}_b$. So if there are more than ten such large units in sample, the expansion estimator will be preferable, but if there are ten or less, the adjusted estimator will be the closer one. Although we still do not know that in fact there are five, we may be fairly certain that there are not more than ten, in which case the adjusted estimator would be the better choice.

Winsorization

14.10 One obvious objection to the stark choice offered in **14.9** between the expansion estimator and the (crudely) adjusted estimator is the sudden transition between the application of the standard sampling weight, g, and the 'add-on' weight of unity. A more gradual progression is provided by using the weight g up to a cut-off value, and beyond that value weights that gradually diminish and tend asymptotically to unity. This has the great advantage of avoiding sudden changes to the survey's time series as units move slightly above or below the chosen cut-off.

Suppose, for instance, that the cut-off value in the hth stratum is set at K_h and that the ith unit in that stratum takes values Y_{hi} that are sometimes above K_h and sometimes below it. A useful and popular way of handling this situation is to *Winsorize* the Y_{hi}, that is, to replace them by $Y_{hi}(K_h)$, where

$$Y_{hi}(K_h) = \begin{cases} Y_{hi} & \text{if } Y_{hi} \le K_h, \\ f_h Y_{hi} + (1 - f_h)K_h & \text{otherwise.} \end{cases} \tag{14.1}$$

Following Gross *et al.* (1986), the choice $f_h = 0$ is said to result in the *Winsorized Type 1 estimator* and the choice $f_h = g_h^{-1}$ in the *Winsorized Type 2 estimator*. Gross *et al.* demonstrated that there was little difference in practice between these estimators; but that as the sample size, n_h, approached the population size, N_h, the contribution of the outlying observation Y_{hi} to the total tended to K_h for the Type 1 estimator and to the correct value, Y_{hi}, for the Type 2 estimator. This led Kokic and Bell (1994) to choose in favour of Winsorization Type 2.

14.11 Winsorization is a value-modification method of adjustment, but, as noted in **14.9**, wherever there is only one survey variable there is an equivalent weight-modification adjustment. For Winsorization Type 2, equivalence is achieved by choosing the modified weight for the *hi*th sample unit to be w_{hi}, where

$$w_{hi} = \begin{cases} g_{hi} & \text{if } Y_{hi} \leq K_h, \\ 1 + (g_{hi} - 1)K_h/Y_{hi} & \text{otherwise.} \end{cases} \tag{14.2}$$

The equivalence between (14.1) and (14.2) is easily seen when the value-modified contribution, $g_{hi}Y_{hi}(K_h)$, is compared with the weight-modified contribution, $w_{hi}Y_{hi}$. If $Y_{hi} \leq K_h$, they are both equal to $g_{hi}Y_{hi}$. Otherwise, they are both equal to $Y_{hi} + (g_{hi} - 1)K_h$.

Equations (14.1) and (14.2) do, however, result in different estimates of total for survey variables other than Y_{hi}, and for all supplementary variables as well. If the value-modification procedure of (14.1) is used, the other variables are Winsorized (or not modified at all) each on its own merit; but if the weight-modification procedure of (14.2) is used, the weights specified by the Winsorization of the Y_{hi} are applied to all variables alike. Brewer always believed that an appropriate survey variable could always be found to Winsorize on, and that using the correspondingly modified weights for all other variables would prevent the formation of internally inconsistent unit records. Whether he was right in this or not, it is convenient to proceed further only with the description of Kokic and Bell's value-modification Winsorization procedure, as the weights w_{hi} of (14.2) can easily be calculated once the K_h of (14.1) have been chosen.

14.12 We therefore describe next how Kokic and Bell optimized the choice of these K_h. They achieved this by minimizing the design MSE of the estimated total, namely

$$\mathrm{E}(\hat{Y}_{\bullet} - Y_{\bullet})^2 = \sum_h N_h(g_h - 1)S_h^2(K_h) + \left[\sum_h \sum_i \{Y_{hi}(K_h) - Y_{hi}\}\right]^2,$$

under the following modelling assumptions:

1. For each h, $\{Y_{hi}, i = 1, \ldots, N_h\}$ is a sequence of uncorrelated and identically distributed variables following model ξ in which $\mathrm{E}_\xi Y_{hi} = \mu_h$ and $\mathrm{V}_\xi Y_{hi} = \sigma_h^2 < \infty$.
2. Y_{hi} possesses a density $g_h(y)$ for all $y > 0$.
3. $\{Y_{hi}; i = 1, \ldots, N_h, h = 1, \ldots, H\}$ is statistically independent of the sample selection process.

The algorithm to minimize the MSE under these three assumptions is a very simple one, and it yields (as Kokic and Bell demonstrated) something close to the best result with real data. Its derivation, however, is a lengthy one, and since it is readily accessible in their paper, only an outline of it will be given here.

The MSE minimized under the three assumptions above is actually the model expectation of the design-based MSE defined above, $\mathrm{MSE}\hat{Y}_{\bullet} = \mathrm{E}_\xi \mathrm{E}(\hat{Y}_{\bullet} - Y_{\bullet})^2$, where the expectation E is taken first (over all possible samples) and then the expectation E_ξ (over all possible realizations of model ξ).

It appears at first sight that, since there are H strata, the search for the optimum needs to be conducted in H-dimensional space, but Kokic and Bell showed that under mild conditions the H expressions $(g_h - 1)(K_{hO} - \mu_h)$, where K_{hO} is the optimal value of K_h, were each asymptotically equal (for large N_h and n_h) to the optimal bias in $\hat{Y}_{\bullet}$. In general, this bias is $B = \sum_h \sum_i \delta_{hi} g_{hi}\{Y_{hi}(K_h) - Y_{hi}\}$ and Kokic and Bell showed that its optimal value was $B_O = \hat{Y}_{\bullet} - Y_{\bullet} = -(n-1)^{-1} \times \sum_h n_h(g_h - 1)(K_{hO} - \mu_h)$, the subscript O indicating that the corresponding value has been optimized. This result reduces the search in H dimensions to one in a single dimension only.

Their search for the optimum was carried out as follows. Since, in practice, B is almost always negative, the authors denoted the quantity $-B$ by L, and $-B_O$ by L_O, both of which are typically positive. They then showed that, if the H asymptotically equal expressions $(g_h - 1)(K_h - \mu_h)$ were regarded as *exactly* equal, it followed that $K_{hO} = (g_h - 1)L_O + \mu_h$ for all h and that $L_O = \sum_h n_h(g_h - 1)\{\mathrm{E}_\xi(Y_h J_h) - K_h \mathrm{E}_\xi J_h\}$.

Writing $Y^*_{hi} = (n_n^{-1} N_h - 1)(Y_{hi} - \mu_h)$, $K^*_h = (n_n^{-1} N_h - 1)(K_h - \mu_h)$ and, in addition, $J^*_h = 1$ if $Y^*_h \geq L$ but $J^*_h = 0$ otherwise, their sample estimate of L_O is the value for which $F(L) = 0$, where

$$F(L) = L\left[1 + \sum_h \sum_i I(Y^*_{hi} \geq L)\right] - \sum_h \sum_i Y^*_{hi} I(Y^*_{hi} \geq L)$$

where $I(Y^*_{hi} \geq L)$ takes the value one if Y_{hi} is greater than or equal to L, and the value zero otherwise. The search for L_O is thus simplified to evaluating $F(L)$ for L set first to the largest value of the Y^*_{hi} and then to successively smaller values until eventually $F(L)$ becomes negative. Linear interpolation between the Y^*_{hi} yielding the last positive value and first negative value of $F(L)$ leads to the optimal sample estimate of L_O.

14.13 The following simple example illustrates how Kokic and Bell's Winsorization can be put into practice. Only a single stratum is considered, since the transformation of the Y_{hi} into Y^*_{hi} allows all strata to be considered simultaneously, and that transformation is required even if there is only a single stratum.

Consider, then, a sample of $n = 10$ units from a population of $N = 110$. The sample fraction is $f = n/N = 1/11$. The sample interval is $g = f^{-1} = 11$. The 10 sample Y-values are:

$$1, 2, 3, 4, 5, 6, 7, 8, 23, 141; \qquad \text{sample take 200, mean 20.}$$

The unbiased expansion estimate for the total is $\hat{Y}_{\bullet} = 11 \times 200 = 2200$. The sample variance is:

$$\begin{aligned} \hat{S}^2 &= (10-1)^{-1}(19^2 + 18^2 + 17^2 + 16^2 + 15^2 + 14^2 + 13^2 + 12^2 + 3^2 + 121^2) \\ &= 9^{-1}(361 + 324 + 289 + 256 + 225 + 196 + 169 + 144 + 9 + 14\,641) \\ &= 9^{-1} \times 16\,614 = 1846. \end{aligned}$$

The estimated variance of the expansion estimate is

$$110 \times (11 - 1) \times 1846 = 2\,030\,600 \cong 1425^2.$$

The estimated standard error of the expansion estimate is therefore approximately 1425, or 64.8% of the estimated total. This completes the preliminary calculations.

14.14 To find the Kokic–Bell minimum MSE estimate of total requires ten steps.

1. Transform the Y-values to Y^*-values by mean-correcting and multiplying by $g-1$. The Y^*-values are:

$$-190, -180, -170, -160, -150, -140, -130, -120, 30, 1210;$$

sample take 0, mean 0.

2. Calculate $F(L)$ for $L = 1210$ (only the largest Y^*-value is Winsorized):

$$F(1210) = 1210(1+1) - 1210 = 2420 - 1210 = 1210.$$

3. Calculate $F(L)$ for $L = 30$ (the two largest Y^*-values are now Winsorized):

$$F(30) = 30(1+2) - (1210+30) = 90 - 1240 = -1150.$$

This is the first negative value for $F(L)$.

4. Interpolate linearly between $L = 1210$ and $L = 30$. (Note that only the largest value of Y^* is definitively Winsorized.) The next trial value of L is

$$L = 30 + \frac{(1210 - 30) \times 1150}{1210 + 1150}$$
$$= 30 + 1180 \times \frac{1150}{2360} = 30 + 575 = 605.$$

(Note that 605 is precisely half of 1210. It is in fact always the case, when only the largest unit is Winsorized, that L is half of the largest transformed value.)

5. Calculate $F(L)$ for $L = 605$:

$$F(605) = 605(1+1) - 1210 = 1210 - 1210 = 0.$$

So $L = 605$ is confirmed as the optimal choice.

6. Calculate the Winsorized value (i.e. find the $Y^*(L)$-value) to replace the largest Y^*-value. For convenience we order the Y^*- values in ascending order of size, so that the largest such value is $Y_n^* = 1210$. Then,

$$fY_n^* = 11^{-1} \times 1210 = 110 \quad \text{and} \quad (1-f)L = 10 \times 11^{-1} \times 605 = 550.$$

So $Y_n^*(605) = 110 + 550 = 660$.

7. Back-transform L to K and $Y_n^*(L)$ to $Y_n(K)$:

$$K = (605/10) + 20 = 80.5 \quad \text{and} \quad Y_n(K) = (660/10) + 20 = 86.$$

Alternatively,

$$Y_n(K) = Y_n(80.5) = (11^{-1} \times 141 + 10 \times 11^{-1} \times 80.5) = 86.$$

8. Calculate the Winsorized estimate of total and estimate its bias. After Winsorization, the 10 sample Y-values are:

$$1, 2, 3, 4, 5, 6, 7, 8, 23, 86; \qquad \text{sample take } 145, \text{ mean } 14.5.$$

(Check: the new sample take is $200 - 141 + 86 = 145$.) The Winsorized estimate of total is therefore $11 \times 145 = 1595$. The estimated bias of the Winsorized estimate of total is $B = 1595 - 2200 = -605$.
9. Compare the values of L and $-B$. We have $L = 605$ and $-B = 605$. This equality of the two absolute values is brought about by the estimation process. The best *estimates* are, in fact, necessarily equal, even though the ideal values are equal only asymptotically.
10. Compare the estimated MSEs of the expansion estimate and of the Winsorized estimate. From Section **14.13**, the estimated MSE and the estimated variance of the unbiased expansion estimate are the same at 2 030 600, and the estimated standard error of that estimate is therefore approximately 1425 or 64.8% of the estimated total. The sample variance after Winsorization is:

$$\begin{aligned}\hat{S}^2 &= (10-1)^{-1}(13.5^2 + 12.5^2 + 11.5^2 + 10.5^2 + 9.5^2 + 8.5^2 + 7.5^2 \\ &\quad + 6.5^2 + 8.5^2 + 31.5^2) \\ &= (10-1)^{-1}(182.25 + 156.25 + 132.25 + 110.25 + 90.25 \\ &\quad + 72.25 + 56.25 + 42.25 + 72.25 + 992.25) \\ &= 1906.5/9 \cong 211.833.\end{aligned}$$

The estimated variance of the Winsorized estimate is therefore approximately $110 \times (11 - 1) \times 211.833 \cong 233\,017$. The estimated standard error of the Winsorized estimate is thus approximately 482.7, or 30.3% of the estimate itself. The square of the estimated bias of the Winsorized estimate is $605^2 = 366\,025$. The estimated MSE of the Winsorized estimate is therefore approximately $233\,017 + 366\,025 = 599\,042 \cong 774^2$, and the estimated root mean squared error of that estimate is therefore approximately 774 or 48.5% of the estimate itself; not much more than half than the original 1425, and appreciably less than the original 64.8%.

Remark 14.14.1 Not only is the estimated variance of the estimate of total substantially decreased by Winsorization; in this example at least, its estimated RMSE is also decreased in relative terms. While this relative decrease in RMSE cannot be guaranteed, it appears to happen in the great majority of cases.

Remark 14.14.2 Kokic and Bell further recommend that the optimum value of L be estimated using previous survey data and supply formulae for doing this.

Spreading the Estimated Bias Back

14.15 For all its attraction, the Winsorized estimator is a biased estimator, and the bias is always downwards. If that estimator is used in stratum after stratum, the estimate for each individual stratum may represent an improvement on every occasion it is used, but with the biases always being in the same direction and the relevant contribution to the MSE being the *square* of that bias, the estimate for the entire population may well end up with a larger MSE than if the expansion estimator had consistently been used instead. (This is true, regardless of whether the Winsorizing is used in its original form to modify individual values only, or in the recast form described above, in which it is used to change the weights instead.)

It seems to us that what should be done (though we have not been able to find any reputable authority offering this suggestion) is to specify the domain within which a large value should be treated as extreme. One such value might, for instance, be regarded as extreme for its individual stratum (defined, for example, by its state, industry and size) but not as extreme for its state by industry classification. In that case, the estimated bias (calculated as the difference between the expansion and adjusted estimate) could be spread proportionately over all the size strata within that classification as an additional component of each stratum's estimate. A group of larger values could be regarded as extreme for the state by industry classification, but not as extreme for a group of related industries within the state, or perhaps for the state as a whole, or even for the entire nation. Except in that last case, the rule would be to use the adjusted estimate at the level for which the extremeness was recognized, but to spread the estimated bias proportionately over the next level up.

Something different is, of course, required where there is no next level up. Several options are nevertheless available even in this instance.

1. The best option is to ensure that there are no such observations defined at this level. Such exceptional observations should hardly ever come as a surprise, and they would not do so if there were competent subject-matter experts around who knew their collections.
2. The next best option is to carry out an investigation after the event to make sure that there are no more such instances. (If carried out competently, there seldom would be any.)
3. Failing both of these, the *assumption* can be made that there are in fact no other such instances. ('If there were, we should have heard of them by now. Yes, we should also have known about this one, and we've taken steps to ensure we won't be caught napping again…')
4. Finally, if, for some good reason such an assumption cannot be made, the last resort would be to regard the large value as extreme even at the national level, but not over an extended time period. At every survey round, the negative bias could then be estimated, and the aim should be to ensure that it was zero more often than not. But even if the worst came to the worst, after a few rounds we should have some idea of what the average bias was going to be, and be able to adjust for it accordingly.

14.16 Early in **14.9** we drew a distinction between weight modification and value modification, and showed that there was a value-modification method that corresponded exactly to any weight-modification method and vice versa, which gave us an excuse to consider either method on its own. We also indicated there that our own preference was for weight modification.

We should warn you that in espousing weight modification to the virtual exclusion of value modification, we have pitched ourselves in what is most probably a minority camp; also that in advocating the spreading out of bias, as we have just done, we are almost certainly in a very small minority. In fact our stance might well be regarded as odd-ball, and we feel the need to explain why we hold it.

First, then, why weight modification as opposed to value modification? Remember that we are dealing here with instances where there is evidence that the values we are considering are genuine. Extreme values that are not genuine typically occur in a single field and are out of kilter with other fields in the same record. They can be detected and appropriately adjusted by competent computer editing, the precise specification of which is outside the scope of this report. Suffice to say that they include (but are not exhaustively described by) arithmetical consistency checks, absolute difference checks, ratio checks within ranges, and coding checks. They are typically highly survey-specific, and require input from people with good subject-matter knowledge.

If, then, we are dealing with extreme values that are *prima facie* genuine, we are in all probability dealing with not just one extreme value within the record, but several at least, and perhaps many. Moreover, since they would probably not be unrelated, it would be unrealistic to modify each extreme value without taking into account extreme values in other fields of the same record. But if the record is to be treated as a whole, it is more straightforward to modify its weight than its individual fields. Weight modification based on the Winsorization of a particularly sensitive variable is a simple and obvious choice; and the simpler and more obvious the choice, the greater the chance of it being generally adopted (Schelling, 1980, pp. 54–67).

Summary and Concluding Remarks

14.17 It is (almost by definition) impossible to deal adequately with all types of extreme values and unusual events in any report of finite length. Nevertheless, we believe we have covered here the major sources of such problems, and we hope that in the course of this review we have conveyed enough of the spirit of what is required to tackle with some confidence unusual circumstances that we have not been able to cover.

The most important distinction is between genuine and spurious instances of such values and events. In order to decide on the category to which any given value or event belongs, the first requirement is a close acquaintance with the population being surveyed. There are almost always relationships between variables within a record that provide clues. For instance, there is typically a fairly stable relationship between the volume and the monetary value of a manufactured product. If volume goes up sharply and value remains the same, it is quite likely that one of the two has been recorded incorrectly. If both are correct, the price per unit must have fallen considerably, and there is almost certainly a simple reason why this should have been so, and someone with a knowledge of the industry should be able to explain it. The question then arises whether the price per unit fell only for a single respondent, or for some, or for most or all of them. Once there is a clear idea of what the possibilities are, an informed decision can usually be made as to which of the extreme observations are genuine and which are spurious. The relevant and recognizable subsets of Section **14.2** and the unusual population units mentioned in **14.3** and **14.4** are examples of genuine rarities. Sections **14.5** and **14.6** deal with the recognition of spurious extreme values.

14.18 Once an extreme value has been recognized as genuine, there are several ways of proceeding. The first is to treat it in the same way as an observation on any other sample unit. This is equivalent to assuming that it is as much representative of a particular part of the population as each other sample unit is representative of some other part. Under that assumption, the usual estimator is unbiased, but has high variance.

A second way to treat it is to remove the extreme-valued sample unit from both the sample and from the population of the stratum in which it is located, and to add its value on separately. This has a long history behind it, but should probably be considered now as out of date. The principal problem with it is the sharp discontinuity between the high estimate yielded as long as the unit remains in the hth sampled stratum with weight g_h, and the much smaller estimate when its observed value is just high enough to exclude it from the hth sampled stratum and add it on with weight unity.

A third way is to Winsorize the individual extreme observed value(s) only, leaving all the other survey and supplementary values unchanged. This gets rid of the sharp discontinuities, but generally distorts the relationships among the variables in those records containing Winsorized observations. The Kokic–Bell procedure for Winsorization is described in **14.10–14.14**.

The fourth way (which we recommend) is to Winsorize on the basis of the variable most prone to extreme values, but, instead of modifying the extreme values themselves, to modify the weight of each affected sample unit in such a manner that the unit's contribution to the sample estimate for that sensitive variable is the same as it would have been had its value for that variable been Winsorized and its weight unchanged. This also gets rid of the sharp discontinuities, while avoiding the distortion of the relationships among the variables.

Response from Supervisor

14.19 Thank you for your comprehensive treatment of an intrinsically difficult topic. Once again your approach has been somewhat unorthodox, but you hail from an unorthodox tradition and I can see that this independence of approach has washed off on you. The important question, as always, is 'Does it work?' and you have clearly signalled where you have your own experience (or others') to back your ideas up, and where you do not. I am prepared to give a trial to some of your speculative ideas, even those on the use of weight modification based on an initial Winsorization and those on spreading back the bias, just as long as you understood that the proof of the pudding will have to be in the eating!

Looking back on the ever lengthening list of reports that you have been writing for me recently, I can see a few gaps, such as the design of longitudinal surveys, that we have not covered, but longitudinal surveys (like the treatment of extreme values) is a notoriously difficult topic to tackle, and I know you have not had contact with anyone with any appreciable experience in that area; so I will spare you that.

The one remaining topic that we cannot afford to ignore, I believe, is that of replicate methods of estimation. It is just too widely used. I remember that at the end of Chapter 11 you indicated that you were not too enthusiastic about them, and I also know that your experience of them has been limited, but at least you need to tell me what they are and why they are so popular.

After that, I intend to leave you alone for a while to pursue your own choice of investigations – subject, of course, to the imperative that we have to take on enough consultation work to be able to survive – and you can see how much you learned yourselves (and taught me) as a result of your dealing with the circus contract. Applications stimulate research, and research expedites applications. Finding the right balance is my job now and I trust will be yours one day. Just never pass up any opportunity to learn.

Exercises

14.1 Consider a stratified sample of $n_1 = 6$ units from a population of $N_1 = 132$ and $n_2 = 4$ from a population of $N_2 = 44$. The sample Y-values are:

Stratum 1	1, 2, 3, 4, 5, 6;	sample take 21, mean 3.5;
Stratum 2	7, 8, 23, 141;	sample take 179, mean 44.75.

Repeat the analysis of Section **14.14**, taking account of the stratification. What are the main similarities? What are the main differences? Comment.

15

Resampling Methods of Variance Estimation: the Jackknife and the Bootstrap

Report to Supervisor: Introduction 283
Jackknifing the Variance 284
Bootstrapping the Variance 285
Some Semi-empirical and Empirical Findings 286
Response from Supervisor 287
Exercise 287

Report to Supervisor: Introduction

15.1 Resampling methods are widely used to provide variance estimates in situations where direct estimators are difficult to derive, of uncertain quality or awkward to handle. You will recall, however, that in **11.16** we were less than enthusiastic about the use of resampling methods for the estimation of variance. We should perhaps commence by briefly restating our reasons.

1. Resampling methods are only useful where no simple, efficient and direct estimator of variance is easily available. In the past, there have been problems with estimating the design variance of the HTE and GREG estimators of total, but with the theory presented in Chapter 9 this should no longer be a problem.
2. If there is an efficient direct estimator available, resampling methods can never improve on it.
3. On the contrary, resampling methods used in practice frequently ignore relevant information, such as that the sample had been selected without replacement, or that the sample had been stratified. Where such information is taken into account, the complexity of the calculations is appreciably increased (Jones, 1974).
4. Resampling methods typically require larger amounts of programming, CPU time, memory and storage than do direct estimation methods.

We would not deny, however, that resampling methods can sometimes be useful, and not only with variance estimation. The jackknife, for instance, was originally suggested as a way of reducing the bias of an estimator, and the bootstrap can also be used for that purpose. Even if the types of sampling that we characteristically use do not seem to call for resampling methods, it is as well to know what they are and what purpose they serve, for the occasion might arise where they would in fact be useful. In what follows below we will limit ourselves to the jackknife and the bootstrap as applied to variance estimation in the context of finite-population sampling.

Jackknifing the Variance

15.2 The jackknife was introduced by Quenouille (1949) as a method for reducing the bias of an estimator. It was Tukey (1958) who suggested that it might be used to estimate variances. Durbin (1959) used it to estimate variances in the context of finite-population sampling. More detailed accounts, such as that by Wolter (1985), are now readily available.

The jackknife variance estimator in most common use (the *delete-one jackknife*) operates as follows. Suppose there is some parameter θ that we wish to estimate from a sample of n values, Y_i, $i = 1, 2, \ldots, n$. The estimate of θ from the whole sample is denoted by $\hat{\theta}$, and the estimate from the sample obtained by dropping the ith sample unit is denoted by $\hat{\theta}_{(i)}$. Next we define what is known as the ith *pseudo-value* by $\hat{\theta}_i = n\hat{\theta} - (n-1)\hat{\theta}_{(i)}$. The mean of these pseudo-values, Tukey's *jackknife estimator* of θ, is denoted by $\hat{\theta}_{JK}$. If $\hat{\theta}$ has a proportionate bias that is $O(n^{-1})$, the proportionate bias of $\hat{\theta}_{JK}$ is only $O(n^{-2})$. Tukey's *jackknife variance estimator*, for both $\hat{\theta}$ and $\hat{\theta}_{JK}$, is $\hat{\mathrm{V}}_{JK}\hat{\theta} = n^{-1}(n-1)\sum_{i=1}^{n}(\hat{\theta}_i - \hat{\theta}_{JK})^2$.

15.3 For a finite population of N units, the population total is $Y_{\bullet} = \sum_i Y_i$ and the population mean is $\bar{Y} = N^{-1}\sum_i Y_i = N^{-1}Y_{\bullet}$. Given an *srswr* or *srswor* sample of n sample units, the mean of the y variable for the entire sample of n observations is $\hat{\bar{Y}} = n^{-1}\sum_{i=1}^{N}\nu_i Y_i$ or $\hat{\bar{Y}} = n^{-1}\sum_{i=1}^{N}\delta_i Y_i$, respectively, and the expansion estimator of $Y_{\bullet}$ is $\hat{Y}_{\bullet} = N\hat{\bar{Y}}$. The pseudo-values $\bar{Y}_i$ are then identical with the original Y_i, so the jackknife variance estimator for the mean is identical in form with the ordinary *srswr* variance for the mean. This is the case regardless of whether the sampling is with or without replacement (*srswr* or *srswor*).

Since the variance estimator that is design-unbiased for *srswor* is smaller than the one for *srswr* by the factor $1-f$, where $f = n/N$, the unadjusted jackknife estimator of variance overestimates the *srswor* variance by the factor $(1-f)^{-1}$ or $N/(N-n)$. So when sampling is *srswor*, the adjustment factor $1-f$ is required.

To estimate the population total we simply multiply the individual observations, Y_i, by N, and the same procedure applies as was used to estimate the mean.

15.4 The same procedure carries over almost unchanged when sampling is carried out with unequal probabilities. In that context, we estimate the population total more frequently than we estimate the population mean, so we shall consider estimation of the population total only.

Consider the case where sampling is $\pi ps wor$. Individual observations that are comparable in size with the population total may be written $Z_i = nY_i\pi_i^{-1}$.

The HTE is $\hat{Y}_{\bullet HT} = \bar{Z} = \sum_{i=1}^{N} \delta_i Y_i \pi_i^{-1}$, the delete-one values of the HTE are $Z_{(i)} = (n - 1)^{-1} \sum_{j(\neq i)=1}^{N} \delta_j Z_j$, the corresponding pseudo-values are $\hat{Z}_i = \sum_{j=1}^{N} \delta_j Z_j - (n - 1)Z_{(i)} = Z_i$, and the jackknife estimator of total is simply $\hat{Y}_{\bullet JK} = \hat{Y}_{HT}$. The jackknife variance estimator is therefore $\hat{V}_{JK} \hat{Y}_{\bullet JK} = n^{-1}(n-1) \times \sum_{i=1}^{N} (Z_i - \hat{Y}_{HT})^2$. The finite-population correction factor is therefore simply omitted unless it is explicitly supplied. For high entropy selection procedures it is usually taken to be $1 - f$ outside the summation sign, but the results of Chapter 9 imply a finite-population correction factor $\{n/(n-1)\}(c_i^{-1} - \pi_i)$ inside the summation sign. Whether that would still be the appropriate factor to apply to the pseudo-values on a case-by-case basis, however, is not immediately clear.

Bootstrapping the Variance

15.5 The bootstrap method (Efron, 1979) was originally designed for use with independent observations. In survey sampling, sampling without replacement gives rise to observations that are not independent, so, as with the jackknife, the question arises as to how to adjust for the finite-population correction when sampling without replacement.

First, however, we consider how the original bootstrap works. Suppose there is a population U with a parameter θ which we seek to estimate by $\hat{\theta}$, and we wish to estimate its variance, $V\hat{\theta}$. Bootstrapping originally involved the following steps.

1. A sample, s, of n independently selected units is drawn from U.
2. Using the data from s, a *resampling population*, U^*, is created, resembling U as closely as possible.
3. A series of *bootstrap samples*, s^*, each one usually also of size n, is drawn independently from U^*.
4. For each bootstrap sample, a bootstrap replicate estimate, $\hat{\theta}_b^* = \hat{\theta}(s_b^*)$, is computed, $b = 1, 2, \ldots, B$, using the same estimator to infer from s_b^* to U^* as was used initially to infer from s to U.
5. If B is large enough, the observed distribution of the $\hat{\theta}_b^*$ approximates the sampling distribution of $\hat{\theta}$, and (if the s^* are each of size n) then $V\hat{\theta}$ can be estimated by $\hat{V}\hat{\theta} = (B-1)^{-1} \sum_{b=1}^{B} (\hat{\theta}_b^* - \bar{\hat{\theta}}^*)^2$, where $\bar{\hat{\theta}}^*$ is the mean of the $\hat{\theta}_b^*$.

If sampling is *srswor* from a finite population, U, the following modifications are needed.

1. The sample, s, of n units, is drawn from U using *srswor*.
2. The series of *bootstrap samples*, s^*, is drawn from U^* in the same way as s was drawn from U, that is, using *srswor*.

If sampling is π*pswor*, corresponding changes are required to steps 1 and 2, and in addition a special procedure must be used at step 2. To cut a longish story short, if the ith population unit of U is included in the sample s, the number of units it contributes to the population U^* must be as nearly as possible equal to the inverse of its inclusion probability, that is, to π_i^{-1}. But since π_i^{-1} is not generally an integer, the fractions left over must only contribute to U^* with probabilities equal to their size. In consequence, the size of U^* will be a random variable, and it would probably be best to force it to be equal to the original size N using the rounding techniques described for numbers of clusters in Chapters 10 and 11.

In addition, it would be possible, occasionally, for a unit with very small inclusion probability to be selected in the sample s, with the consequence that the population U^* would be dominated by a very large number of very small units. To prevent this happening (and, in any case, to avoid the possibility of very large raising factors giving rise to estimates with very high variance), experienced sampling statisticians usually set a minimum value to the probability of inclusion in sample for any population unit. The minimum set may vary depending on the situation, but we imagine it would typically be in the range 0.001 to 0.01.

It will be seen, in any case, that the construction of the population U^* can sometimes involve a certain amount of common sense. The application of the approaches set down in Chapter 14 for dealing with atypical and unexpected situations is likely to be useful in such circumstances.

Some Semi-empirical and Empirical Findings

15.6 In the postscript to our report in Chapter 9 (Section **9.13**) we presented a small amount of semi-empirical and empirical data that suggested but did not conclusively demonstrate the following inferences.

1. Direct estimation of variance is usually less biased than resampling inference.
2. Resampling methods can nevertheless produce more stable variance estimates (perhaps particularly so in the presence of extreme and influential observations). Consequently, resampling methods may be appropriate for small domains and direct methods for large domains.
3. Bootstrapping unequal probability samples (in addition to being a delicate operation that should be approached with caution, as indicated in **15.5**) is unlikely to produce better estimates than the direct estimation methods.
4. When using the delete-one jackknife (and presumably also other jackknives) the unadjusted estimator pays no attention as to whether sampling is with or without replacement and therefore overestimates the variance by a factor that is approximately $N/(N-n)$. We do not know whether a better adjustment factor than $(N-n)/N$ is yet available.

In summary, we are not yet convinced about the value of resampling methods, and believe that they have been oversold; but in the same way as we were prepared to give a hearing to prediction-based inference, we are prepared to give a hearing to resampling methods also. The case is far from closed.

Response from Supervisor

15.7 Well, that's life. Never completely free from loose ends. But I think you've still earned that respite I promised you. Enjoy.

Exercise

15.1 Examine Tables 9.6 and 9.7.

(a) To what extent (if any) do they provide support for the consultants' scepticism regarding the use of resampling methods?
(b) Are there any ways in which resampling methods might have been used more effectively in the context of the postscript to Chapter 9?

Epilogue

The Most Important Topic Left Out

The Other Statistical Inference Controversy 288
Statistical Inference under Tractable Distributions 288
The Inference Problem When the Distributions are Intractable 291

The Other Statistical Inference Controversy

It may seem strange that this book, which is so concerned with the question of statistical inference in the context of survey sampling, should have scarcely raised the even more fundamental issue of statistical inference in general. My excuse is that in this particular field it hardly ever matters, and there are two reasons why. One applies chiefly in the context of samples of individuals and households, while the other is more relevant to samples of businesses and institutions. I will limit myself to considering the differences between frequentist and Bayesian inference. (Other inferential approaches exist, but few statisticians follow them.)

Statistical Inference under Tractable Distributions

When sampling individuals and households, the population units are small and comparatively homogeneous. For samples that are large enough to produce useful statistics (and there are few samples of less than 500 individuals that do that) the central limit theorem and the normal distribution are already well on the way to taking over. Now, except where it comes to hypothesis testing, the inferences that Bayesians make about samples from the normal distribution are very similar to those that statisticians in the frequentist tradition of Neyman and Pearson make. An introduction to the Bayesian approach to estimation and confidence (or credibility) intervals, written by my colleague, Borek Puza, is presented in the Postscript that follows this Epilogue.

Hypothesis testing is, by contrast, a crucial area of difference between Bayesian and frequentist inference. Given the same data, the Bayesian approach is substantially less likely to reject a null hypothesis than the frequentist. There are at least two substantial reasons for this. The first is that frequentists work in terms of areas under the probability density function, while Bayesians work in terms of its ordinates. Ratios of ordinates are generally less spectacular than ratios of areas. (Bayesians like to say that they make inferences in terms of the likelihood of events that have been observed, while the frequentists make inferences in terms of the low probability of events that haven't even happened. It must be admitted that they have a point.)

The other (and at least equally important) reason why the Bayesian is substantially less likely to reject a null hypothesis than the frequentist, is that Bayesian hypothesis tests have to specify a probability distribution over the alternative hypothesis. It is often difficult to specify a distribution that is sufficiently general to be a worthy alternative, and yet still have sufficient prior probability in the region where the observations are likely to fall for their likelihoods to be able to transform that prior into a respectable posterior probability. In fact, Bayesian hypothesis testing has been more than a bit problematical for more than four decades, even where the normal distribution is the only one involved. (If you are interested in how I believe it should be tackled, see Brewer, 1999c.)

But there is at least one situation where the nature of the alternative hypothesis is relatively unimportant, even for a Bayesian analysis. That is where the Bayesian can see at a glance that the data provide *no* evidence *against* the null hypothesis. If the frequentist analysis is simultaneously rejecting the null hypothesis, that leads to an instructive paradox.

Consider, for example, the following situation. An instrument measures position with an error that is uniformly distributed between -1 cm and $+1$ cm. It measures the position of a certain point as being at $+0.9999$ cm from the origin. The precise null hypothesis is that the point lies exactly at the origin. A frequentist and a Bayesian are asked what inference is to be drawn from that measurement.

The frequentist reasons this way: if the null hypothesis is true, an event has occurred with a (two-sided) probability of 0.0002 or less. By any reasonable criterion, this is an impressively rare event, and the null hypothesis should therefore be roundly rejected.

But the Bayesian sees things quite differently. Given that observation, the likelihood associated with the point being anywhere in the interval between -0.0001 cm and $+1.9999$ cm is the same, at 0.5. Outside those limits, the likelihoods are all zero. The location of the null hypothesis is exactly at the origin, 0.0000. It therefore lies *within* the region where the likelihood is 0.5. There is no point anywhere on the real line that has any greater likelihood. Indeed, everywhere on the real line outside that favoured interval, the likelihood is zero; so whatever prior probability was associated with that very large region has now been converted to a posterior probability of zero. Hence, if the prior probability associated with the null hypothesis was P_0, its posterior probability is at least P_0 now, and almost inevitably a good deal greater than P_0. In summary, the available data contain no evidence against the null hypothesis, but conclusive evidence against most of the interval associated with the alternative hypothesis. If the value $1 - P_0$ was insufficient to reject the null hypothesis before the observation was taken, the posterior probability associated with the alternative hypothesis (whatever that now may be) must still be insufficient to reject it.

What are we to make of this paradox? There could hardly be any greater conflict between the two conclusions. I suggest that both statisticians are partly right and partly wrong. The frequentist is right to say that, on the evidence he has available, either an extremely rare event has occurred or the null hypothesis is wrong.

He correctly smells a rat. But the Bayesian is also correct to say that, in terms of the situation as stated, there is no evidence against the null hypothesis.

The trouble lies, I suggest, with 'the evidence available', or equivalently with 'the situation as stated'. Both statisticians believed what they were told, that the machine's error distribution was uniform between -1 cm and $+1$ cm. It is that information (or rather that assumption) that leads to the paradox. Starting without it, what would you (the reader) conclude, if you were told simply that the machine could not be out by more than a centimetre, that the machine's reading was $+0.9999$ cm, and that it was strongly suspected that the relevant point was really at the origin? Would you not guess that the machine had a tendency to get stuck at the upper end, or perhaps either end, of its permissible readings? So suppose the error distribution was not uniform, but U-shaped. The frequentist might then conclude that a reading of $+0.9999$ cm was quite compatible with a p-value much larger than 0.0002, maybe even something close to $p = 0.5$. But even in the actual case, where he *was* told that the error distribution was uniform, he was still right in smelling a rat.

And the Bayesian was partly wrong. Bayesians tend to work within the situation they believe exists (or at least believe that they believe exists), and just allow Bayesian logic to move them around within it. The Bayesian in this paradox was complacently claiming that there was no evidence against the null hypothesis, because his axioms and logic were so easily capable of absorbing the 'situation as stated' and coming to a neat conclusion within it that happened to be right for the wrong reason. He had so neglected his olfactory talent, that he had become incapable of smelling the rat.

What I conclude from this paradox is that both the frequentist and Bayesian approaches have their place, and that it can be a very useful thing to know that they are disagreeing. My conjecture is that when they disagree sharply, there is likely to be something wrong with their shared assumptions.

There is something of an analogy here with what happens when randomization-based and prediction-based estimates of variance differ sharply. If all is well, and the estimator is unbiased, or nearly so, under both approaches, then the design expectation of the model variance and the model expectation of the design variance should be nearly the same. If their estimates differ sharply, then something is wrong. Perhaps the sample is atypical. Perhaps the model is misleading. Perhaps both. Perhaps neither, but something else I haven't thought of yet is causing the problem. Whatever it is or isn't, it needs to be looked into. (Know your collection!)

But the analogy cannot be pressed too far. Sample estimators can be devised that make sense under both sampling approaches simultaneously. I doubt that any test statistic could ever be devised that had the same signification for frequentist and Bayesian alike. The most that could be achieved in that direction, I believe, is a way of translating from one language to the other: 'If the frequentist is saying this, the Bayesian would be saying that' and vice versa. If a common distribution is shared, like the normal, then it is possible to convert a p-value into a likelihood ratio, and the converse also holds. But I doubt that anything more will ever be possible than a polite exchange of views, and maybe that is a good thing. We might need the residual friction to stimulate our imaginations!

The Inference Problem When the Distributions are Intractable

When sampling individuals and households, it might well be useful to have both the frequentist and the Bayesian approaches to inference up our sleeves, but I strongly suspect that when sampling businesses and institutions we can seldom profitably use either. The problem here is the intractable natures of the real-life finite populations, which are always springing surprises on the unsuspecting analyst. (That problem is not actually limited to samples of businesses and institutions. A population consisting of a million subsistence farmers and one secretive miserly billionaire would indubitably wreck the most carefully designed wealth survey.)

Putting it another way, what we typically face with such surveys are populations that have large but unknown skewnesses and kurtoses. They are finite, so *all* their moments are also finite, but we never know when or even whether the central limit theorem will take over. It is safer to assume that it hasn't, rather than that it has.

Frequentist sampling statisticians occasionally make a point of constructing confidence intervals based on the normal distribution, and testing to see whether they contain the nominal 5% beyond 1.96 standard errors (or whatever the relevant figure is from the appropriate t distribution). In my experience they seldom come close to it, and my solution is not to bother about it.

Confidence intervals are weird animals in any case. We tie ourselves in semantic knots to define them. Alexander (1994) does so in this way:

> Keep in mind that the particular sample we selected was one of many possible samples. . . . Different samples would give different results.
>
> If many samples were selected, then for approximately 95% of the samples, the confidence interval which would be calculated would contain the result that would be obtained from surveying the entire population.
>
> It sounds like someone's worst nightmare from Freshman Statistics [he comments] but it does two things:
>
> (a) It gives the reader a concrete image to reinforce the notion that there is uncertainty because of sampling error.
> (b) It precisely and completely states the fact upon which we expect the readers to base their statistical inferences about sampling error . . .
>
> I have to admit [he concludes] that what people would really like to know is the probability that the population value is in the confidence interval, which isn't exactly what we non-Bayesians can tell them.

In this short passage, Alexander exposes the two major difficulties that frequentists have with their public relations; namely, that 'people' find their concepts difficult to follow, and that if they actually take the trouble to understand them, they often decide that they are not what they really want.

Sometimes even some of us who claim to be statisticians forget what those concepts mean, and treat confidence intervals as though they were Bayesian credibility intervals. They aren't, of course, and because they aren't, they aren't really useful either, which is what tempts us to forget the fact. (As it happens, the *t* distribution derived as a confidence interval in Chapter 5 can also be viewed as a Bayesian credibility interval based on an improper uniform prior, but the two kinds of interval are not generally equivalent.)

Outside the statistical profession, an even larger proportion of people treat confidence intervals as though they were credibility intervals – 'If there are 19 chances in 20 of a true value lying within its 95% confidence interval, there must be 19 chances in 20 that the true value I'm interested in lies within this particular 95% confidence interval.' Call them the naïve Bayesians (or, perhaps more accurately the naïve fiducialists). Then there are the science-blinded, who use confidence intervals because everybody else does, confident chiefly that they will not get into trouble for doing so. Finally, there are the resigned pragmatists, an elite group who know very well that confidence intervals are not telling them what they really want to know, but also know that they *will* get into trouble if they *don't* use them.

So why don't I use more Bayesian credibility intervals in my sampling work? Simply because I'm usually not sure enough about what I believe regarding the population I am sampling from. Instead I fall back on the fact that I can produce estimates of variance, sometimes even unbiased estimates of variance. I don't pretend to know in detail what those variances might imply, and for that matter I don't think anybody else does. But I do know that the smaller those variances are, the better off my clients will be, and the better off I will be in consequence. Variances alone may not be very helpful in what is usually called statistical inference, but they are excellent at setting off alarm bells. Call me a pragmatist by all means, but I am not a resigned pragmatist. I know what is achievable, and I work contentedly within those constraints. And that is why there is almost nothing in this book about the most fundamental issue in statistical inference.

Postscript

Bayesian Methods for Estimation

Borek Puza

Example 1 294
Example 2 294

In this Postscript we will illustrate the Bayesian approach to estimation and confidence intervals (or 'credibility intervals', as they are sometimes termed in that context). Bayesian methods were introduced in the Epilogue, mainly in relation to hypothesis testing (which is the other main area of inference).

The Bayesian approach involves postulating a probability model for the data, wherein all quantities, including model parameters, are treated as random variables. This approach is an alternative to the frequentist, and in many situations leads to inferences that are identical or very similar.

The main reason why one might be tempted to choose the Bayesian approach over the frequentist is that the former is typically more convenient for dealing with complicated situations. In particular, Bayesian methods are highly suitable for incorporating prior information (which is often problematic for frequentists). Furthermore, there exist strategies (see below) for solving very complex Bayesian models with surprising ease.

In what follows we present two examples of how the Bayesian paradigm can be used to estimate the total weight of the herd of 50 elephants (see Appendix B). The first example assumes no information other than the weights of the five sample elephants. The second example incorporates knowledge of which elephants are bulls and which are cows (stratification), as well as the 48 eye estimates relative to the unknown weights of Sambo and Kara (covariate information). It will be of interest to compare the resulting inferences with those obtained using earlier strategies. Details of the Bayesian calculations (which may appear more complicated than they really are) can be found in Appendix C.

For an introduction to Bayesian theory the reader is referred to Box and Tiao (1973), Lee (1989) and Press (1989). For applications to survey sampling in particular, see Ericson (1969, 1988), Royall and Pfeffermann (1982) and Bolfarine and Zacks (1992). Details of some mathematical tools and software that are useful when dealing with complex Bayesian models can be found in Tanner (1993), Gelman *et al.* (1995), Gilks *et al.* (1996), Best *et al.* (1996) and Spiegelhalter *et al.* (1996).

Example 1

Suppose that we know only the weights of the $n=5$ sample elephants and the fact that they were obtained via *srswor* from the $N=50$ elephants in the herd. Then the following is a plausible Bayesian model which may be used as a basis for inference:

$$
\begin{aligned}
&(Y_i \mid \mu, \theta) \sim \text{i.i.d. } N(\mu, 1/\theta), \qquad i = 1, \ldots, N; \\
&f(\mu, \theta) \propto 1/\theta, \qquad -\infty < \mu < \infty, \quad \theta > 0.
\end{aligned}
$$

Here Y_i refers to the weight (in tonnes) of the ith elephant in the herd. It is postulated that these weights are conditionally independent and normally distributed random variables. The parameters of the underlying normal distribution, μ (the mean) and θ (the inverse variance, or 'precision') are assigned a joint prior distribution that is commonly accepted as being appropriate in the case of *a priori* ignorance (a further discussion of such 'uninformative' priors can be found in the given references).

The data in this context may be taken as the sample vector $Y_s = (Y_1, \ldots, Y_n) =$ (4.765, 3.032, 3.328, 3.427, 2.910), and the inferential target is the population total $\dot{Y} = Y_1 + \cdots + Y_N$ (which equals 194, by Appendix B). It can be shown (see Appendix C) that the posterior distribution of $\dot{Y}$ is given by

$$\left(\frac{\dot{Y} - a}{b} \,\middle|\, Y_s \right) \sim t(n-1),$$

where

$$a = N\bar{Y}_s, \qquad b^2 = \frac{N^2}{n}\left(1 - \frac{n}{N}\right) S_s^2,$$

in which

$$\bar{Y}_s = \frac{1}{n}\sum_{i=1}^{n} Y_i, \qquad S_s^2 = \frac{1}{n-1}\sum_{i=1}^{n} (Y_i - \bar{Y})^2$$

are the sample mean and sample variance, respectively. From this result an obvious point estimate of $\dot{Y} = 194$ is the posterior mean $E(\dot{Y} \mid Y_s) = a = 174$ (this is also the posterior mode and median). Also, a 99% interval estimate for $\dot{Y}$ is $(a \pm t_{0.025}(49)b) = (105, 243)$. It will be observed that these estimates are identical, both numerically and in form, to the first estimates computed in this book (see Chapter 1).

Example 2

We will now examine a more complicated scenario, where the sex of each elephant is known and there are available 48 eye estimates relative to the unknown weights of the 'reference' elephants Sambo and Kara (see Appendix B). We begin with some redefinitions for notational convenience.

Let Y_{ij} be the weight (in tonnes) of the jth elephant in the ith gender group (stratum), where $i = 1$ (males), 2 (females), $j = 1, \ldots, N$ and $N = 25$ (not 50). We will suppose that the sample units in each group are listed first, and the 'reference' elephant is listed last. Thus the male sample weights are Y_{11}, Y_{12} (Combo and Flimbo) and the female sample weights are Y_{21}, Y_{22}, Y_{23} (Linda, Pamela and Sara), Sambo's weight is Y_{1N}, and Kara's weight is Y_{2N}. The other weights are $Y_{13}, \ldots, Y_{1,N-1}$ (males) and $Y_{24}, \ldots, Y_{2,N-1}$ (females), in any fixed order (see Appendix B).

Next, let X_{ij} be the estimated number of reference elephants corresponding to Y_{ij}, where $i = 1, 2$ and $j = 1, \ldots, N - 1$. Thus for example, $X_{12} = 0.60$, meaning that Flimbo's weight has been estimated as 60% of Sambo's weight, i.e. $Y_{12} \cong 0.60 Y_{1N}$. Note that Y_{1N} is not known since Sambo was not selected into the sample.

Also let $y_{ij} = \log Y_{ij}$ and $x_{ij} = \log X_{ij}$ for all i, j.

Finally, let

$$
\begin{aligned}
y_i &= (y_{i1}, \ldots, y_{iN}), & y &= (y_1, y_2), \\
x_i &= (x_{i1}, \ldots, x_{i,N-1}), & x &= (x_1, x_2), \\
n_1 &= 2, \quad n_2 = 3, & & \\
y_{is} &= (y_{i1}, \ldots, y_{1n_i}), & y_s &= (y_{1s}, y_{2s}), \\
y_{ir} &= (y_{i,n_i+1}, \ldots, y_{1N}), & y_r &= (y_{1r}, y_{2r}).
\end{aligned}
$$

With these definitions, the following is a plausible Bayesian model for the 50 weights and 48 eye estimates:

$$
\begin{aligned}
&(x_{ij} \mid y, \phi, \theta, \mu_1, \mu_2) \sim \perp N(y_{ij} - y_{iN}, 1/\phi), \qquad i = 1, 2, \quad j = 1, \ldots, N - 1; \\
&(y_{ij} \mid \phi, \theta, \mu_1, \mu_2) \sim \perp N(\mu_i, 1/\theta), \qquad i = 1, 2, \quad j = 1, \ldots, N; \\
&f(\phi, \theta, \mu_1, \mu_2) \propto 1/(\phi\theta), \qquad \phi > 0,\ \theta > 0,\ -\infty < \mu_1 < \infty, -\infty < \mu_2 < \infty.
\end{aligned}
$$

In this hierarchical model, the 50 log-weights, y_{ij}, are conditionally independent and normally distributed with common variance $1/\theta$ and mean either μ_1 (males) or μ_2 (females). Also the 48 log-estimates, x_{ij}, are conditionally independent and normally distributed with common variance $1/\phi$. The model parameters, ϕ, θ, μ_1 and μ_2, are assigned an uninformative joint prior distribution (similar to the one in Example 1).

The mean of each x_{ij} in the model is specified as $y_{ij} - y_{iN}$. This is appropriate since X_{ij} is an estimate of Y_{ij}/Y_{iN}, and hence $\log X_{ij} = x_{ij}$ is an estimate of $\log(Y_{ij}/Y_{iN}) = \log Y_{ij} - \log Y_{iN} = y_{ij} - y_{iN}$.

The data may be written (x, y_s) (two vectors consisting of 48 and 5 elements, respectively), and the quantity of interest is the total weight of the 50 elephants, $\dot{Y} = \sum_{i=1}^{2} \sum_{j=1}^{N} Y_{ij}$, where $Y_{ij} = \mathrm{e}^{y_{ij}}$. For inference we require the posterior density, $f(\dot{Y} \mid x, y_s)$. Given this density, a point estimate of $\dot{Y}$ is the posterior mean,

$$
\hat{\dot{Y}} = \mathrm{E}(\dot{Y} \mid x, y_s) = \int_0^\infty \dot{Y} f(\dot{Y} \mid x, y_s)\, \mathrm{d}\dot{Y}
$$

(note that $\dot{Y} > 0$ with probability 1); and a 99% interval estimate for $\dot{Y}$ is (L, U), where L and U satisfy the equation

$$0.005 = \int_0^L f(\dot{Y} \mid x, y_s) \mathrm{d}\dot{Y} = \int_U^\infty f(\dot{Y} \mid x, y_s) \, \mathrm{d}\dot{Y}.$$

Unfortunately, the required posterior density, $f(\dot{Y} \mid x, y_s)$, is very difficult to evaluate analytically. However, the computational problems can be sidestepped via the Monte Carlo method; see Tanner (1993). This method involves making use of a large random sample, $\dot{Y}_1, \ldots, \dot{Y}_M$, from the posterior distribution of $\dot{Y}$. The Monte Carlo estimate of $\hat{\dot{Y}}$, and hence also of $\dot{Y}$, is then the average $\bar{\dot{Y}} = (\dot{Y}_1 + \cdots + \dot{Y}_M)/M$, and a 99% interval estimate of $\dot{Y}$, is $(q_{0.005}, q_{0.995})$, where q_p denotes the empirical p-quantile of $\dot{Y}_1, \ldots, \dot{Y}_M$. These point and interval estimates are consistent, in that they converge to the 'exact' estimates, $\hat{\dot{Y}}$ and (L, U) (see above), as M approaches infinity. (Confidence intervals can also be computed for the Monte Carlo estimates themselves, but these are of little practical importance if M is very large.)

The required sample, $\dot{Y}_1, \ldots, \dot{Y}_M \sim$ i.i.d. $f(\dot{Y} \mid x, y_s)$, can be obtained using Markov chain Monte Carlo (MCMC) methods, in particular a Metropolis–Hastings algorithm known as the Gibbs sampler. Details regarding these techniques can be found in the references mentioned earlier.

The Gibbs sampler was applied in our situation to generate a sample of size $M = 10\,000$. Exactly how this was done is outlined in Appendix C. The resulting point estimate of the total weight of the herd, $\dot{Y} = 194$, was $\bar{\dot{Y}} = 195$, with associated 99% interval estimate (181, 203). These estimates may be compared with the estimates obtained in Chapter 5, namely 198 and (178, 217).

We see that the two point estimates are very similar. Also, the Bayesian interval estimate is asymmetric and somewhat narrower than its counterpart. (As regards precision, the point estimate was in fact 195.30, with associated Monte Carlo 99% confidence interval for $\hat{\dot{Y}}$ equal to (195.20, 195.40).)

Note that we could 'refine' the above procedure by assigning separate variances to the male and female log-weights. This would involve replacing the variance $1/\theta$ by $1/\theta_i$ and specifying a relationship, either exact or stochastic, between θ_1 (males) and θ_2 (females). However, such a modification would probably result in little difference to our final conclusions.

Appendix A

Basu's Original Elephant Fable

The circus owner is planning to ship his 50 adult elephants and so he needs a rough estimate of their total weight. As weighing an elephant is a cumbersome process, the owner wants to estimate the total weight by weighing just one elephant. Which elephant should he weigh? So the owner looks back on his records and discovers a list of the elephants' weights taken 3 years ago. He finds that 3 years ago Sambo, the middle-sized elephant, was the average (in weight) elephant in his herd. He checks with the elephant trainer who reassures him (the owner) that Sambo may still be considered to be the average elephant in the herd. Therefore the owner plans to weigh Sambo and take $50\,y$ (where y is the present weight of Sambo) as an estimate of the total weight $Y = Y_1 + \cdots + Y_{50}$ of the 50 elephants. But the circus statistician is horrified when he learns of the owner's purposive sampling plan. 'How can you get an unbiased estimate of Y this way?' protests the statistician. So together they work out a compromise sampling plan. With the help of a table of random numbers they devise a plan that allots a selection probability of 99/100 to Sambo and equal probabilities of 1/4900 to each of the other 49 elephants. Naturally Sambo is selected, and the owner is happy. 'How are you going to estimate Y?' asks the statistician. 'Why? The estimate ought to be $50\,y$ of course', says the owner. 'Oh! No! That cannot possibly be right', says the statistician. 'I recently read an article in the *Annals of Mathematical Statistics* where it is proved that the Horvitz–Thompson estimator is the unique hyperadmissible estimator in the class of all generalized polynomial unbiased estimators.' 'What is the Horvitz–Thompson estimator in this case?' asks the owner, duly impressed. 'Since the selection probability in our plan was 99/100,' says the statistician, 'the proper estimate of Y is $100\,y/99$ and not $50\,y$.' 'And how would you have estimated Y', inquires the incredulous owner, 'if our sampling plan made us select, say, the big elephant Jumbo?' 'According to what I understand of the Horvitz–Thompson estimation method,' says the unhappy statistician, 'the proper estimate of Y would then have been $4900\,y$, where y is Jumbo's weight.' That is how the statistician lost his circus job (and perhaps became a teacher of statistics!).

Appendix B

The Circus's 50 Indian Elephants

	BULLS					COWS			
	NUMBERS		WEIGHTS			NUMBERS		WEIGHTS	
Name	Bulls' list	Full list	Actual (kg)	Estimated (Sambos)	Name	Cows' list	Full list	Actual (kg)	Estimated (Karas)
Anembo	1	2	4552	0.90	Amanda	1	1	3567	1.20
Bembo	2	3	4643	0.95	Brenda	2	4	3270	1.10
Combo*	3	5	4675	0.95	Cora	3	6	2971	1.00
Dumbo	4	8	5480	1.15	Delila	4	7	3028	1.00
Embo	5	9	4380	0.90	Edna	5	10	2588	0.85
Flimbo*	6	11	3032	0.60	Freda	6	12	2860	0.95
Gumbo	7	14	4299	0.85	Greta	7	13	2801	0.90
Hambo	8	15	4936	1.00	Hilda	8	16	2896	0.95
Ianambo	9	17	4307	0.85	Inana	9	18	3144	1.05
Jumbo	10	20	5917	1.25	Jemima	10	19	3338	1.15
Korombo	11	22	4646	0.95	Kara	11	21	3002	1.00
Limbo	12	23	5470	1.15	Linda*	12	24	3328	1.10
Mumbo	13	26	4635	0.95	Maia	13	25	2842	0.95
Nimbo	14	27	4625	0.95	Nora	14	28	3148	1.05
Olombo	15	29	4459	0.90	Olivia	15	30	3078	1.00
Potombo	16	32	4418	0.90	Pamela*	16	31	3427	1.10
Rambo	17	33	5106	1.10	Rebecca	17	34	3012	1.00
Sambo	18	35	4801	1.00	Sara*	18	36	2910	1.00
Timbo	19	38	3900	0.80	Tanya	19	37	3382	1.10
Urambo	20	40	4203	0.90	Una	20	39	2760	0.90
Vimbo	21	42	5385	1.15	Vera	21	41	2738	0.90
Wombo	22	44	4980	1.05	Wanda	22	43	3350	1.10
Xembo	23	45	5414	1.15	Xena	23	46	3017	1.00
Yalumbo	24	47	5225	1.10	Yenta	24	48	2754	0.90
Zombo	25	50	4415	0.90	Zenobia	25	49	3109	1.05

*Sample elephants. Weights known to narrator.

Appendix C

Details of Calculations in the Postscript

Borek Puza

Proof of the Result in Example 1 299
Outline of the Gibbs Sampler in Example 2 301

Proof of the Result in Example 1

The following shows how the result in Example 1 of the Postscript was obtained. We begin by noting that the joint posterior distribution of μ and θ is given by

$$f(\mu,\theta \mid Y_s) \propto f(\mu,\theta) f(Y_s \mid \mu,\theta) \overset{\mu,\theta}{\propto} \frac{1}{\theta} \prod_{i=1}^{n} \frac{1}{\sqrt{1/\theta}} \exp\left\{-\frac{(Y_i-\mu)^2}{2/\theta}\right\}$$

$$= \theta^{(n/2)-1} \exp\left\{-\frac{\theta}{2} \sum_{i=1}^{n} (Y_i-\mu)^2\right\}$$

$$= \theta^{(n/2)-1} \exp\left\{-\frac{\theta}{2}\left[(n-1)S_s^2 + n(\mu-\bar{Y}_s)^2\right]\right\}.$$

Hence

$$f(\theta \mid Y_s) = \int f(\mu,\theta \mid Y_s)\,\mathrm{d}\mu \overset{\theta}{\propto} \theta^{(n/2)-1} \exp\left\{-\frac{\theta}{2}(n-1)S_s^2\right\}$$

$$\times \sqrt{\frac{1}{\theta}} \int_{-\infty}^{\infty} \frac{1}{\sqrt{1/(n\theta)}\sqrt{2\pi}} \exp\left\{-\frac{(\mu-\bar{Y}_s)^2}{2/(n\theta)}\right\} \mathrm{d}\mu$$

$$= \theta^{((n-1)/2)-1} \exp\left\{-\frac{\theta}{2}(n-1)S_s^2\right\}$$

(since the last integral equals 1), which implies that $(\theta \mid Y_s) \sim \text{Gamma}\left(\frac{1}{2}(n-1), \frac{1}{2}(n-1)S_s^2\right)$. Also,

$$f(\mu \mid \theta, Y_s) \propto f(\mu,\theta \mid Y_s) \overset{\mu}{\propto} \exp\left\{-\frac{(\mu-\bar{Y}_s)^2}{2/(n\theta)}\right\};$$

hence $(\mu \mid \theta, Y_s) \sim N(\bar{Y}_s, 1/(n\theta))$.

Now the non-sample total $\dot{Y}_r = Y_{n+1} + \cdots + Y_N$ has a conditional distribution given by $(\dot{Y}_r \mid Y_s, \mu, \theta) = (\dot{Y}_r|\mu, \theta) \sim N(m\mu, m/\theta)$, where $m = N - n$ (the non-sample size). Hence $f(\dot{Y}_r \mid Y_s, \theta) = \int f(\dot{Y}_r \mid Y_s, \mu, \theta) f(\mu \mid Y_s, \theta)\,\mathrm{d}\mu$ must be proportional to the exponent of a quadratic in $\dot{Y}_r$. Thus $(\dot{Y}_r \mid Y_s, \theta) \sim N(u, v)$, where

$$\begin{aligned}
u &= \mathrm{E}(\dot{Y}_r \mid Y_s, \theta) = \mathrm{E}\{\mathrm{E}(\dot{Y}_r \mid Y_s, \mu, \theta) \mid Y_s, \theta\} = \mathrm{E}\{m\mu \mid Y_s, \theta\} = m\bar{Y}_s \\
v &= \mathrm{V}(\dot{Y}_r \mid Y_s, \theta) = \mathrm{E}\{\mathrm{V}(\dot{Y}_r \mid Y_s, \mu, \theta) \mid Y_s, \theta\} + \mathrm{V}\{\mathrm{E}(\dot{Y}_r \mid Y_s, \mu, \theta) \mid Y_s, \theta\} \\
&= \mathrm{E}\left\{\frac{m}{\theta} \,\middle|\, Y_s, \theta\right\} + \mathrm{V}\{m\mu \mid Y_s, \theta\} = \frac{m}{\theta} + \frac{m^2}{n\theta}.
\end{aligned}$$

Consequently, $(\dot{Y}_r \mid Y_s, \theta) \sim N(m\bar{Y}_s, k/\theta)$, where

$$k = m + \frac{m^2}{n} = \frac{N^2}{n}\left(1 - \frac{n}{N}\right).$$

It follows that the posterior density of $\dot{Y}_r$ is

$$\begin{aligned}
f(\dot{Y}_r \mid Y_s) &= \int f(\dot{Y}_r \mid Y_s, \theta) f(\theta \mid Y_s)\,\mathrm{d}\theta \\
&\overset{\dot{Y}_r}{\propto} \int_0^\infty \frac{1}{\sqrt{1/\theta}} \exp\left\{-\frac{(\dot{Y}_r - m\bar{Y}_s)^2}{2k/\theta}\right\} \theta^{((n-1)/2)-1} \exp\left\{-\frac{\theta}{2}(n-1)S_s^2\right\} \mathrm{d}\theta \\
&= \int_0^\infty \theta^{(n/2)-1} \exp\left\{-\frac{\theta}{2}\left[\frac{(\dot{Y}_r - m\bar{Y}_s)^2}{k} + (n-1)S_s^2\right]\right\} \mathrm{d}\theta \\
&\overset{\dot{Y}_r}{\propto} \left\{\frac{1}{2}\left[\frac{(\dot{Y}_r - m\bar{Y}_s)^2}{k} + (n-1)S_s^2\right]\right\}^{-n/2}.
\end{aligned}$$

But $\dot{Y} = n\bar{Y}_s + \dot{Y}_r$, so that $\dot{Y}_r - m\bar{Y}_s = (\dot{Y} - n\bar{Y}_s) - (N - n)\bar{Y}_s = \dot{Y} - N\bar{Y}_s$. Therefore

$$\begin{aligned}
f(\dot{Y} \mid Y_s) &\propto \left\{\frac{1}{2}\left[\frac{(\dot{Y} - N\bar{Y}_s)^2}{k} + (n-1)S_s^2\right]\right\}^{-n/2} \overset{\dot{Y}}{\propto} \left\{1 + \frac{(\dot{Y} - N\bar{Y}_s)^2}{k(n-1)S_s^2}\right\}^{-n/2} \\
&= \left\{1 + \frac{1}{n-1}\left(\frac{\dot{Y} - N\bar{Y}_s}{\sqrt{\frac{N^2}{n}\left(1 - \frac{n}{N}\right) S_s^2}}\right)^2\right\}^{-((n-1)+1)/2}.
\end{aligned}$$

It follows that

$$\left(\frac{\dot{Y} - N\bar{Y}_s}{\sqrt{\frac{N^2}{n}\left(1 - \frac{n}{N}\right) S_s^2}} \,\middle|\, Y_s\right) \sim t(n-1),$$

as required.

Outline of the Gibbs Sampler in Example 2

The Gibbs sampler in Example 2 of the Postscript involves the conditional distributions of the unknown quantities y_r, ϕ, θ, μ_1 and μ_2. These distributions are given by:

$$y_{ij} \sim N\left(\frac{\theta\mu_i + \phi(x_{ij} + y_{iN})}{\theta + \phi}, \frac{1}{\theta + \phi}\right), \qquad j = n_i + 1, \ldots, N-1, \ i = 1, 2;$$

$$y_{iN} \sim N\left(\frac{\theta\mu_i + \phi[(y_{i1} + \cdots + y_{i,N-1}) - (x_{i1} + \cdots + x_{i,N-1})]}{\theta + (N-1)\phi}, \frac{1}{\theta + (N-1)\phi}\right),$$
$$i = 1, 2;$$

$$\phi \sim \text{Gamma}\left(N - 1, \exp\left\{\frac{1}{2}\sum_{i=1}^{2}\sum_{j=1}^{N-1}[x_{ij} - (y_{ij} - y_{iN})]^2\right\}\right);$$

$$\theta \sim \text{Gamma}\left(N, \exp\left\{\frac{1}{2}\sum_{i=1}^{2}\sum_{j=1}^{N}(y_{ij} - \mu_i)^2\right\}\right);$$

$$\mu_i \sim N\left(\bar{y}_i, \frac{1}{N\theta}\right), \qquad i = 1, 2,$$

where $\bar{y}_i = (y_{i1} + \cdots + y_{iN})/N$. Each of these distributions is derived from the joint density of all quantities in the model, namely

$$\begin{aligned} f(x, y, \phi, \theta, \mu_1, \mu_2) &= f(x \mid y, \phi, \theta, \mu_1, \mu_2) f(y \mid \phi, \theta, \mu_1, \mu_2) f(\phi, \theta, \mu_1, \mu_2) \\ &\propto \prod_{i=1}^{2}\prod_{j=1}^{N-1}\frac{1}{\sqrt{1/\phi}}\exp\left\{-\frac{[x_{ij} - (y_{ij} - y_{iN})]^2}{2(1/\phi)}\right\} \\ &\quad \times \prod_{i=1}^{2}\prod_{j=1}^{N}\frac{1}{\sqrt{1/\theta}}\exp\left\{-\frac{(y_{ij} - \mu_i)^2}{2(1/\theta)}\right\} \times \frac{1}{\phi\theta}. \end{aligned}$$

Thus, for example, the conditional density of θ is

$$\begin{aligned} f(\theta \mid x, y, \phi, \mu_1, \mu_2) &\propto f(x, y, \phi, \theta, \mu_1, \mu_2) \\ &\overset{\theta}{\propto} \theta^{N-1}\exp\left\{-\theta\left[\frac{1}{2}\sum_{i=1}^{2}\sum_{j=1}^{N}(y_{ij} - \mu_i)^2\right]\right\}, \end{aligned}$$

which implies that

$$(\theta \mid x, y, \phi, \mu_1, \mu_2) \sim \text{Gamma}\left(N, \exp\left\{\frac{1}{2}\sum_{i=1}^{2}\sum_{j=1}^{N}(y_{ij} - \mu_i)^2\right\}\right).$$

The conditional distribution of ϕ can be obtained in a similar fashion. Each of the other conditional distributions requires that the square of an exponent be completed.

In our simulation, arbitrary 'starting values' of ϕ, θ, μ_1 and μ_2 were chosen. Then the above conditional distributions were sampled from, in the given sequence. At each draw all variables but one were fixed at their latest value. This was done 11 000 times in total. The last $M = 10\,000$ values of y_r were then used to compute the required M values of $\dot{Y}$, according to $\dot{Y} = T(y_s, y_r)$, where we define $T(c_1, \ldots, c_q) = e^{c_1} + \cdots + e^{c_q}$. The first 1000 iterations were 'discarded' as the 'burn-in', meaning a stage at which stochastic equilibrium has not yet occurred.

References

Aires, N. (2000) *Techniques to Calculate Exact Inclusion Probabilities for Conditional Poisson Sampling and Pareto πps Sampling Designs*. Doctoral thesis, Department of Mathematical Statistics, Chalmers University of Technology and Göteborg University, Göteborg, Sweden.

Aires, N. (2001) Comparisons between conditional Poisson sampling and Pareto sampling designs. In *ICES-II, Proceedings of the Second International Conference on Establishment Surveys*. Contributed paper in Section 46 on the included CD. American Statistical Association, Alexandria VA.

Alexander, C.H. (1994) Comment in the discussion of Smith (1994), 21–28.

Asok, C. and Sukhatme, B.V. (1976) On Sampford's procedure of unequal probability sampling without replacement. *Journal of the American Statistical Association*, **71**, 912–918.

Atmer, J., Thulin, G. and Bäcklund, S. (1975) Coordination of samples with the JALES technique. *Statistisk Tidskrift*, **13**, 443–450 (in Swedish with English summary).

Australian Bureau of Statistics (2000) Sample design for population surveys in the ABS. Transparencies for in-house training courses. ABS internal document.

Australian Bureau of Statistics (2001) *Labour Statistics: Concepts, Sources and Methods*. Cat. no. 6102.0. ABS, Canberra. http://www.abs.gov.au.

Basu, D. (1971) An essay on the logical foundations of survey sampling, Part One (with discussion). In V.P. Godambe and D.A. Sprott (eds), *Foundations of Statistical Inference*. Holt, Rinehart and Winston, Toronto, pp. 203–242.

Best, N.G., Spiegelhalter, D.J., Thomas, A. and Brayne, C.E.G. (1996) Bayesian analysis of realistically complex models. *Journal of the Royal Statistical Society, Series A*, **159**, 323–342.

Bolfarine, H. and Zacks, S. (1992) *Prediction Theory for Finite Populations*. Springer-Verlag, New York.

Box, G.E.P. (1979) Robustness in the strategy of scientific model building. In G.N. Wilkinson and R.L. Launer (eds), *Robustness in Statistics*. Academic Press, New York, pp. 201–236.

Box, G.E.P. and Tiao, G.C. (1973) *Bayesian Inference in Statistical Analysis*. Addison-Wesley, London.

Brewer, K.R.W. (1979) A class of robust sample designs for large scale surveys. *Journal of the American Statistical Association*, **74**, 911–915.

Brewer, K.R.W. (1995) Combining design-based and model-based inference. In B.G. Cox, D.A. Binder, B.N. Chinnappa, A. Christianson, M.J. Colledge and P.S. Kott (eds), *Business Survey Methods*. Wiley, New York, pp. 589–606.

Brewer, K.R.W. (1999a) Design-based or prediction-based inference? Stratified random vs stratified balanced sampling. *International Statistical Review*, **67**, 35–47.

Brewer, K.R.W. (1999b) Cosmetic calibration for unequal probability samples. *Survey Methodology*, **25**, 205–212.

Brewer, K.R.W. (1999c) Testing a precise null hypothesis using reference posterior odds. *Revista de la Real Academia de Ciencias Exactas Físicas y Naturales (Review of the Royal Academy of Sciences)*, **93**, 303–310. (This English-language volume is entitled *Bayesian Methods in the Sciences*.)

Brewer, K.R.W. (2001) Deriving and estimating an approximate variance for the Horvitz–Thompson estimator using only first order inclusion probabilities. In *ICES-II, Proceedings of the Second International Conference on Establishment Surveys*. Contributed paper in Section 30 on the included CD. American Statistical Association, Alexandria, VA.

Brewer, K.R.W. and Gregoire, T.G. (2001) Estimators for use with Poisson sampling and related selection procedures. In *ICES-II, Proceedings of the Second International Conference on Establishment Surveys*. American Statistical Association, Alexandria VA, pp. 279–288. (Also available as invited paper in Section 4 on the included CD.)

Brewer, K.R.W. and Hanif, M. (1970) Durbin's new multistage variance estimator. *Journal of the Royal Statistical Society, Series B*, **32**, 302–311.

Brewer, K.R.W. and Hanif, M. (1983) *Sampling with Unequal Probabilities*, Lecture Notes in Statistics 15. Springer-Verlag, New York.

Brewer, K.R.W. and Tam, S.-M. (1990) Is the assumption of uniform intra-class correlation ever justified? *Australian Journal of Statistics*, **32**, 411–423.

Brewer, K.R.W., Early, L.J. and Joyce, S.F. (1972) Selecting several samples from a single population. *Australian Journal of Statistics*, **14**, 231–239.

Brewer, K.R.W., Early, L.J. and Hanif, M. (1984) Poisson, modified Poisson and collocated sampling. *Journal of Statistical Planning and Inference*, **10**, 15–30.

Cassel, C.M., Särndal, C.-E. and Wretman, J. (1976) Some results on generalized difference estimation and generalized regression estimation for finite populations. *Biometrika*, **63**, 615–620.

Cochran, W.G. (1953) *Sampling Techniques*. Wiley, New York.

Cochran, W.G. (1963) *Sampling Techniques*, 2nd edn. Wiley, New York.

Cochran, W.G. (1977) *Sampling Techniques*, 3rd edn. Wiley, New York.

Deville, J.-C. (1999) Variance estimation for complex statistics and estimators: Linearization and residual techniques. *Survey Methodology*, **25**, 193–203.

Durbin, J. (1959) A note on the application of Quenouille's method of bias reduction to the estimation of ratios. *Biometrika*, **46**, 477–480.

Durbin, J. (1967) Design of multistage surveys for the estimation of sampling errors. *Applied Statistics*, **15**, 152–164.

Efron, B. (1979) Bootstrap methods: Another look at the jackknife. *Annals of Statistics*, **7**, 1–26.

Ericson, W.A. (1969) Subjective Bayesian models in sampling finite populations (with discussion). *Journal of the Royal Statistical Society, Series B*, **31**, 195–233.

Ericson, W.A. (1988) Bayesian inference in finite populations. In P.R. Krishnaiah and C.R. Rao (eds), *Handbook of Statistics, Vol. 6*. Elsevier Science Publishers, Amsterdam, pp. 213–246.

Furnival, G.M., Gregoire, T.G. and Grosenbaugh, L.R. (1987) Adjusted inclusion probabilities with 3P sampling. *Forest Science*, **33**, 617–631.

Gelman, A., Carlin, J.B., Stern, H.S. and Rubin, D.B. (1995) *Bayesian Data Analysis*. Chapman & Hall, London.

Gilks, W.R., Richardson, S. and Spiegelhalter, D.J. (eds) (1996) *Markov Chain Monte Carlo in Practice*. Chapman & Hall, London.

Godambe, V.P. (1955) A unified theory of sampling from finite populations. *Journal of the Royal Statistical Society, Series B*, **17**, 269–278.

Godambe, V.P. and Joshi, V.M. (1965) Admissibility and Bayes estimation in sampling finite populations, 1. *Annals of Mathematical Statistics*, **36**, 1707–1722.

Goodman, R. and Kish, L. (1950) Controlled selection – a technique in probability sampling. *Journal of the American Statistical Association*, **45**, 350–372.

Gregoire, T.G. (1999) Composite and calibration estimation with Grosenbaugh's 3p sampling. In L. Arvanitis (ed.), *Proceedings of the Symposium of Forest Biometricians Honoring Dr Lewis R. Grosenbaugh, May 12–13 1997*. University of Florida Press, Gainesville, pp. 45–67.

Grosenbaugh, L.R. (1964) Some suggestions for better sample-tree-measurement. In *Proceedings of the Society of American Foresters*, Oct. 1963. Society of American Foresters, Boston, MA and Bethesda, MD.

Grosenbaugh, L.R. (1965) Three-pee sampling theory and program THRP for computer generation of selection criteria. USDA Forest Service Research Paper PSW-21.

Gross, W.F., Bode, G., Taylor, J.M. and Lloyd-Smith, C.W. (1986) Some finite population estimators which reduce the contribution of outliers. In I.F. Francis, B.F.J. Manly and F.C. Lam (eds), *Proceedings of the Pacific Statistical Conference*, Auckland, NZ, 20–24 May 1985. North-Holland, Amsterdam.

Hájek, J. (1958) Some contributions to the theory of probability sampling. In *Bulletin of the International Statistical Institute: Proceedings of the 30th Session (Stockholm)*, Vol. 36, Book 3. ISI, The Hague, pp. 127–134.

Hájek, J. (1964) Asymptotic theory of rejection sampling with varying probabilities from a finite population. *Annals of Mathematical Statistics*, **35**, 1491–1523.

Hájek, J. (1981) *Sampling from a Finite Population*. Marcel Dekker, New York.

Hansen, M.H. and Hurwitz, W.N. (1943) On the theory of sampling from finite populations. *Annals of Mathematical Statistics*, **14**, 333–362.

Hansen, M.H., Hurwitz, W.N. and Madow, W.G. (1953) *Sample Survey Methods and Theory*, 2 Vols. Wiley, New York. Reprinted 1993.

Hansen, M.H., Madow, W.G. and Tepping, B.J. (1983) An evaluation of model-dependent and probability-sampling inferences in sample surveys. *Journal of the American Statistical Association*, **78**, 776–793.

Hartley, H.O. and Ross, A. (1954) Unbiased ratio estimates. *Nature*, **174**, 270–271.

Hartley, H.O. and Rao, J.N.K. (1962) Sampling with unequal probabilities and without replacement. *Annals of Mathematical Statistics*, **33**, 350–374.

Hinde, R. and Young, D. (1984) *Synchronised Sampling and Overlap Control Manual*. Statistical Services Branch, Australian Bureau of Statistics, Canberra.

Horvitz, D.G. and Thompson, D.J. (1952) A generalization of sampling without replacement from a finite universe. *Journal of the American Statistical Association*, **47**, 663–685.

Huff, D. (1954) *How to Lie with Statistics*. Gollancz, London.

Isaki, C.T. and Fuller, W.A. (1982) Survey design under the regression superpopulation model. *Journal of the American Statistical Association*, **77**, 89–96.

Johnson, A.E. (1995) Business surveys as a network sample. In B.G. Cox, D.A. Binder, B.N. Chinnappa, A. Christianson, M.J. Colledge and P.S. Kott (eds), *Business Survey Methods*. Wiley, New York, pp. 219–233.

Jones, H.L. (1974) Jackknife estimation of functions of stratum means. *Biometrika*, **61**, 343–348.

Keyfitz, N. (1951) Sampling with probabilities proportional to size: Adjustment for changes in the probabilities. *Journal of the American Statistical Association*, **46**, 105–109.

Kokic, P.N. and Bell, P.A. (1994) Optimal Winsorizing cutoffs for a stratified finite population estimator. *Journal of Official Statistics*, **10**, 419–435.

Kröger, H., Särndal, C.-E. and Teikari, I. (1999) Poisson mixture sampling: A family of designs for coordinated selection using permanent random numbers. *Survey Methodology*, **25**, 3–11.

Kyburg, H.E. (1987) The basic Bayesian blunder. In I.B. MacNeill and G.J. Umphrey (eds), *Foundations of Statistical Inference*. Reidel, Dordrecht, pp. 219–232.

Lahiri, D.B. (1951) A method of sample selection providing unbiased ratio estimators. In *Bulletin of the International Statistical Institute: Proceedings of the 27th Session (New Delhi/Calcutta)*, Vol. 33, Part II. ISI, The Hague, pp. 133–140.

Lee, P.M. (1989) *Bayesian Statistics: An Introduction*. Oxford University Press, New York.

Mickey, M.R. (1959) Some finite population unbiased ratio and regression estimators. *Journal of the American Statistical Association*, **54**, 594–612.

Midzuno, H. (1952) On the sampling system with probability proportional to sum of sizes. *Annals of the Institute of Statistical Mathematics*, **3**, 99–107.

Nathan, G. (1976) An empirical study of response and sampling errors for multiplicity estimates with different counting rules. *Journal of the American Statistical Association*, **71**, 808–815.

Neyman, J. (1934) On the two different aspects of the representative method: The method of stratified sampling and the method of purposive selection. *Journal of the Royal Statistical Society*, **97**, 558–606.

Ogus, J.L. and Clark, D.F. (1971) *The Annual Survey of Manufactures: A Report on Methodology*. U.S. Bureau of the Census Technical Paper No. 24. U.S. Government Printing Office, Washington, DC.

Ohlsson, E. (1990) *Sequential Sampling from a Business Register and its Application to the Swedish Consumer Price Index*. R&D Report 1990:6. Stockholm: Statistics Sweden.

Ohlsson, E. (1995) Coordination of samples using permanent random numbers. In B.G. Cox, D.A. Binder, B.N. Chinnappa, A. Christianson, M.J. Colledge and P.S. Kott (eds), *Business Survey Methods*. Wiley, New York, pp. 153–169.

Patterson, H.D. (1950) Sampling on successive occasions with partial replacement of units. *Journal of the Royal Statistical Society, Series B*, **12**, 241–255.

Paxson, M.C., Dillman, D.A. and Tarnai, J. (1995) Improving response to business mail surveys. In B.G. Cox, D.A. Binder, B.N. Chinnappa, A. Christianson, M.J. Colledge and P.S. Kott (eds), *Business Survey Methods*. Wiley, New York, pp. 303–316.

Press, S.J. (1989) *Bayesian Statistics: Principles, Models and Applications*. Wiley, New York.

Quenouille, M.H. (1949) Approximation tests of correlation in time series. *Journal of the Royal Statistical Society, Series B*, **11,** 18–84.

Quenouille, M.H. (1956) Notes on bias in estimation. *Biometrika*, **43**, 353–360.

Rand Corporation (1955) *A Million Random Digits with 100,000 Normal Deviates*. Free Press, Glencoe, IL.

Rao, J.N.K. and Vijayan, K. (1977) On estimating the variance in sampling with probability proportional to aggregate size. *Journal of the American Statistical Association*, **72**, 579–584.

Rosén, B. (1997a) Asymptotic theory for order sampling. *Journal of Statistical Planning and Inference*, **62**, 135–158.

Rosén, B. (1997b) On sampling with probability proportional to size. *Journal of Statistical Planning and Inference*, **62**, 159–191.

Rosén, B. (2001) A user's guide to Pareto πps sampling. In *ICES-II, Proceedings of the Second International Conference on Establishment Surveys*, American Statistical Association, Alexandria VA, pp. 289–299. (Also available as invited paper in Section 4 on the included CD.)

Royall, R.M. (1970) On finite population sampling theory under certain regression models. *Biometrika*, **57**, 377–387.

Royall, R.M. (1971) Linear regression models in finite population sampling theory (with discussion). In V.P. Godambe and D.A. Sprott (eds), *Foundations of Statistical Inference*. Holt, Rinehart and Winston, Toronto, pp. 259–279.

Royall, R.M. and Herson, J. (1973a) Robust estimation in finite populations. I. *Journal of the American Statistical Association*, **68**, 880–889.

Royall, R.M. and Herson, J. (1973b) Robust estimation in finite populations. II: Stratification on a size variable. *Journal of the American Statistical Association*, **68**, 890–893.

Royall, R.M. and Pfeffermann, D. (1982) Balanced samples and robust Bayesian inference in finite population sampling. *Biometrika*, **69**, 401–409.

Saavedra, P. (1995) Fixed sample size PPS approximations with a permanent random number. In *Proceedings of the Section on Survey Research Methods*. American Statistical Association, Alexandria, VA, pp. 697–700.

Sampford, M.R. (1967) On sampling without replacement with unequal probabilities of selection. *Biometrika*, **54**, 499–513.

Sánchez-Crespo, J.L. (1997) A sampling scheme with partial replacement. *Journal of Official Statistics*, **13**, 327–339.

Särndal, C.-E. (1996) Efficient estimators with simple variance in unequal probability sampling. *Journal of the American Statistical Association*, **91**, 1289–1300.

Särndal, C.-E. and Wright, R.L. (1984) Cosmetic form of estimators in survey sampling. *Scandinavian Journal of Statistics*, **11**, 146–156.

Särndal, C-E., Swensson, B. and Wretman, J. (1992) *Model Assisted Survey Sampling*. Springer-Verlag, New York.

Schelling, T.C. (1980) *The Strategy of Conflict*. Harvard University Press, Cambridge, MA.

Sen, A.R. (1953) On the estimate of the variance in sampling with varying probabilities. *Journal of the Indian Society of Agricultural Statistics*, **5**, 119–127.

Shao, J. and Tu, D. (1995) *The Jackknife and Bootstrap*. Springer-Verlag, New York, Section 1.3.

Sigman, R.S. and Monsour, N.J. (1995) Selecting samples from list frames of businesses. In B.G. Cox, D.A. Binder, B.N. Chinnappa, A. Christianson, M.J. Colledge and P.S. Kott (eds), *Business Survey Methods*. Wiley, New York, pp. 133–152.

Smith, T.M.F. (1994) Sample surveys 1975–1990: An age of reconciliation? (With discussion). *International Statistical Review*, **62**, 5–34.

Spiegelhalter, D.J., Thomas, A., Best, N.G. and Gilks, W.R. (1996) *BUGS: Bayesian Inference Using Gibbs Sampling, Version 0.5*. Medical Research Council Biostatistics Unit, Cambridge.

Tam, S.-M. and Chan, N.N. (1984) Screening of probability samples. *International Statistical Review*, **52**, 301–308.

Tanner, M.A. (1993) *Tools for Statistical Inference: Methods for the Exploration of Posterior Distributions*, 2nd edn. Springer-Verlag, New York.

Thulin, G. (1976) Co-ordination of samples in enterprise statistics (SAMU). Implementation of the JALES technique. *Statistisk Tidskrift*, **14**, 209–222 (in Swedish with English summary).

Tillé, Y. (1996) Some remarks on unequal probability sampling designs without replacement. *Annales d'Economie et de Statistique*, **44**, 177–189.

Tschuprow, A. (1923) On the mathematical expectation of the moments of frequency distributions in the case of correlated observations. *Metron*, **2**, 646–680.

Tukey, J.W. (1958) Bias and confidence in not quite large samples (abstract). *Annals of Mathematical Statistics*, **29**, 614.

Turner, A.G. (1996) *The United Nations Common Code of Statistical Practice*, ST/ESA/STAT/Technical Notes/No. 5, June 1996. http://www.un.org/Depts/unsd/demotss/tcnjun96/tony.htm.

United Nations Statistical Office (1964) *Recommendations for the Preparation of Sample Survey Reports*. Statistical Papers, Series C, No. 1, Rev. 2.

Valliant, R., Dorfman, A.H. and Royall, R.M. (2000) *Finite Population Sampling and Inference: A Prediction Approach*. Wiley, New York.

Wolter, K.M. (1985) *Introduction to Variance Estimation*. Springer-Verlag, New York.

Yates, F. and Grundy, P.M. (1953) Selection without replacement from within strata with probability proportional to size. *Journal of the Royal Statistical Society, Series B*, **15**, 235–261.

Index

a priori probability 258
across-stratum ratio estimation 52–7
Aires, N. 146, 259, 260, 262
Alexander, C.H. 291
allocation ratios 35–6, 37
anticipated variances 92, 171–2
  generalized regression estimator (GREG) 135–8
  Horvitz–Thompson estimators (HTE) 154–8
  multistage without replacement 226–8
Asok, C. 147–8, 152, 153
asymptotic approximations 44–8, 100
atypical units 270–1
Australian Bureau of Statistics (ABS) 177, 205, 208, 209, 256
  survey redesign 269–70
Australian farm surveys 108–9
averages of ratios estimators 42, 43
  Horvitz–Thompson (HT) 63–4

balanced samples 82, 102, 271
Bayesian inference 104, 288–91, 293–6
Bell, P.A. 274–5
benchmark vectors 132
Bernoulli sampling 74, 247, 249
best linear unbiased estimator (BLUE) 21, 25, 111
best linear unbiased predictor (BLUP)
  combined inferences (*πpswor*) 127–8
  combined inferences (*srswor*) 125–6
  prediction-based inference 21, 25
  simple regression estimation 118
best predicted value (BPV) of population total 21
bias
  actual bias 46–8, 50–1
  birth biases 247, 257–9
  co-dependence bias 115, 119
  relative bias 44–6, 100
  spreading it back 278–80
  variance of across-stratum ratio estimator 55
bootstrap resampling 228–9, 285–6
Box, G.E.P. 103
Brewer, K.R.W.
  approximation to HTE 148–52
  atypical units 270–1
  coefficient of heteroscedasticity 203
  collocated sampling 256
  extreme values 271–4
  high-entropy estimators 170
  Horvitz–Thompson ratio estimator (HTRE) 254–5
  linear regression models 20
  Poisson sampling 248–9
  randomization and prediction inferences 102–4
  small case weights 133–4
  subsets 268–70
  low-entropy variance estimator 160
  Winsorization 275

calibration term 124, 170
  see also cosmetically calibrated estimators
Capital Expenditure Survey 269
case weights 110–11, 116, 131, 162
  unacceptably small 133–5
Census Collector's District (CD) 179
central limit theorem 288
classical ratio estimator (CRE) 96
  actual bias and variance approximations 46–8
  as best linear unbiased estimator (BLUE) 111
  bias 43–4
  BLUP 126
  Cochran consistency 42–3
  combined inferences 126
  design-based inference 41–3
  Horvitz–Thompson ratio estimator (HTRE) 254–5
  randomization bias 100–1
  in ratio prediction model 85–6
  relative bias and variance approximations 44–6
  synthetic estimation 119
  two-phase sampling 235
clusters 190–1
  additional notation 194
  optimal levels 199
  optimum alternative 205
  optimum clustering equation 204–5
  selection of 195

size 178, 179
variance component 198
co-dependence bias 115, 119
Cochran consistent estimators 42, 43, 48
Cochran, W.G. 42, 44, 50, 62
coefficient of heteroscedasticity 87
choice of 137, 142, 200–1
estimation 203
modelling 111
coefficient of variation 33
collocated sampling 256
combined inferences
anticipated variances 135–8, 154–8, 171–2, 226–8
best linear unbiased predictor (BLUP) 125–8
classical ratio estimator (CRE) 126
cosmetically calibrated estimators 104
design variances 171–2
Horvitz–Thompson ratio estimator (HTRE) 255
multistage sampling without replacement 219–23
regression estimation 125–6
short-cut variance estimation 171–2
simple random sampling without replacement (*srswor*) 123–7
unequal probability samples ($\pi pswor$) 127–8
composite estimator 236
conditional Poisson sampling (CPS) 259–60
conditioned estimators 194, 198, 216, 254–5
confidence intervals 5–6, 91–3, 291–2
consistent estimators 42; *see also* Cochran consistent estimators
cosmetically calibrated estimators (CCEs) 104, 127–8, 132
GREG and PRED forms 128–9, 133, 171
unacceptably small case weights 133–4
cost parameters 203–5
covariance
in bias formula for classical ratio estimator (CRE) 44
design-based 9
in variance formula for Horvitz–Thompson ratio estimator (HTRE) 254–5
prediction-based 23
coverage rules 184–5
credibility intervals 291–2

degrees of freedom 162
'delete and add on' procedure 273
design-based inference
generalized regression estimator (GREG) 128–9
mean squared error (MSE) 275–8
non-response 235
randomization modelling 81–3, 96, 97
regression estimation 123–4
Representative Principle 103, 118, 132
design bias
across-stratum 54–6
asymptotic formula for actual 46–8, 50–1, 99
asymptotic formula for relative 44–6, 100
spreading it back 278–80
design covariance 9, 44
design expectations
srswor 9, 10–12
srswr 15
design-unbiased estimators
MSE 24–5
srswor 8–14
srswr 14–18
design variances
across-stratum ratio estimation 53–4
and anticipated variance formula 171–2
anticipated variance a substitute for 136
asymptotic formula for actual 46–8
asymptotic formula for relative 44–6
combined inferences 171–2
estimators compared 167–70
generalized regression estimator (GREG) 135–8, 161–2
Hansen–Hurwitz (HH) estimator 66–9, 72, 73–4
multistage without replacement 225–8
poststratified estimation 34
relative design variances 44–6
Sen–Yates–Grundy (SYG) variance estimator 71, 148, 161, 260
srswor 9, 11–14
srswr 15–16
Taylor series approximation 44–5, 51
two-phase estimator 235
two-stage samples 191–3
see also Horvitz–Thompson estimator (HTE)
Deville, J.-C. 167
difference estimator 161
direct and indirect inference 103
domain estimates 118–19
Donadio, M.E. 167, 170
doubly unbiased estimators 243
dummy stages of selection 177, 184
Durbin, J. 284

empty samples 256
end-effect 220
endcurves 263
endpoints 257
enterprises 246
entropy 260
  see also high-entropy estimators
equal probability selection method (*epsem*) 176
  with replacement 177–83
  without replacement 209–12
  self-weighting 186–8
exchangeability symmetry 10–11, 22–3
expectation operators 20
  see also design expectations
extreme values 271–4
  bias 278–80
  genuine 272–4, 281
  spreading estimated bias back 278–80
  spurious 271–2, 280
  subsets 268–70
  Winsorization 274–8

F statistic 111
final stage selection 183–5, 212
final stage variance 194, 200, 215–16
finite-population correction factors 147–8, 152–3, 159, 285–6
  anticipated variance 157–9
  bootstrap variance estimator 285–6
  design-based 148–54
  GREG 162
  model-assisted 154–6
  multistage sampling 219
first-phase sample, total estimation 232–3
first-stage variance 193, 198, 215, 216, 225–6
Fisher, Sir Ronald 268
Foreman, Ken 7, 176
frequentist inference 288–90, 291
Fuller, W.A. 91, 92, 136, 243

generalized regression estimator (GREG) 128–9
  design variances 135, 161–2, 170–2
  unacceptably small case weights 133–4
Gibbs sampler 295
Godambe, V.P. 97
Gregoire, T.G.
  coefficient of heteroscedasticity 203
  collocated sampling 256
  correction factors 152
  Horvitz–Thompson ratio estimator (HTRE) 254–5
  synthetic estimation 119
  variance estimator 160
Gross, W.F. 274

Hájek, J. 153, 167, 248, 260
Hansen–Hurwitz (HH) estimators 65–9, 72
Hansen, M.H. 176, 203
Hartley, H.O. 147–8, 152, 153
Hartley–Ross unbiased estimator 56
heteroscedastic models 121
high-entropy estimators 146–8, 153, 170
Hinde, R. 257, 259
homoscedastic error term 107, 111–12
Horvitz–Thompson estimator (HTE) 63–4
  anticipated variance 136, 156–8
  design variance approximations 148–54
  design variance approximations
    usefulness 154–6
  design variances 69–71, 135, 159–61
  equal inclusion probabilities 124
  GREG form 129, 133
  jackknife variance estimator 284–5
  natural variance 146
  Poisson sampling 74–7, 252–3
  Representative Principle 103
  understanding 105
  variance 69–71
Horvitz–Thompson ratio estimator (HTRE) 253, 254–5
household consumption 109
household survey *see* multistage sampling with replacement
hypothesis testing 111, 288–91

identically and independently distributed (i.i.d.) random variables 22
imputation 32–3, 200–1
inclusion counter 14–15
inclusion probabilities
  case weights 133
  chosen 154
  conditional 96, 186
  equal 124, 247
  evaluation 135
  high-entropy estimators 147–8, 153
  Poisson sampling 248, 252
  probability of selection 176
  proportional to size ($\pi pswor$) 69–71, 127–8, 210–11, 248, 284–5, 285–6
  unequal 96, 127–8, 248
  upper limits 133
inconsistent estimators 43
independence 22–3
indicator variates 8–9, 21

individual mean
  prediction-based 20, 24
  ratio prediction model 83–5
individual population units
  BLUP 118
  combined inferences 125
  cosmetically calibrated estimators 129–30
individual variance
  multivariate regression model 140–2
  prediction-based 23–5
  ratio prediction model 83, 84, 86–90
  univariate regression model 139–40
informative samples 19, 26
intractable distributions 291–2
inverse and direct inference 99, 103
Isaki, C.T. 91, 92, 136, 243

jackknife resampling 228–9, 284–5
Johnson, A.E. 244
joint inclusion probabilities 11, 71–2

Keyfitz technique 61–2, 63, 64, 211
Kokic, P.N. 274–5
Kott, P.S. 140, 152
Kröger, H. 248
Kyburg, H.E. 99, 103–4

Labour Force Survey 175, 177–83
Lahiri–Midzuno unbiased ratio estimator 60–3
Langrangian 204
linear regression models *see* regression estimation
low-entropy estimators 147

Markov chain Monte Carlo (MCMC) 296
mean-corrected sum of squares, *srswor* 7
mean squared error (MSE) 23–5
  Kokic–Bell minimum 277–8
  random systematic selection 210
  ratio estimators 43
  relative design 46
  two-step ratio estimator 255
  Winsorization 275
Midzuno, H. 61
Million Random Digits (Rand) 4
model-assisted survey sampling 102
modified Poisson sampling 77–8, 256
Monsour, N.J. 266
Monte Carlo forest experiment 163–7
multilevel schemes 266
multistage sampling with replacement
  cost parameters 203–4
  equal probability selection 177–9
  estimation formulae 188–91
  generalized population variance 202–3
  imputation 200–1
  individual stages of variance 197–8
  probability of selection 176
  sample estimator of total variance 198, 200
  suitability of 174–5
  total variance estimation 196–7
  variance estimation 191–6
  variance reconsidered 199–203
multistage sampling without replacement
  combined inference estimation of total 219–23
  design-unbiased estimators 217–19
  equal probability selection 209–12
  estimation formulae 212–13
  resampling methods 228–9
  sample estimator of total variance 216
  variance estimation 214–19
  variances of total 223–8

Nathan, G. 244
natural relationship 100
network sampling 244
Neyman, J. 35, 101, 288
non-informative sampling 22–3
non-response 238–44
non-sample sum 129
normal distribution theory 100–1
notional strata 159–61
null hypothesis 288–91

order sampling 260–5
ordered systematic sampling 159–61
ordinary least squares (OLS) regression 99–101, 107
  circumstances against 109–12
  circumstances for 108–9
overlap ranges 257

panel sampling 265–6
Pareto sampling Pπ*ps* 153, 262–5
permanent random number (PRN) sampling 247
  alternatives 265
persons associated with dwellings 183–5
π*pswor* sampling *see* random systematic selection (π*pswor*)
pilot samples 4
Poisson sampling
  alternatives 256–9
  conditional 259–60
  estimation formulae 252–3
  practical use of 248
  ratio estimators for unequal samples 74–9
  rotation and control 248–52

Pomix sampling 248
population mean
  jackknife variance estimator 284
  prediction-based theory 25
  ratio estimators 45, 46
  srswor 7, 9–10
  srswr 15
  and unweighted sample mean 117
population standard deviation, *srswor* 7
population total
  BLUP 21, 25, 127
  BPV 21
  cosmetically calibrated estimators 127, 222
  definition of 9
  design-based inference 42
  design-unbiased estimator 10
  Hansen–Hurwitz (HH) estimator 65, 72, 73–4
  Horvitz–Thompson (HT) estimator 63–4, 103
  Horvitz–Thompson (HT) estimator under Poisson 74, 75–7, 252–3
  jackknife variance estimator 284
  Lahiri–Midzuno unbiased ratio estimator 61
  regression estimators 108, 115, 124–5
population variances
  multistage sampling with replacement 199–203
  multistage sampling without replacement 223–8
  poststratified 31–4
  ratio prediction model 89–92
  srswor 7–8, 12, 13
  srswor, two-phase sampling 233–5
  srswr 15–16
posterior distribution 294–5
poststratified estimation 29–34
  population total 31
  sample dependence 31
  stratum mean 30
  stratum total 30
  variances under prediction-based approach 31–3
  variances under *srswor* 30
prediction-based inference
  and design-based inference 80–3
  general regression model 129
  model expectations 23
  model-unbiased estimators 23–5
  model variances 23, 25
  and non-response 239–42
  and poststratified estimation 31, 38
  regression estimation 125
  simple regression estimator 117
  srswor 18–21, 23–6
  srswr 25–6
prediction variances
  combined inferences 102, 172
  generalized regression estimator (GREG) 171
  individual sample units 83, 139–43
  linear estimators based on a probability sample 138–9
  multistage sampling without replacement 223–5
  poststratified estimation 31, 34
  ratio prediction model 89–91
  sample variance 84–6
  srswor 20–1, 23–5
  srswr 25–6
  two-phase estimator 241–2
primary sampling units (PSUs) 177–9
probability of selection 176, 186–8
probability proportional to size with replacement (*ppswr*) 65–6, 101
proportionate variability 111
pseudo-values 284–5
Puza, B. 288

Quenouille, M.H. 284

random selection procedures 4–5
random systematic selection (π*pswor*)
  bootstrap variance 285–6
  combined inferences 127–8
  correction factor 147–8
  household survey 210–11
  HTE variance 69–71
  jackknife resampling 284–5
  Poisson sampling 248
randomization-based and prediction-based inferences 101–4
randomization bias 100–1
randomness 146–8, 260
Rao, J.N.K. 63, 147–8, 152, 153
ratio estimation (design-based)
  across-stratum 52–7
  actual bias and variance 46–8
  asymptotic approximations 44–8
  exact bias of ratio estimator 43–4
  normality 51–2
  numerical results 48–52
  relative bias and variance 44–6
  supplementary variables 40–1
ratio estimation (prediction-based)
  ratio prediction model 83–93

ratio estimation (unequal probability samples)
  Horvitz–Thompson and Hansen–Hurwitz estimators of total 63–74
  Lahiri–Midzuno unbiased ratio estimator 60–3
  Poisson sampling 74–9
ratio prediction model 83–93
ratio relationship 100
rejective sampling 260
relative bias 44–6, 100
relative covariance 45, 100
relative standard deviation 33
relative variance 44–6, 100
repeated sampling 236–8
replicated samples 45
Representative Principle 103, 118, 132
resampling estimators 170
  bootstrap variance estimator 285–6
  jackknife variance estimator 284–5
  multistage without replacement 228–9
  use of 283–4, 286
resampling population 285
residual random variables 20, 107, 111–12
response 187–8
root mean squared errors (RMSEs) 120, 278
Rosén, B. 153, 167, 262
rotation 236–8
  and control 248–52, 255, 265–6
Royall, Richard 101–2

Saavedra, P. 262
Sampford, M.R. 147
sample fractions 4
sample frame, construction of 174–5, 177
sample indicators *see* indicator variates
sample mean
  Bayesian model 294
  model variance 23–5
  prediction-based theory 21
  ratio prediction model 83–4
  srswor 9, 10–13, 30
  srswr 15
  weighted 117
sample size 4
  adequacy of 8
  bias 119
  fixed size 70–1, 148
    notation 9
  fixed *or* predetermined 70–1, 148, 259
  prediction models 103
  random *or* variable 136, 163–7
  small samples 80–3, 171–2
  smallest possible 158–9
  stratified sampling 35, 37, 50
sample sum 61
sample variance
  Bayesian model 294
  prediction-based 23–5
  ratio prediction model 84–6
  srswor 13–14, 30–3
  srswr 16
  Winsorization 276
Särndal, C.-E. 104, 127, 135, 161
Second International Conference on Establishment Surveys (ICES-II) 146
second-phase sample 232
secondary sampling units (SSUs) 179–80
selecting the sample, manner of 19, 26
selection intervals 257
selection probabilities 61–3, 147–8
self-representing areas (SRAs) 177
self-weighting 186–8
Sen–Yates–Grundy (SYG) variance estimator 71, 148, 161, 260
sequential Poisson sampling 261–2
serpentine ordering 205
Sigman, R.S. 266
simple random sampling with replacement (*srswr*)
  equal weights 14–18
  jackknife variance estimator 284
  multistage sampling 175, 176
  and prediction-based inference 20, 25–6
  and *srswor* compared 4–5, 14, 17, 18, 26–7
simple random sampling without replacement (*srswor*) 8–14
  averages of ratios estimators 42, 43
  bootstrap variance estimator 285
  combined inferences 123–7, 156–8
  equal weights 18–21, 23–6
  jackknife variance estimator 284
  multistage sampling 175, 181–2
  sample estimator of anticipated variance of HTE under 156–8
  and stratification 36
  two-phase sampling 232–5
  using poststratification 29–34
simple regression estimation 107–8
  circumstances against 109–12
  circumstances for 108–9
  coefficient 111, 113, 114–15
  combined inferences 125–6
  combined inferences with unequal probabilities 127–8

simple regression estimation *cont.*
design-based inference 116–17, 123–4
estimator properties 112–19
general model 128–33
intercept term 107, 109–12, 114–15, 119–20
prediction-based inference 117–19, 125
ratio prediction model 83
regressor variables 109–12
synthetic estimation 118–19
see also generalized regression estimator (GREG)
size, measure of 262
standard deviation 33, 91
standard errors
ratio estimators 44
srswor 6
srswr 16
stratification 36
startlines 264
startpoints 257
Stocks Survey 269
stratification 29
allocation ratios 35–6, 37
atypical units 270–1
Bayesian model 294–5
multistage sampling 177–8
multistage sampling with replacement 205, 208
notional strata 159–61
poststratified estimation 29–34
and prediction-based inference 31, 38
Representative Principle 103
sample design 34–7
by size 81
and *srswor* 36
stratum mean 30
stratum total 30, 83
stratum variances 30–4
prediction-based 89–91
subpopulation estimates 118–19
subsets, relevant and recognizable 268–70
Sukhatme, B.V. 147–8, 152, 153
sum of squares 7
superpopulation mean 25
superpopulation models 102
supplementary variables
balanced samples 82
finding 40–1
intercept term 110
more than one 128–33
survey coverage 185–6
survey scope 185–6
synchronized sampling 256–9
synthetic estimation 80, 118–19

t distributions 6
Tam, S.-M. 20
tertiary sample units (TSUs) 180–1
Tillé, Y. 152
tracking, need for 246–7
Tschuprow, A. 35
Tukey, J.W. 284
two-level schemes 266
two-phase sampling 232–6
srswor and non-response 242–4
two-phase sampling, two variables 235
non-response 238–42
sample rotation 236–8

UN guidelines 186
unequal probability samples
combined inferences 127–8
HH estimator 65–9
HTE estimator 63–4, 69–70
jackknife variance estimator 284–5
Lahiri–Midzuno estimator 60–3
Poisson sampling 74–8
Sen–Yates–Grundy (SYG) variance estimator 71
US Bureau of the Census (USBC) 205

value modification 273
Winsorization 274–8
variables
identically and independently distributed (i.i.d.) random variables 22
indicator variates 8–9, 21
supplementary variables 40–1, 82, 110, 128–33
two-phase sampling, two variables 235, 236–8, 238–42
Vijayan, K. 63

weight modification 273, 275, 279–80
weighted averages 236
weighted least squares (WLS) 113
weighted sample mean 117
weighted samples 128
Winsorization 274–8
Wolter, K.M. 284
Wright., R.L. 104, 127

Young, D. 257, 259